Hospital Medicine Handbook

Recognition, Rescue, and the Discipline of Doing Less

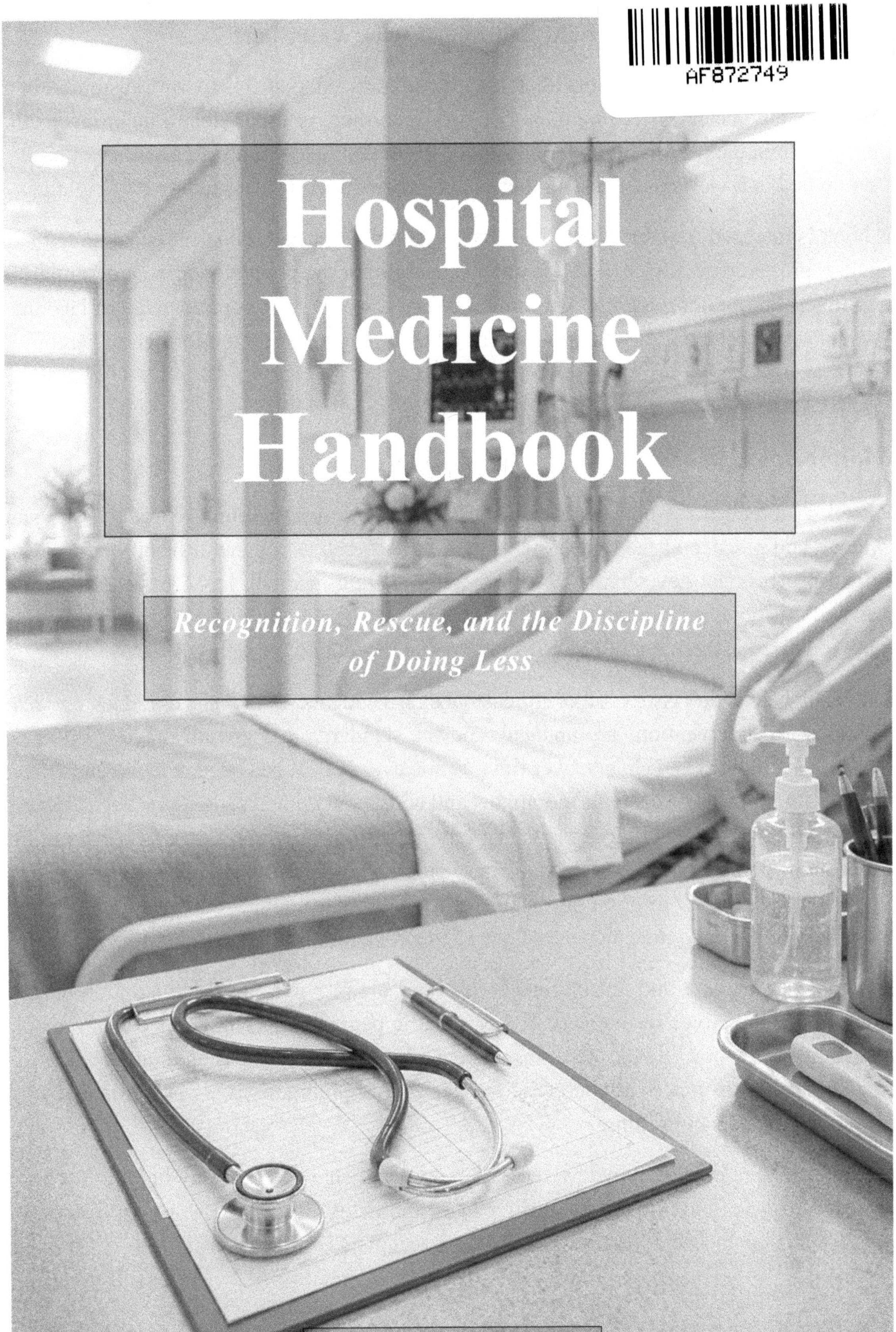

Cidaar Publishing

This book is intended for educational and informational purposes. It does not constitute medical, legal, or professional advice, and it is not a substitute for the clinical judgment of a qualified practitioner. The author makes no warranties as to the accuracy or completeness of its contents and assumes no liability for any actions taken in reliance on the information herein.

Disclaimer

This book is intended for educational and informational purposes only. It reflects the state of knowledge and practice at the time of writing and is offered as a general resource for advanced study and professional development. It does not constitute medical, legal, or other professional advice, and it is not a substitute for the clinical judgment of a qualified healthcare provider or for the individualized assessment of any particular patient, situation, or setting.

The field of healthcare is one of continual change. Evidence evolves, guidelines are revised, medications and interventions are updated, and the standards that govern practice differ across regions and institutions and change over time. While every effort has been made to ensure that the information in this book is accurate, complete, and consistent with accepted practice at the time of publication, the author and publisher make no representations or warranties, express or implied, as to its accuracy, completeness, currency, or fitness for any particular purpose. Readers are strongly encouraged to verify all information against current primary sources, professional guidelines, institutional policies, and the guidance of qualified colleagues before applying it in practice.

The examples, scenarios, and illustrations in this book are provided for teaching purposes and are not intended as directives for the care of any specific patient. Any clinical decision remains the responsibility of the practitioner, who must exercise independent professional judgment in light of the individual circumstances of each case and the laws, regulations, and standards that apply in their own jurisdiction and setting.

To the fullest extent permitted by law, the author and publisher disclaim any liability for any loss, injury, or damage of any kind arising, directly or indirectly, from the use or application of the contents of this book. Use of this book constitutes acceptance of these terms.

DEDICATION

This book is for the people who taught me what it is written about.

For the clinicians who showed me that medicine is mostly attention: noticing the observation that does not fit, the patient who is not progressing, the family who has not understood. For the nurses who called early and were usually right. For the trainees who asked the question I could not answer and sent me back to find out.

And above all for the patients. You did not choose to be there. You were frightened, you were interrupted, you were examined by strangers, and you trusted us anyway. Much of what is in these pages was learned from moments when we could have done better for you.

I hope this helps someone do better for the next one.

TABLE OF CONTENTS

INTRODUCTION

How to Use This Book

Who this book is for

This handbook is written for anyone who takes responsibility for a patient in a hospital bed. That includes medical students meeting inpatient medicine for the first time, residents and registrars carrying a bleep overnight, advanced practice clinicians, and consultants and attendings who have been doing this for twenty years and want a considered account of what the evidence currently supports.

The material is pitched at an advanced level throughout. It assumes basic physiology and pharmacology and does not rehearse them. Where a topic is genuinely contested, the contest is described rather than resolved by assertion, because a clinician who knows why an area is uncertain will practise better in it than one who has memorised a position.

Why a book organised this way

Hospital medicine is unusual among specialties in defining itself by a place rather than by an organ, a disease, or an age range. The claim embedded in that choice is that the hospital is a distinct clinical environment with its own physiology, its own tempo, its own failure modes, and its own body of expertise. This book takes that claim seriously and organises itself accordingly.

The consequence is that a substantial portion of the content is not disease-specific at all. Chapters on transitions of care, on clinical reasoning, on systems and safety, and on communication sit alongside chapters on respiratory failure and gastrointestinal bleeding, and they sit there because the evidence indicates that they account for at least as much preventable harm.

How the book is structured

Part I, Foundations of Inpatient Practice, establishes the specialty, the reasoning discipline that underpins diagnosis, the transitions at which information is lost, and the systems methodology for changing the environment in which all of it occurs.

Part II, Medical Consultation, covers the consultative role and perioperative medicine, from the structure of a consultation through risk assessment, comorbidity management, and postoperative complications.

Part III, The Undifferentiated Patient, addresses the presentations that arrive without a diagnosis attached: cardinal symptoms, altered mental status, fever, and the fluid, electrolyte, and acid-base disturbances that underlie a great many of them.

Part IV, Organ-System Emergencies on the Ward, covers acute deterioration by system, written for the clinician who is present when it happens rather than for the specialist who arrives afterwards.

Part V, Populations, Values, and the End of the Hospital Course, addresses the patients for whom standard care produces worse outcomes, and the care of the dying.

What this book argues

Three positions recur across the twenty chapters, and readers should recognise them as arguments rather than as neutral summary.

The consequential failures in inpatient medicine are rarely failures of knowledge. They are failures of transition, of recognition, of communication, and of attention. The diagnosis transmitted as a conclusion rather than as a question. The deterioration observed and not escalated. The medication stopped correctly and never restarted. The conversation deferred because there was always a reason to wait. These recur in almost every chapter, and they are correctable.

A great deal of confident practice does not survive contact with evidence. Aggressive fluid resuscitation in pancreatitis, bridging anticoagulation, prophylactic revascularisation before surgery, deep hypothermia after cardiac arrest, high-dose perioperative beta-blockade, prolonged antibiotic courses, and antipsychotics for delirium were all standard within recent professional memory and are now known to be unhelpful or harmful. Where this book departs from what a reader was taught, it generally says so and gives the reason.

Doing less is frequently the harder and better decision. The reasoning behind withholding a test, stopping an antibiotic, declining to lower a blood pressure, and not offering an intervention is developed throughout, because the incentives in a hospital run consistently in the other direction and the harms of overtreatment are diffuse, delayed, and attributable to no one.

How to use it

Each chapter is self-contained and can be read alone. Each opens with learning objectives and a short overview stating the chapter's argument, and closes with a summary of the points that carry the most clinical weight, review questions suitable for teaching or self-assessment, and a source list.

The cross-references are a feature rather than a formality. Clinical problems do not respect chapter boundaries, and where a topic is developed elsewhere the reference is specific to the section. A reader following the management of a single complex patient will find themselves moving between parts, which reflects the work rather than a defect of organisation.

The figures illustrate reasoning rather than anatomy. They are, deliberately, diagrams of decisions, mechanisms, and frameworks, because that is where the difficulty in this material lies.

What this book is not

It is not a formulary. Drug doses are omitted in several chapters, and this is deliberate rather than an oversight. Doses for status epilepticus, for opioid conversion, for perioperative corticosteroid supplementation, and for several other high-risk situations vary between institutions and are revised, and a wrong number printed in a book is more dangerous than no number at all. Where a dose is required, take it from a current local protocol, and involve pharmacy.

It is not jurisdiction-neutral. Admission status rules, capacity and detention law, surrogate decision-making frameworks, controlled drug regulation, post-acute care structures, and antimicrobial resistance patterns all differ substantially between health systems. Where a section describes one system's arrangements, it says so, and the underlying clinical logic is stated separately from the administrative machinery so that it transfers.

It is not current indefinitely. Several sections describe evidence that changed within the last few years and will change again. The source lists name the primary literature so that a reader can check whether a position still holds.

It is not a substitute for judgement, for local guidance, or for asking someone. No book is, and one written for a specialty defined by uncertainty under time pressure should say so plainly.

A closing note

The patient in the bed did not choose to be there, is frightened, and is frequently unable to advocate for themselves. The clinician standing at the end of that bed is the person who will decide what happens next, often on incomplete information and often at an inconvenient hour.

Everything that follows is in service of making that decision better.

CHAPTER 1: The Hospitalist Model: Scope, Systems, and Professional Identity

Learning Objectives

After studying this chapter, the reader should be able to:

1. Explain the historical, economic, and clinical forces that produced site-based specialisation, and articulate the three mechanisms by which the hospitalist model generates value.
2. Distinguish the four operating domains of contemporary hospitalist practice and describe the competencies specific to each.
3. Describe the non-linear relationship between clinical workload and quality of care, and identify the cognitive mechanisms that mediate it.
4. Differentiate consultation from comanagement, evaluate the evidence base for comanagement in specific populations, and construct a written scope agreement.
5. Apply the principal techniques of influence available to a clinician who holds responsibility without positional authority.
6. Distinguish burnout from moral injury on the basis of mechanism, and match each to interventions with a plausible route to effect.
7. Recognise how bedside conduct and documentation practice function as clinical instruments that measurably alter downstream care.

Chapter Overview

Hospital medicine is the fastest-growing specialty in the modern history of internal medicine, and it is also the one whose defining boundary is the least intuitive. This chapter establishes the conceptual foundation on which the rest of the handbook rests: what a hospitalist is, why the role exists in the structural form it does, what work it actually comprises, and how a person occupying it should think about capacity, authority, sustainability, and conduct.

Readers approaching this material as students should note that the content of this chapter is not preliminary or ceremonial. The most consequential errors in inpatient medicine are rarely errors of knowledge. They are errors of handoff, of workload, of unclear responsibility, of documentation, and of a clinician operating past the point at which careful reasoning remains possible. Those failure modes are the subject matter of this chapter, and they are the reason the chapters that follow can be written at all.

1.1 Origins and the Structural Logic of Site-Based Specialisation

1.1.1 The problem that produced the specialty

Every medical specialty defines itself by a boundary, and the choice of boundary reveals what the specialty believes to be the most important source of variation in outcomes. Cardiology claims an organ system, and in doing so asserts that organ-specific pathophysiology is the dominant axis of expertise. Paediatrics claims an age range, asserting that developmental physiology reorganises everything else. Oncology claims a disease process. Emergency medicine, notably, claims a phase of illness.

Hospital medicine claims a place.

This is a strange assertion on its face, and it is worth taking seriously rather than treating as a historical accident. The claim embedded in site-based specialisation is that the hospital is not merely a location where medicine happens but a distinct clinical environment with its own physiology, its own failure modes, its own information architecture, and its own tempo, and that mastery of that environment constitutes a body of expertise independent of organ or disease.

The claim was not made in the abstract. It emerged from a specific and well-documented convergence of pressures in the American health system during the late 1980s and 1990s, and versions of the same convergence have since produced parallel developments in Canada, the United Kingdom, Australia, the Netherlands, Brazil, Japan, and across much of Asia and the Gulf.

Four pressures mattered most.

Ambulatory intensification. Office-based internal medicine was becoming a full-time occupation in a way it had not previously been. Panel sizes grew, documentation requirements grew, preventive care obligations grew, and reimbursement models rewarded ambulatory throughput. A primary care physician who once rounded on two hospitalised patients before a nine o'clock clinic increasingly found that a single deteriorating inpatient could consume the entire morning, and that the morning had no financial or scheduling slack to give.

Inpatient acuity compression. Simultaneously and independently, the inpatient population was becoming sicker per bed-day. Procedures that once required admission moved to ambulatory settings. Length of stay fell steadily across nearly all diagnosis groups. The arithmetic consequence is often stated but rarely absorbed: when the well patients leave the denominator, the remaining inpatient population is, by construction, more acute. The average ward patient at the turn of the century required a level of active management that would have been unusual in a general ward twenty years earlier, and the trend has continued.

The rise of measured quality. Public reporting, accreditation requirements, and payment models tied to readmission, mortality, and safety events created institutional demand for physicians who could be held accountable for inpatient processes. A physician present in the building daily can be enrolled in a quality initiative. A physician present for forty minutes each morning cannot.

Information system centralisation. As clinical information migrated into institution-specific electronic systems, fluency in a particular hospital's information environment became a genuine skill with genuine time costs. The physician who uses the system for thirty hours a week develops competencies the physician who uses it for three hours a week does not.

The mismatch these pressures produced can be stated in one sentence: the physician least present in the hospital was managing the patients whose care most required continuous presence.

1.1.2 Naming and formalisation

The term entered the literature in 1996, when Robert Wachter and Lee Goldman described in the *New England Journal of Medicine* an emerging class of physicians whose practice was defined by the inpatient setting. The paper was descriptive rather than prescriptive. It named a phenomenon that was already occurring in scattered form, principally in staff-model health maintenance organisations and academic centres, where the economics of physician time had already forced the separation.

Formalisation followed rapidly by the standards of medical specialisation. A professional society was established. Core competencies were articulated, defining the domain across clinical conditions, procedures, and healthcare systems. Focused practice recognition pathways were created within existing board certification structures rather than through a separate primary board, which is itself a meaningful structural fact: hospital medicine positioned itself as a practice focus within internal medicine, family medicine, and paediatrics rather than as a departure from them.

Growth was extraordinary. From a few hundred practitioners in the mid-1990s, the field expanded to tens of thousands within two decades, and hospitalists now provide the majority of general medical inpatient care in most American hospitals of meaningful size. The comparable trajectory in other health systems has been slower but directionally identical, and where it has been slower the limiting factor has usually been workforce structure rather than any dispute about the underlying logic.

1.1.3 The three mechanisms of value

Site-based specialisation is frequently described, including by its practitioners, as a matter of convenience or scheduling. That description is both incomplete and strategically damaging, because a service justified by convenience is defensible only until someone offers a cheaper convenience. The value generated by the model rests on three distinct mechanisms, and each is independently demonstrable.

Mechanism one: volume and pattern density. A physician who manages forty pneumonias in a month develops calibration that a physician managing four in a month cannot. This is not merely a claim about factual recall. It is a claim about the structure of expert reasoning. Expertise in diagnosis is substantially a matter of well-populated illness scripts, and scripts are populated by repetition with feedback. The hospitalist sees the pneumonia that turns out to be organising pneumonia, the pneumonia that turns out to be heart failure, and the pneumonia that turns out to be an aspiration event in an unrecognised bulbar palsy. Having seen each of these, the pattern space is richer, and the discordant detail is more likely to be noticed.

Volume also produces procedural competence where procedures are within scope, and, more subtly, produces calibrated pessimism. Clinicians who have watched a specific illness trajectory forty times develop accurate priors about which patients will deteriorate at hour thirty-six. That prior is not written in any guideline.

Mechanism two: temporal availability. The value of a clinical decision is not constant across the day. A decision made at eleven in the morning permits a study to be performed that afternoon, a consultant to be reached before their clinic ends, a family meeting to occur before evening, and a discharge to be executed the following morning. The same decision made at six in the evening does none of these things. Availability is therefore not simply about responsiveness to emergencies. It is about occupying the position in the day at which decisions still have downstream room to operate.

This mechanism compounds. A single decision deferred by six hours may cost half a day of stay. Three such deferrals across an admission may cost two days, with all the attendant exposure to hospital-acquired harm that additional days carry. The relationship between physician presence and length of stay, which is one of the more consistent findings in the hospitalist outcomes literature, is largely this mechanism made visible.

Mechanism three: systems fluency. This is the least discussed and, in practice, often the most powerful. The experienced hospitalist knows which radiologist will accommodate an add-on study today, how the utilisation review process actually functions rather than how it is described in policy, which discharge pathway to a skilled nursing facility will collapse on a Friday afternoon, which nurse manager to call when a bed assignment is wrong, and which order set contains a default that must be overridden.

None of this is medical knowledge in the conventional sense. All of it determines whether medical knowledge reaches the patient. Systems fluency is what distinguishes a hospitalist from a very available and very competent general internist, and it is the component that transfers least readily between institutions. A hospitalist who changes hospitals loses perhaps two months of effectiveness to the reacquisition of local systems knowledge, a phenomenon obvious to anyone who has done it and almost never discussed in recruitment.

1.1.4 The trade-off at the core of the model

The model purchases these three mechanisms with a single currency: longitudinal relationship.

This is not an incidental cost or an implementation problem to be engineered away. It is the definitional trade. The hospitalist meets the patient for the first time at the moment of greatest vulnerability, without the accumulated context of years of ambulatory encounters, without knowledge of what this patient's baseline function actually looks like, without the trust that permits a difficult recommendation to be accepted quickly, and without the tacit understanding of what this particular person would want if things went badly.

Almost every quality and safety preoccupation of hospital medicine follows directly from this severance. Medication reconciliation exists because the hospitalist does not know what the patient takes. Structured handoff exists because the hospitalist does not carry the patient across time personally. Discharge summary standards exist because the information must be transmitted rather than retained. Advance care planning documentation exists because the physician who knew the patient's values is not in the building.

Framing these as bureaucratic burdens misunderstands them. They are the load-bearing structure that makes the model safe. A hospitalist who performs medication reconciliation carelessly has not skipped an administrative task; they have removed a wall.

1.1.5 Variants of the model

The specialty is not monolithic, and readers entering practice should understand the principal structural variants because they generate different professional experiences.

Academic hospitalists typically work in teaching hospitals with resident teams, with clinical time protected in some proportion for education, research, quality work, or administration. Direct patient volume is often lower, indirect supervisory load higher, and the census is filtered through a teaching structure that adds both safety redundancy and communication latency.

Community hospitalists carry higher direct volume, work without resident intermediaries, and typically maintain broader procedural and critical care scope because subspecialty support is thinner. The clinical breadth demanded in a two-hundred-bed community hospital without in-house intensivist coverage exceeds that demanded in most academic settings, a fact that academic training frequently fails to convey to its graduates.

Nocturnists work dedicated night schedules. The role solves a real staffing problem and pays a premium, and it carries documented physiological costs that are discussed in section 1.6.

Comanagement and service-line hospitalists focus on defined surgical or subspecialty populations, discussed in section 1.4.

Rural hospitalists occupy the widest scope of all, frequently covering emergency department support, intensive care, and procedural work, with transfer logistics as a core daily competency.

The competencies discussed throughout this handbook apply across all variants. The proportions differ.

1.2 The Hospitalist's Four Domains: Clinical, Systems, Educational, Stewardship

Practising hospitalists distribute their working effort across four domains. The domains overlap in time and in personnel, but they make different cognitive demands, are rewarded by different institutional mechanisms, and are learned through different routes. Trainees typically perceive only the first, which is one reason the transition from residency to attending practice is experienced as a discontinuity rather than a graduation.

1.2.1 The clinical domain

The clinical domain covers the direct diagnosis and management of hospitalised adults. Its scope is broader than any single organ specialty and, in most practices, includes general internal medicine, medical consultation to surgical and procedural services, a variable but often substantial component of critical care, primary palliative care, and bedside procedures.

The distinguishing feature of clinical hospital medicine is not any particular disease. It is **undifferentiated breadth under time pressure with incomplete information**. Consider the structure of a typical admission. A patient arrives with fever, confusion, and a chart that is either absent, in a different institution's system, or so voluminous as to be functionally opaque. The family is not present. The patient cannot give a history. The differential spans infection, drug effect, metabolic derangement, intracranial process, and decompensation of a chronic condition that has not yet been named. A decision about empiric therapy must be made within an hour, before any subspecialist would consider the consultation appropriate, and that decision will constrain everything that follows.

This is the characteristic clinical situation of hospital medicine, and it explains why the specialty invests so heavily in diagnostic reasoning as an explicit discipline, addressed in Chapter 2. Subspecialty consultation is enormously valuable, but it is valuable *after* the problem has been sufficiently framed to know which subspecialist to call. Framing the problem is hospitalist work.

Three clinical sub-competencies deserve early naming.

Recognition of deterioration. The ability to identify the patient who will decompensate in the next twelve hours is a distinct skill from the ability to diagnose. It relies on trajectory rather than cross-section, on nursing report as a primary data source, and on physiological trend rather than absolute value. Chapter 4 addresses the systems built around this recognition, and Chapters 13 and 14 address the physiology.

Diagnostic parsimony and its limits. Hospitalists learn early to seek a single unifying explanation, and learn later that in the older patient with five chronic conditions the unifying explanation is frequently wrong. Hickam's dictum displaces Occam's razor as comorbidity accumulates. Knowing which principle applies to the patient in front of you is a skill in its own right.

Tolerance of diagnostic uncertainty. A substantial fraction of medical admissions are discharged without a confirmed diagnosis, having improved. Managing this responsibly, meaning distinguishing acceptable diagnostic closure from premature closure, and communicating the difference honestly to the patient and the receiving clinician, is a core competency rather than a failure.

1.2.2 The systems domain

The systems domain comprises everything the hospitalist does to the hospital rather than to an individual patient: order set design, clinical pathway development, quality improvement projects, throughput and capacity management, participation in committees and governance, informatics work, and the negotiation of interdepartmental agreements.

This work is not peripheral. It is arguably where the specialty generates the majority of its population-level value, for a straightforward arithmetic reason. A hospitalist personally manages perhaps eight hundred to twelve hundred admissions per year. A hospitalist who improves the institution's sepsis recognition pathway affects every septic patient admitted to that institution, including those admitted by every other clinician, including those admitted at three in the morning by someone tired, and including those admitted five years from now after the original author has left.

The systems domain also explains an otherwise puzzling demographic fact: hospitalists occupy hospital executive and quality leadership positions at rates far exceeding their share of the medical staff. The reason is structural rather than characterological. Hospitalists are the only physicians who routinely observe the entire inpatient system operate, across services, across shifts, and across the boundary between clinical and administrative process. They see where it fails because they are standing in the failure.

Competence in this domain requires a genuinely different skill set from clinical work: measurement literacy, understanding of variation, familiarity with improvement methodology, facility with data presentation, and the political skills addressed in section 1.5. Chapter 4 treats the methodology in detail.

1.2.3 The educational domain

Wherever trainees are present, and for a large fraction of hospitalists that is most working days, the hospitalist is a teacher. This is true regardless of academic appointment and regardless of whether teaching is compensated.

Teaching in the inpatient environment differs from classroom instruction in three ways that matter practically. It is **opportunistic**, arising from whatever patient happens to present rather than from a curriculum. It is **compressed**, occurring in gaps of two to five minutes rather than in scheduled hours. And it is **public**, conducted in front of patients, families, nurses, and other trainees, which raises the stakes of both learner error and teacher error.

The techniques adapted to this environment are learnable and are not absorbed reliably by observation alone. The most useful include:

- **Structured microteaching**, in which the teacher elicits a commitment from the learner, probes for the reasoning behind it, reinforces what was done well, corrects one specific error, and states one general principle. This structure fits inside three minutes and produces more durable learning than a ten-minute lecture.
- **Think-aloud modelling**, in which the attending narrates their own diagnostic reasoning including the uncertainty, the discarded hypotheses, and the reasons for discarding them. Learners cannot acquire reasoning from conclusions alone, and expert reasoning is otherwise invisible.
- **Calibrated autonomy**, meaning the deliberate, progressive granting of decision-making latitude matched to demonstrated competence rather than to postgraduate year. Under-granting produces dependent trainees; over-granting produces harm. Both are common.
- **Feedback that is specific, behavioural, and proximate.** Feedback delivered a week later about general performance changes nothing. Feedback delivered the same afternoon about a specific observed behaviour changes practice.

A further educational obligation is often overlooked. The hospitalist teaches nurses, pharmacists, therapists, and students of those disciplines continuously, usually without noticing, and the tone of that teaching substantially determines whether those colleagues will call early when something is wrong. A hospitalist who is short with a nurse at two in the morning has not simply been rude; they have raised the threshold at which they will next be warned about a deteriorating patient. This is a safety issue, and it is treated as one in section 1.7.

1.2.4 The stewardship domain

The fourth domain concerns responsible use of finite resources: diagnostic tests, antimicrobials, blood products, imaging, intensive care beds, specialist attention, and, importantly, the patient's own time, comfort, and tolerance for intervention.

Stewardship is frequently framed as cost containment. This framing is a category error and should be resisted, both because it is inaccurate and because it invites the reasonable suspicion that patients are being rationed for institutional benefit. The clinical argument for stewardship is considerably stronger than the financial one.

Consider the cascade generated by a single low-value test. A computed tomography study of the abdomen ordered without a clear question in a patient with nonspecific pain identifies an adrenal nodule of no clinical significance. This finding generates biochemical evaluation, a repeat study at six months, patient anxiety that persists for years, an incidental radiation dose, and in a small proportion of cases a biopsy with its own complication rate. The initial test answered no question and initiated a sequence of harms, none of which would have occurred had the question been formulated before the order was placed.

The same logic applies across the domain. Unnecessary antibiotics generate resistance, *Clostridioides difficile*, and adverse drug reactions, addressed in Chapter 18. Unnecessary transfusion carries immunological and volume risk, addressed in Chapter 17. Unnecessary telemetry generates alarm fatigue and immobility. Unnecessary continuous pulse oximetry in a stable ward patient generates nocturnal interruption and, through it, delirium, addressed in Chapter 10.

Stewardship therefore reduces to a single discipline, applied consistently: **formulate the question before ordering the test, and know in advance what each possible result will change.** If no result changes management, the test is not indicated regardless of how reasonable it seems.

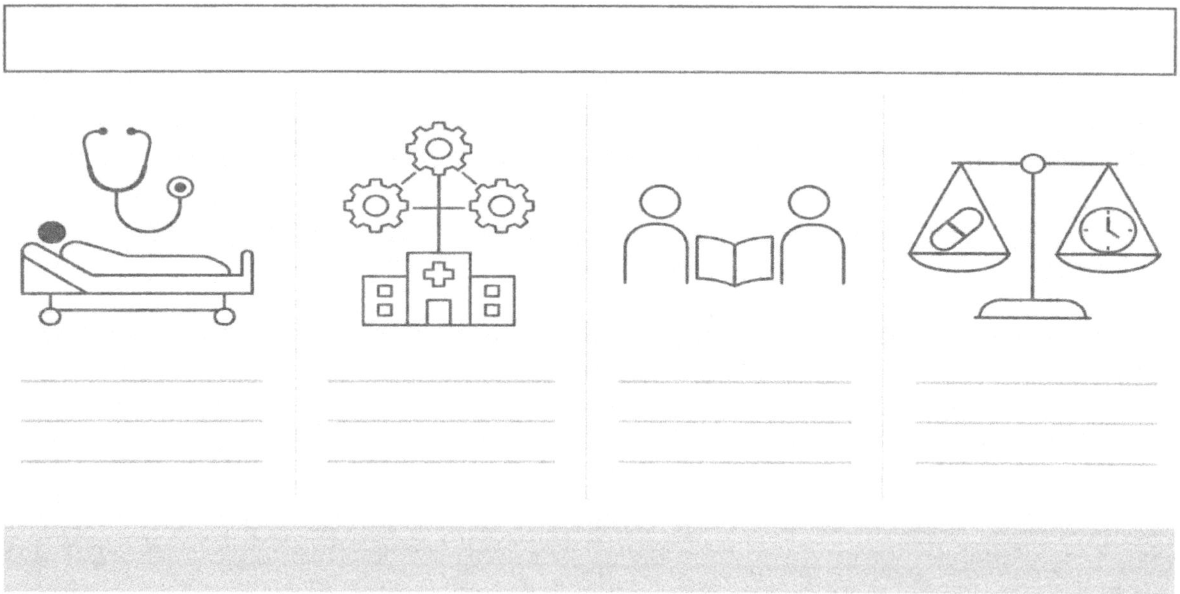

1.3 Workload, Cognitive Load, and the Census-Quality Relationship

1.3.1 The shape of the curve

The relationship between the number of patients a hospitalist carries and the quality of care those patients receive is not linear, and the shape of the curve has direct clinical and political consequences.

At very low census, hospitalists are safe but inefficient. Fixed costs, meaning travel between units, system login and navigation, familiarisation with a unit's staff and layout, and the overhead of participating in rounds and meetings, are distributed across few patients.

As census rises, performance improves on most measures. Batching becomes possible. Familiarity with the units deepens. The physician is already in the building when the next admission arrives. This is the range in which the hospitalist model demonstrates its efficiency advantages, and it is the range in which most institutional staffing models are nominally designed to operate.

Beyond a threshold, several things degrade at once, and they degrade non-independently. Time per patient falls. Interruption frequency rises. Documentation is deferred to the end of the day, when recall is degraded. Communication with families is compressed or omitted. Most importantly, and least visibly, the physician's reasoning shifts from a mixed analytic and intuitive mode toward almost purely heuristic pattern-matching.

Observational work across multiple health systems has consistently found that length of stay and cost per case begin to rise once physician census passes roughly the mid-teens, with the effect strongest when hospital occupancy is low, meaning when throughput pressure is not the constraining factor. Measures of diagnostic thoroughness, family communication, and documentation quality deteriorate in the same range. Readers should treat the specific threshold as institution-dependent rather than universal, since case mix, team structure, geographic distribution of patients, and the availability of advanced practice colleagues all shift it substantially.

1.3.2 The cognitive mechanism

The reason the relationship is non-linear rather than proportional is cognitive rather than temporal, and understanding the mechanism matters because it determines which interventions can possibly work.

Human working memory holds a small number of active elements. Clinical reasoning about a complex inpatient requires holding, simultaneously, the current problem representation, the differential diagnosis with its relative probabilities, the pending data and what each result would imply, the therapeutic plan and its contingencies, and the disposition trajectory. That is already close to capacity for a single patient.

A hospitalist carrying eighteen patients is not performing eighteen units of the work they performed for nine. They are operating a system in which most patients' models are, at any moment, not loaded. Each patient encounter requires reconstruction of the mental model from the record, and reconstruction is lossy. The detail that does not make it into the reconstruction is precisely the sort of detail that revises a diagnosis: the sister's remark about a fall three weeks ago, the transient hypotension at four in the morning, the fact that the creatinine has drifted upward across three days without crossing any alert threshold.

This is also why **interruption** is so corrosive and why interruption frequency is a better predictor of error than raw census in some analyses. Every interruption forces a model reconstruction. A hospitalist interrupted eleven times during a single admission note is not simply delayed; they have rebuilt the patient's model eleven times, and the eleventh version is not the same as the first.

The predictable clinical signatures of overload follow directly:

- **Anchoring on the referral diagnosis**, because generating an independent differential requires cognitive resource that is unavailable.
- **Premature closure**, because reopening a closed question requires reloading a model.
- **Failure to reconcile discordant data**, because noticing discordance requires holding the expectation alongside the observation.
- **Deferred and degraded documentation**, which then propagates the degraded model to the next clinician.
- **Omission of the discretionary act**: the family call, the medication review, the walk back to re-examine. These are omitted first because they are never explicitly required.

That last point deserves emphasis. Overload does not usually present as a wrong decision. It presents as an absent one.

1.3.3 Interventions with a plausible mechanism

Because the mechanism is cognitive, effective interventions are those that reduce the number of model reconstructions or reduce the cost of each one.

Geographic cohorting places a physician's patients on one or two units. It reduces travel, increases incidental contact with the nurses caring for those patients, and permits opportunistic reassessment. The evidence is favourable but not unambiguous, because rigid cohorting can worsen bed assignment efficiency and create census imbalance between teams. Implementation should preserve some flexibility.

Unit-based interdisciplinary rounds with defined participation and a structured format front-load communication into a single predictable window rather than distributing it across the day as pages and calls. The intervention converts many small interruptions into one scheduled block, which is precisely the correct transformation given the mechanism.

Explicit deferral protocols. Overloaded clinicians triage whether or not they intend to. The choice is between triage as a deliberate act and triage as drift. Making deferral explicit, meaning naming which tasks are being postponed and to when, converts an invisible risk into a managed one and creates a record that can be handed off.

Census caps with functioning overflow. A cap is only meaningful if the overflow pathway genuinely exists and is genuinely activated. A cap that is routinely exceeded because the alternative is an unstaffed patient is not a cap; it is a statement of preference.

Reduction of non-clinical load. Documentation burden, prior authorisation, and inbox management consume cognitive resource that is not distinguishable, physiologically, from the resource required for diagnosis. Scribes, ambient documentation technology, and note template reform are workload interventions even though they are usually classified as administrative ones.

Team structure. Pairing a physician with an advanced practice clinician in a defined division of labour, rather than as an undifferentiated additive, raises effective capacity without proportionally raising the number of models any one person must hold.

1.3.4 Census as a safety parameter

The practical conclusion of this section is a professional one. Census is not merely a staffing preference or a compensation variable. It is a patient safety parameter with a demonstrable mechanism and a measurable effect, and it belongs in the same conversation as nurse staffing ratios, alarm limits, and pharmacy verification.

Hospitalists therefore have a legitimate and arguably obligatory role in advocating for workload standards, and should make that argument in safety language rather than in workload language. The two arguments are received completely differently by hospital leadership, and only one of them is accurate.

1.4 Comanagement Models and the Negotiated Scope of Responsibility

1.4.1 Consultation and comanagement are different in kind

Traditional medical consultation is advisory. A consultant is asked a question, evaluates the patient, renders an opinion, writes recommendations, and the requesting service decides whether to implement them. Authority and responsibility remain with the primary service. The consultant's obligations are bounded by the question asked.

Comanagement is a different arrangement altogether. In comanagement, the hospitalist shares primary responsibility with the surgical or subspecialty service. The hospitalist writes orders directly, carries accountability for medical outcomes, participates in disposition decisions, and is expected to identify and act on problems that no one has asked about. The relationship is concurrent and continuous rather than episodic.

The distinction matters because the two arrangements have different failure modes and require different agreements, and because they are frequently confused in practice, with one service believing it is consulting while the other believes it is comanaging. That mismatch is a recurring source of harm and is discussed further below. Chapter 5 develops the consultation relationship in full; this section addresses comanagement specifically.

1.4.2 Where comanagement is established

Comanagement has become standard practice in several populations, and the pattern of adoption is informative. It has spread furthest where three conditions coincide: the patient population carries substantial medical comorbidity, the primary service's operative and procedural obligations limit ward availability, and the medical complications are both common and time-sensitive.

The archetype is **hip fracture in the older adult**, where orthogeriatric comanagement is now the standard of care in many health systems. Neurosurgical, spine, vascular, and complex oncological surgical populations have followed. Comanagement of solid organ transplant recipients, of patients admitted for complex haematological therapy, and of certain neurological populations is increasingly common.

1.4.3 What the evidence actually shows

The evidence base for comanagement is mixed in a specific and instructive way, and hospitalists should be able to describe it accurately rather than advocate for the model uncritically.

Process measures improve reliably. Venous thromboembolism prophylaxis rates, glycaemic control, delirium screening and prevention, appropriate antimicrobial selection, medication reconciliation completion, and management of chronic disease during the admission all improve consistently under comanagement across published series. This finding is robust and unsurprising, since these are precisely the processes a medical physician attends to and a busy operative service does not.

Satisfaction improves reliably. Nursing satisfaction, surgeon satisfaction, and patient-reported communication measures improve in most studies. Surgeons in particular value the model, since it returns their time to operative work and provides a responsive medical presence.

Mortality effects are small or absent in most populations, with an important exception. In general surgical and mixed populations, comanagement has not consistently demonstrated mortality benefit. In **frail older adults with hip fracture**, however, orthogeriatric comanagement models show consistent reductions in complications, and several models demonstrate mortality benefit. The distinguishing feature of that population is worth naming, because it generalises: the medical comorbidity burden is high, the complications are predictable, the time window for intervention is short, and the patients cannot advocate for themselves.

Length of stay effects are inconsistent, improving in some series and unchanged in others, with results depending heavily on whether the comanagement service has authority over disposition.

The synthesis for practice is this: comanagement reliably improves the reliability of medical process, and translates into outcome benefit specifically where the population is frail, the complications are predictable, and the primary service is structurally unavailable. Institutions should target the model accordingly rather than applying it universally.

1.4.4 The dominant failure mode: diffusion of responsibility

The recurrent, predictable, and occasionally lethal failure of comanagement is **ambiguity about who is responsible for what**.

The mechanism is familiar from social psychology and entirely applicable here. When two parties both have plausible responsibility for a task, and neither has been assigned it explicitly, the probability that neither performs it is substantially higher than the probability that either would fail if solely responsible. Two services both assuming the other is managing anticoagulation produces a patient on no anticoagulation. Two services both assuming the other has spoken to the family produces a family who has spoken to no one. Two services both assuming the other will decide about discharge produces a patient who stays an extra day.

Related failure modes:

- **The comanagement relationship as a dumping mechanism**, in which the primary service disengages entirely and the hospitalist becomes responsible for decisions requiring surgical judgment they cannot supply.
- **Order conflict**, in which two services write contradictory orders, most dangerously for analgesia, anticoagulation, and fluids.
- **Escalation ambiguity at night**, when the covering hospitalist and the covering surgical resident each believe the other is primary for an acute event.
- **Consultation creep**, in which a service requests a bounded consultation and then progressively behaves as though comanagement had been agreed, without any conversation having occurred.

1.4.5 Constructing a written comanagement agreement

The remedy is unglamorous and effective: a written agreement, negotiated between service leaders in advance, specific enough to resolve real disputes, and reviewed periodically. An unwritten comanagement relationship reliably degrades into a resentful one, because in the absence of a document each party's memory of the arrangement drifts toward its own convenience.

A functional agreement addresses, at minimum:

1. **Population.** Which patients are comanaged, by which criteria, and who applies the criteria.
2. **Admission attribution.** Which service is the admitting service of record, and how that maps to billing and to the medical record's designation of the responsible physician.
3. **Acute deterioration.** Who responds, in what order, and who leads the response.
4. **Analgesia.** Who prescribes it, who adjusts it, and who manages opioid-related complications. This is the single most common source of order conflict and should be settled explicitly.
5. **Anticoagulation and antithrombotics.** Who decides on prophylaxis, therapeutic anticoagulation, interruption, and resumption after operation, and who is responsible for the resumption actually occurring.
6. **Diagnostic studies.** Who orders which categories, and who is responsible for reviewing and acting on results, including incidental findings.
7. **Consultation authority.** Who may call additional consultants, and whether notification of the other service is required.
8. **Family communication.** Who conducts routine updates, who conducts goals-of-care conversations, and how the two services avoid contradicting each other.
9. **Disposition.** Who decides readiness for discharge, who arranges it, and who writes the summary.
10. **Escalation of disagreement.** The named individuals to whom an unresolved clinical disagreement is escalated, and the expectation that escalation is a normal professional act rather than an accusation.

The tenth item is the one most often omitted and most often needed. A comanagement relationship without a defined escalation pathway resolves disagreements by whoever is more insistent, which is not a clinical criterion.

1.4.6 Professional conduct within comanagement

Two behavioural norms substantially determine whether a comanagement relationship functions.

The first is **staying inside your judgment**. The hospitalist who overrules a surgical decision on surgical grounds, or who discusses operative risk with a family without the surgeon present, damages the relationship and frequently misinforms the patient. The correct move is to raise the concern to the surgeon directly and, if unresolved, to escalate through the named pathway.

The second is **proactive rather than reactive presence**. The value of comanagement is generated by the problems identified before anyone notices them: the drifting creatinine, the missed home medication, the early delirium. A comanaging hospitalist who functions reactively, addressing only what is asked, has recreated consultation at higher cost.

1.5 Leadership Without Formal Authority

1.5.1 The structural position

Almost all hospitalist influence is exercised without positional power. The hospitalist cannot direct the nurse, who reports through nursing administration. Cannot direct the pharmacist, the physical therapist, the case manager, or the radiologist. Cannot compel a consultant to see the patient today rather than tomorrow. Cannot instruct the surgeon. Cannot allocate a bed. Cannot change the discharge pathway.

And yet the care plan depends on every one of these people, and the hospitalist is the person whose name is on the plan.

This gap between responsibility and authority is the defining political fact of hospitalist practice. It is experienced by new attendings as a persistent low-grade frustration, and it is not resolvable by seniority, because senior hospitalists face the same structure. It is resolvable only by developing the specific competencies that produce influence in its absence.

1.5.2 Framing

The single most useful technique is **framing a request in terms of the other party's goals rather than your own.**

Compare two versions of the same request to a radiologist for an add-on study.

The first: "I need the CT today, it has been pending since this morning." This frames the request around the requester's need and implicitly assigns fault. The predictable response is defensive.

The second: "I have a patient I think has an early anastomotic leak. If she does, she needs to go back to theatre tonight, and if she does not, I can send her home tomorrow. Is there any way to get her scan into today's list?" This frames the request around the clinical question, supplies the reason urgency exists, and offers the other party a role in a decision rather than a task.

The same transformation applies across every relationship. To a nurse: not "please check the vitals more often" but "I am worried she is going to drop her pressure overnight and I would rather we catch it early." To a case manager: not "we need to discharge this patient" but "this patient is at high risk of a hospital-acquired infection every extra day she is here; what is blocking the placement?"

This is not manipulation, and it should not be executed as a script. It is accurate communication. The reason the second version works is that it contains the information the other party actually needs in order to prioritise correctly, and the first version withholds it.

1.5.3 Escalation discipline

A second competency is knowing which disagreements to absorb and which to escalate, and escalating in a manner that preserves the relationship you will need next week.

Most disagreements should be absorbed. The consultant's preference for a different antibiotic within a reasonable range, the nurse's request for a different timing, the case manager's insistence on a particular form: absorbing these builds credit and costs almost nothing.

A disagreement should be escalated when the difference is material to patient safety, when it has resisted direct discussion, and when the delay of further discussion itself carries risk. When escalating, three practices reduce damage: escalate the issue rather than the person; inform the other party that you are escalating before you do it; and state the clinical stake explicitly rather than the procedural grievance.

The hospitalist who never escalates is unsafe. The hospitalist who escalates weekly becomes ineffective, because the escalation pathway prices in the sender.

1.5.4 Credit allocation and the currency of a system without payment

In a system where you cannot pay, promote, or discipline anyone, the only durable currency is credit and reciprocity.

Consistently attributing improvement to the team is therefore both accurate and strategically necessary. The pharmacist who caught the interaction, the nurse who called early, the therapist who identified the unsafe gait: naming these people in rounds, in the note, and to their managers costs nothing and compounds. The hospitalist who does this reliably finds, within a year, that people call them early, accommodate their requests, and warn them about problems before those problems become emergencies.

The inverse also compounds. A reputation for irritability functions as a tax levied on every future interaction, and it is levied most heavily at the moments of greatest need, which are at night, when the caller is deciding whether the situation is worth waking you for.

1.5.5 From informal influence to formal role

Formal leadership positions in hospital medicine, meaning group director, quality officer, service line lead, chief medical officer, follow from demonstrated informal influence far more often than from credentials. The sequence is generally: reliable clinical performance, then successful completion of a visible improvement project, then committee participation, then formal role.

For readers who intend to pursue this trajectory, three practical notes. Choose an early project that is small, measurable, and genuinely wanted by someone with authority, because a completed small project is worth more than an abandoned ambitious one. Learn to present data to non-clinical audiences, which is a distinct and teachable skill. And develop at least a working literacy in the institution's finances, because clinical arguments that are indifferent to cost are systematically discounted, whether or not that is fair.

1.6 Burnout, Moral Injury, and Career Sustainability

1.6.1 Why the risk is elevated in this specialty

Hospital medicine carries elevated occupational distress risk, and the reasons are structural rather than a reflection on the people who choose it.

High turnover without longitudinal reward. The hospitalist invests intensely in a patient for four days and then never learns what happened. The emotional labour is expended; the reward of knowing that the person went back to their life is withheld. Over years, this asymmetry accumulates.

Circadian disruption. Night and swing shift work produces measurable physiological consequences including sleep architecture disruption, metabolic and cardiovascular risk, and mood effects, and the cognitive impairment of sustained night work is comparable in magnitude to meaningful degrees of alcohol intoxication. Rotating schedules that repeatedly shift the circadian phase are worse than fixed night schedules in most analyses.

Documentation and administrative burden. A substantial proportion of the working day is spent on the record rather than the patient, and much of that work serves billing, legal, and regulatory purposes rather than clinical communication. The mismatch between why a physician entered medicine and how they spend their afternoon is a well-documented driver of disengagement.

Density of death without relationship. Hospitalists are present at a great many deaths, usually of people they met a few days earlier. The relational context that ordinarily makes accompanying a death meaningful rather than merely distressing is absent by design.

Repeated exposure to system failure. The hospitalist stands at the point where the health system's structural failures become visible: the patient who cannot be discharged because no facility will take them, the readmission that was inevitable, the uninsured patient whose treatment plan is determined by their coverage.

1.6.2 Burnout and moral injury are not the same construct

This distinction is clinically and practically important, and conflating the two has done real damage.

Burnout, as originally described in occupational psychology, comprises emotional exhaustion, depersonalisation, and a reduced sense of personal accomplishment. Its principal driver is the sustained mismatch between demand and resource. Its remedies are therefore load-related: fewer patients, more time, better systems, adequate recovery.

Moral injury, a construct imported from military psychology and applied to clinical work by Talbot and Dean, describes the distress that arises from being repeatedly prevented from doing what one knows to be right, or from participating in acts that violate one's moral commitments. The hospitalist who discharges a patient knowing they will return, who withholds an indicated therapy because of coverage, who provides aggressive care they believe is causing suffering, or who cannot obtain the placement a patient needs, is not experiencing a resource shortfall. They are experiencing a values violation.

The practical consequence is that the two require different interventions, and matching the wrong intervention to the wrong problem predictably increases cynicism. Responding to moral injury with resilience training communicates, accurately, that the institution has diagnosed the physician rather than the system. Clinicians recognise this immediately, and the resulting contempt for wellness programming is not irrational.

1.6.3 Interventions and their evidence

Intervention studies in physician distress consistently find that **organisational interventions outperform individual ones**, though both have measurable effects and the two are complementary rather than competing.

Organisational interventions with evidence or strong mechanism:

- Workload limits with functioning overflow, as discussed in section 1.3.
- Schedule predictability, adequate recovery intervals after night blocks, and avoidance of rapid phase rotation.
- Reduction of documentation burden through scribes, ambient documentation, note template reform, and elimination of redundant required fields.
- Meaningful physician participation in decisions that affect practice, which appears to operate through restored agency rather than through the content of any particular decision.
- Local leadership behaviour, which in large studies is among the strongest single predictors of group-level burnout. The behaviour of the immediate supervisor matters more than institution-wide programmes.

Individual interventions with evidence:

- Facilitated small-group programmes with protected time, which have demonstrated durable effects where the time is genuinely protected and paid.
- Mindfulness-based and cognitive behavioural programmes, with modest but real effect sizes.
- Peer support programmes following adverse events, addressed as the second victim phenomenon in Chapter 4.

The critical qualifier is that individual interventions must not be deployed as substitutes for organisational ones. Where they are, they fail and they discredit the underlying methods.

1.6.4 Designing a durable career

A full clinical hospitalist load sustained without variation for thirty years is uncommon, and readers should plan on that basis rather than discovering it at year eight.

Most durable careers in hospital medicine incorporate a **second domain**, drawn from section 1.2: quality and safety, education, administration, informatics, research, palliative care, or perioperative medicine. The second domain provides intellectual variation, a growth trajectory that does not require leaving clinical work, protection against the monotony of high-volume ward medicine, and eventually a partial off-ramp from full-time nights and weekends.

Practical guidance for the first five years:

- Protect sleep with the seriousness of a clinical intervention, because it is one.
- Choose a second domain early enough to build credibility in it, but late enough to be clinically competent first. The second or third year of practice is typical.
- Maintain relationships outside medicine deliberately, since shift work erodes them passively.
- Distinguish, when distressed, whether the problem is load or values, and direct the response accordingly.
- Treat persistent symptoms of depression, anxiety, or substance use as the medical conditions they are, and seek care. Physician reluctance here is well documented, frequently rationalised as licensure concern, and materially dangerous.

1.7 Professionalism at the Bedside and in the Electronic Record

Two settings deserve specific attention, because they are where the professionalism of a hospitalist is most often tested and where the consequences of failure are most concrete.

1.7.1 At the bedside

The hospitalist meets a frightened person at their least dignified moment, as a stranger, without the credit of prior acquaintance, and must establish a working relationship in minutes. This must be done repeatedly, several times a day, on the worst days of other people's lives.

Practices that measurably improve this encounter are unglamorous and well established:

- **Sit down.** Seated clinicians are perceived as having spent substantially longer at the bedside than standing clinicians who spent the same actual time. The effect is robust across settings.
- **Introduce the role explicitly.** Most patients do not know what a hospitalist is and reasonably assume their own physician has abandoned them. A single sentence resolves this: "I am the doctor who works here in the hospital. I will be seeing you every day this week, and I will send everything back to your own doctor when you go home."
- **Name the discontinuity honestly.** When your block ends, tell the patient. Discovering on day five that the physician they trusted has been replaced without warning damages trust more than the handoff itself does.

- **Ask what they are most worried about**, which is a different question from what brought them in, and frequently produces the information that changes the plan.
- **Speak to the nurse before entering the room**, which takes ninety seconds and prevents the common failure of contradicting information the patient was given an hour earlier.

1.7.2 In the record

Clinical documentation now serves at least five constituencies simultaneously: clinical communication, billing justification, medico-legal defence, quality measurement, and, under open-notes access legislation, the patient themselves. These purposes pull in different directions, and the resulting compromise has degraded the note as a communication instrument in most institutions.

Three obligations follow for the individual hospitalist.

Do not propagate what you have not verified. Copy-forward practice transmits errors indefinitely. A note describing left leg swelling, carried unchanged for nine days after the swelling resolved, is a false statement in a legal document that will eventually inform a clinical decision. The standard is straightforward: anything asserted in today's note was verified today, or is explicitly attributed and dated.

Write for the next clinician, not for the auditor. The single most valuable element of a hospitalist note is a current, honest assessment: what is actually going on, what remains uncertain, what would change the plan, and what should worry the person covering tonight. This is precisely the element most often omitted in favour of imported data. A note containing four pages of laboratory values and no reasoning has transmitted nothing.

Attend to language, because it changes care. Controlled studies have demonstrated that stigmatising language in the medical record, including terms such as difficult, noncompliant, and drug-seeking, alters subsequent clinicians' attitudes toward the patient and their analgesic prescribing decisions, even when the clinical facts presented are identical. Negative descriptors appear disproportionately in the records of Black patients and patients with substance use disorders, which means the practice is also a mechanism of documented disparity. Chapter 19 develops this further.

Because patients now read these notes routinely, a simple operational standard resolves most cases: **write nothing you would not say to the patient's face, and assert nothing you have not confirmed today.** This is not a constraint on candour. Difficult clinical realities can and should be documented; they are documented in behavioural, specific, non-pejorative terms. "Declined the recommended anticoagulation after discussion of risks; plans to reconsider" is more clinically useful than "noncompliant," and it is also true.

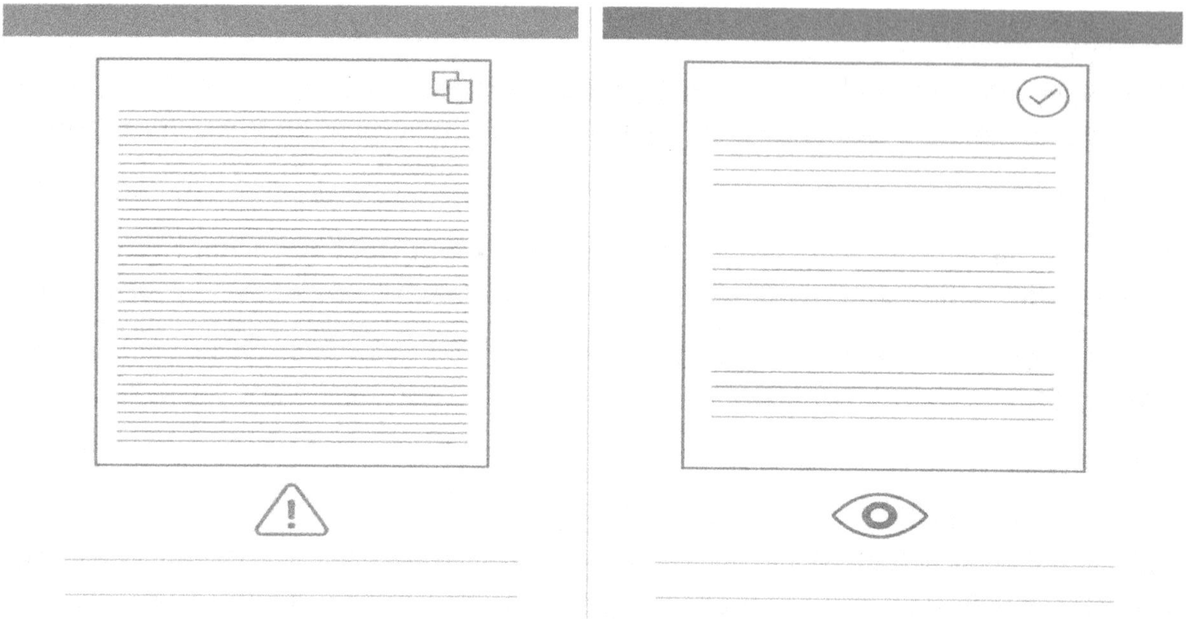

1.7.3 Professionalism toward colleagues as a safety practice

A final point closes the loop with section 1.2.3. The manner in which a hospitalist treats nurses, pharmacists, therapists, students, and covering colleagues is not solely a matter of courtesy. It sets the threshold at which those colleagues will contact them with a concern.

A hospitalist who is curt at two in the morning has, in a single interaction, raised the bar the nurse will apply before the next call. The next call may be the one about the patient who is deteriorating. Disruptive behaviour by physicians is associated with measurable increases in adverse events for exactly this reason, and the mechanism runs through suppressed communication rather than through any direct act.

This is the strongest available argument for civility, and it is worth stating in these terms precisely because it does not depend on anyone's temperament. Whatever a clinician's disposition, the information they receive is a function of how safe others feel bringing it.

Chapter Summary

- Hospital medicine specialises by **site**, asserting that the hospital is a distinct clinical environment requiring dedicated expertise. The model emerged from ambulatory intensification, inpatient acuity compression, quality accountability, and information system centralisation.
- Value is generated through three mechanisms: **volume and pattern density**, **temporal availability**, and **systems fluency**. The last transfers least readily between institutions and is the least discussed.

- The model purchases these mechanisms with **longitudinal relationship**. Medication reconciliation, structured handoff, and discharge summary standards are the load-bearing structures that compensate for that loss, not administrative burdens.
- Practice spans four domains: **clinical**, **systems**, **educational**, and **stewardship**. Population-level impact often arises from the systems domain rather than from direct care.
- The **census-quality relationship is non-linear**, mediated by working memory and interruption-driven model reconstruction. Overload presents as omitted decisions rather than wrong ones. Census is a patient safety parameter and should be argued as one.
- **Comanagement** differs from consultation in kind. It reliably improves process measures and satisfaction, and improves outcomes specifically in frail populations with predictable complications. Its dominant failure mode is diffusion of responsibility, remedied only by a specific written agreement that includes a defined escalation pathway.
- Hospitalists hold **responsibility without authority**. Influence derives from framing requests around others' goals, disciplined escalation, and consistent credit allocation.
- **Burnout and moral injury are distinct constructs** with distinct remedies. Treating moral injury as a resilience deficit predictably increases cynicism. Organisational interventions outperform individual ones, and local leadership behaviour is among the strongest predictors of group distress.
- **Bedside conduct and documentation language measurably alter downstream clinical decisions.** Stigmatising descriptors change subsequent prescribing. Civility toward colleagues determines the threshold at which you are warned about a deteriorating patient.

Review Questions

1. A hospital administrator proposes increasing average hospitalist census from fourteen to nineteen patients, arguing that the group has capacity because rounds finish by noon. Construct the safety argument against this proposal, specifying the mechanism by which quality would degrade and the clinical signature you would expect to observe first.

2. An orthopaedic service requests comanagement of all arthroplasty patients. Identify the four elements of a written agreement most likely to prevent harm in this specific population, and justify each.

3. Distinguish burnout from moral injury using a clinical example drawn from discharge planning. State which intervention category applies to each and why the alternative would fail.

4. A resident's note describes a patient as "a difficult historian, noncompliant with prior therapy, likely drug-seeking." Rewrite the clinically relevant content in language that is accurate, specific, and non-pejorative, and explain what evidence supports the rewriting.

5. You are the sole hospitalist covering a patient whose surgical service has not responded to two pages regarding a possible anastomotic leak. Describe your escalation sequence and the framing you would use at each step.

CHAPTER 2: Clinical Reasoning and Diagnostic Excellence

Learning Objectives

After studying this chapter, the reader should be able to:

1. Describe dual-process theory as applied to clinical reasoning, and state the principal empirical objections to its use as a model of diagnostic error.
2. Construct a problem representation using semantic qualifiers, and explain how illness scripts are stored, retrieved, and refined.
3. Apply Bayesian reasoning quantitatively, using pretest probability, likelihood ratios, and the test and treatment thresholds, to decide whether a diagnostic test is indicated.
4. Classify diagnostic error by mechanism, and reconstruct the sequence by which a missed diagnosis typically occurs.
5. Evaluate cognitive debiasing strategies against the evidence for their effectiveness, and identify which interventions have demonstrated effect and which have not.
6. Appraise a guideline or systematic review rapidly, identifying the specific failure modes that most often mislead inpatient clinicians.
7. Apply the principles of diagnostic stewardship to test selection, and explain how reducing test volume can increase diagnostic accuracy.

Chapter Overview

Chapter 1 argued that the characteristic clinical situation of hospital medicine is undifferentiated breadth under time pressure with incomplete information. This chapter addresses the discipline required to operate in that situation well.

The framing matters. Diagnostic reasoning is often taught as though it were a byproduct of knowledge, on the assumption that a clinician who knows enough medicine will diagnose accurately. The evidence does not support this. Diagnostic error occurs at meaningful rates among clinicians whose factual knowledge is not in question, and the errors cluster around identifiable features of the reasoning process rather than around gaps in content. Knowledge is necessary and insufficient.

The chapter proceeds from cognitive architecture to formal probability, then to failure and its remedies, then to the appraisal of external evidence, and finally to the practical discipline of test selection. The order is deliberate: stewardship in section 2.7 is the applied consequence of everything preceding it, and it is unintelligible without the probability discussed in section 2.3.

Two warnings apply throughout. First, much of the cognitive psychology imported into medical education has been oversold, and readers should hold the frameworks in this chapter as useful models rather than as established mechanism. Second, the numerical examples given are illustrative and drawn from published estimates that vary considerably between populations. Verify any figure against a current source before applying it to a specific patient.

2.1 Dual-Process Theory and Its Limits in Real Wards

2.1.1 The standard account

The dominant framework for describing clinical reasoning divides cognition into two modes, conventionally labelled System 1 and System 2.

System 1 is fast, automatic, associative, and effortless. It operates by pattern recognition. The experienced clinician who glances at a patient from the doorway and forms an immediate impression of sepsis is using System 1. It requires no deliberate attention, produces an answer almost instantly, and runs continuously whether or not it is invited.

System 2 is slow, deliberate, analytic, and effortful. It operates by explicit rule application, hypothesis generation, and sequential reasoning. The clinician who lists a differential, weighs each item against the available data, and calculates a risk score is using System 2. It requires working memory, is easily disrupted by interruption, and is metabolically and attentionally expensive.

The standard account holds that expertise consists largely in the development of accurate System 1 pattern recognition, that System 2 serves as a monitor and corrective, and that diagnostic error arises predominantly when System 1 produces a wrong answer and System 2 fails to catch it. On this account, the remedy for error is to slow down, engage the analytic system, and check the intuitive answer.

This framework has been enormously influential in medical education, and it has genuine explanatory power. It accounts for why expertise does not feel like reasoning, why fatigue and interruption degrade diagnosis specifically rather than generally, and why the same clinician can be brilliant at eight in the morning and unreliable at two the following morning.

2.1.2 The empirical objections

Readers should nonetheless understand the substantial criticism this framework has attracted, because the criticism has direct practical consequences.

Intuitive reasoning is not systematically less accurate than analytic reasoning. This is the most damaging finding for the standard account. Experimental work by Norman, Eva, and colleagues has repeatedly shown that forcing clinicians to reason slowly and analytically does not reliably improve diagnostic accuracy, and in some conditions worsens it. Experts asked to think aloud and justify each step sometimes perform worse than experts allowed to answer immediately. If the intuitive system were the primary source of error, this should not occur.

Most diagnostic errors are errors of knowledge organisation rather than errors of speed. When missed diagnoses are analysed carefully, the failure is frequently that the correct diagnosis was never generated as a possibility at all. Slowing down does not help a clinician consider a diagnosis they do not possess in retrievable form. The problem is the contents of memory, not the speed of access to it.

The two systems are not cleanly separable. The distinction is a useful description of subjective experience, but attempts to identify two distinct processing architectures have not succeeded. Most real clinical reasoning appears to be a blend, with pattern recognition generating candidates that are then evaluated with varying degrees of deliberateness, iteratively and rapidly.

The framework generates a false remedy. If error is caused by insufficient System 2, the remedy is to slow down and reflect. The evidence for the effectiveness of generic "slow down" interventions is weak, as discussed in section 2.5. Meanwhile the framework directs attention away from remedies that do work, principally the accumulation of well-organised experience and the redesign of the information environment.

2.1.3 What to retain and what to discard

The pragmatic position, and the one adopted throughout this handbook, is as follows.

Retain the descriptive vocabulary. It is genuinely useful to be able to say to a trainee that they anchored on the referral diagnosis, or that their immediate impression deserves a second look. The words describe something real about clinical experience even if the underlying architecture is not as advertised.

Retain the observation that **conditions degrade reasoning**. Fatigue, interruption, high census, emotional arousal, and time pressure all impair diagnostic performance, and this is one of the best-supported findings in the field. Chapter 1, section 1.3, addressed the mechanism.

Discard the belief that slowing down is a general-purpose remedy. It is not. Deliberation applied to a wrong hypothesis produces a more elaborately justified wrong hypothesis, which is worse than an unjustified one because it is harder to dislodge.

Discard the belief that expertise consists in suppressing intuition. Expert intuition is the product of accurate pattern learning and is the most valuable diagnostic instrument most clinicians possess. The task is to calibrate it, not to override it.

Replace the general remedy with a specific one: **the value of deliberate reasoning lies in generating alternatives, not in re-examining the original answer.** The productive question is not "am I sure?" but "what else could produce exactly this picture?" This distinction recurs throughout section 2.5.

2.1.4 Practical application on the ward

Three habits follow directly.

Notice the moment of closure. There is an identifiable subjective instant at which a clinician stops considering and starts confirming. It usually occurs early, frequently within the first minutes of an encounter, and often before the examination. Simply noticing this moment, without necessarily doing anything about it, appears to be one of the more useful metacognitive skills available.

Separate data gathering from hypothesis evaluation in high-stakes cases. Once a hypothesis is active, data gathering becomes selective in favour of it. Deliberately completing the history and examination before committing to an interpretation reduces this, at the cost of time.

Treat degraded conditions as a formal indication for external checks. When tired, interrupted, or overloaded, the correct response is not to try harder. It is to invoke something external: a checklist, a colleague, a second look at the imaging with the radiologist, or an explicit statement to the covering clinician that the diagnosis is provisional. Section 2.5 develops this point, which is among the few debiasing recommendations with a defensible evidence base.

2.2 Illness Scripts, Semantic Qualifiers, and Problem Representation

2.2.1 How diagnostic knowledge is actually organised

If diagnostic accuracy depends more on the organisation of knowledge than on the speed of reasoning, the structure of that organisation becomes the central question.

The dominant model holds that clinicians store diagnostic knowledge as **illness scripts**: structured mental representations of diseases that are organised for clinical use rather than for pathophysiological completeness. A script is not a textbook entry. It is a compressed, experience-shaped package containing:

- **Predisposing conditions.** Who gets this, in what context, after what exposure. This is epidemiology as it presents at the bedside rather than as it appears in a population study.
- **Pathophysiological insult.** A brief causal account, usually simplified, sufficient to generate expectations about what else should be present.
- **Clinical consequences.** The expected findings, their typical sequence, their timing, and importantly their expected *absence*.

The compression is the point. A student's knowledge of pulmonary embolism is extensive, detailed, and organised by mechanism, which makes it slow to retrieve and difficult to match against a patient. An experienced clinician's script for pulmonary embolism is smaller, organised by presentation, and includes elements no textbook contains: what the patient's breathing sounds like from the doorway, how the anxiety of hypoxia differs from the anxiety of panic, and the specific quality of the pleuritic pain.

Scripts are refined by three processes: repeated exposure, feedback about outcome, and, critically, **exposure to near misses and atypical presentations**. The third is why a clinician who has once missed an aortic dissection has a permanently richer dissection script than one who has not. It is also an argument for structured case review, since deliberately reviewing others' misses is the only way to acquire this refinement without inflicting the miss on your own patient.

2.2.2 Semantic qualifiers

Skilled diagnosticians describe patients differently from novices, and the difference is measurable and teachable.

Semantic qualifiers are paired, abstract, opposing descriptors that transform raw clinical data into terms that match how diseases are stored. Common pairs include acute versus chronic, sudden versus gradual, constant versus intermittent, progressive versus stable, unilateral versus bilateral, proximal versus distal, painful versus painless, focal versus diffuse, and provoked versus unprovoked.

The distinction between novice and expert language is illustrated by two descriptions of the same patient.

Novice: "This is a 63-year-old man who has had some trouble with his legs for a while, he says it started maybe a few weeks ago, and it has been getting worse, and now he is having trouble climbing the stairs at home, and he mentioned some tingling."

Expert: “This is a 63-year-old man with a subacute, progressive, symmetric, proximal weakness with associated distal sensory symptoms.”

The second version contains less information and is far more useful. Every raw detail has been converted into a qualifier, and the resulting statement maps directly onto a small set of illness scripts. A clinician hearing the second version can generate a differential immediately. A clinician hearing the first cannot, because the data have not been rendered into the form in which diagnostic knowledge is stored.

Research by Bordage and colleagues demonstrated that the density of semantic qualifiers in a clinician’s case description correlates with diagnostic accuracy. This is one of the more directly actionable findings in the field, because the skill is explicitly teachable: require trainees to present in qualifier form, and correct them when they revert to narrative.

2.2.3 The problem representation

The **problem representation** is a one-sentence or two-sentence abstract summary of the case, constructed from semantic qualifiers, that states the diagnostic question in the terms in which it will be answered.

Its canonical form is: *demographic and relevant risk context* plus *temporal and qualitative characterisation of the syndrome* plus *the discriminating features*.

Consider a worked example. A 78-year-old woman is admitted with confusion. The raw data include a three-day history, a urinary tract infection treated as an outpatient, a background of mild cognitive impairment, recent addition of oxybutynin, a fall two weeks ago, a sodium of 128, and a temperature of 37.6 degrees Celsius.

A weak problem representation: “Elderly woman with confusion and a urinary tract infection.”

A strong problem representation: “A 78-year-old woman with baseline mild cognitive impairment presenting with a subacute, fluctuating encephalopathy, in the context of a recent anticholinergic exposure, a recent unwitnessed fall, and a mild hyponatraemia, without focal neurological deficit or significant fever.”

The second version has done nearly all of the diagnostic work. It has named the syndrome correctly as delirium rather than as infection. It has surfaced three competing explanations, each of which requires a different action. It has explicitly documented two negatives that matter. A clinician handed this sentence can construct the correct plan; a clinician handed the first will order a urine culture and stop.

Three practical rules govern good problem representations.

Name the syndrome, not the assumed cause. “Encephalopathy” is a syndrome; “urosepsis” is a hypothesis. Embedding the hypothesis in the representation guarantees anchoring.

Include informative negatives. The absence of a finding that a leading hypothesis predicts is diagnostic information and belongs in the summary.

Revise it explicitly when data change. The problem representation is a living object. A hospitalist who states the revised representation aloud on day three, when the sodium has corrected and the confusion has not, has performed the single most valuable reasoning act of the admission.

2.2.4 Script failure and the illusion of breadth

Two failure modes of script-based reasoning deserve naming, because both are common and neither is obvious.

The impoverished script. A clinician possesses a diagnosis in factual memory but not in retrievable clinical form. They can define thyroid storm on an examination and will not recognise it at the bedside, because the stored representation is a definition rather than a script. This is the dominant failure mode in early practice and explains why reading about a disease is a poor substitute for encountering it. The partial remedy is deliberate case exposure: structured review of real cases with their trajectories, which builds script structure in a way that reading definitions does not.

The overweighted script. Recently or memorably encountered diagnoses become disproportionately retrievable, which is the availability heuristic operating on script access. The hospitalist who diagnosed a pulmonary embolism yesterday will consider pulmonary embolism more readily today, which is helpful when it is present and harmful when it is not.

Both failures point toward the same corrective discipline, developed in section 2.3: once a hypothesis is generated, its plausibility must be assessed against something external to the ease with which it came to mind.

2.3 Bayesian Reasoning: Pretest Probability, Likelihood Ratios, and Test Thresholds

2.3.1 Why formal probability is unavoidable

Sections 2.1 and 2.2 described how hypotheses are generated. This section addresses how they should be evaluated, and it is the technical core of the chapter.

The central insight is that **a test result does not establish a diagnosis; it revises a probability.** This is not a philosophical nicety. It has direct consequences at the bedside, and failure to internalise it produces a specific and recognisable pattern of error: the clinician who treats a positive result as confirmation in a patient who was never likely to have the disease, and the clinician who abandons a diagnosis on a negative result in a patient in whom it remains probable.

Both errors are avoidable with a small amount of arithmetic that can be performed in the corridor.

2.3.2 The three quantities

Pretest probability is the probability that the patient has the disease before the test is performed. It comes from prevalence in the relevant population, adjusted by history and examination. It is an estimate, and it is the single most important number in the calculation, because the same test result yields wildly different conclusions at different starting points.

Sources of pretest probability, in descending order of reliability: a validated clinical decision rule for this population; published prevalence in a comparable population; institutional data; and, last and least reliable, personal impression. Clinicians systematically overestimate the probability of dramatic diagnoses and underestimate the probability of common ones, so the personal estimate should be anchored to published data wherever any exist.

The likelihood ratio expresses how much a given finding or test result changes the probability. It is defined as the probability of that result in patients with the disease divided by the probability of that result in patients without it.

A positive likelihood ratio above 1 raises the probability; below 1 lowers it. The practical interpretation:

Likelihood ratio	Approximate effect on probability
10 or above	Large increase, often decisive
5 to 10	Moderate increase
2 to 5	Small increase
1 to 2	Minimal, rarely worth acting on
1	No information at all
0.5 to 1	Minimal decrease
0.2 to 0.5	Small decrease
0.1 to 0.2	Moderate decrease
0.1 or below	Large decrease, often decisive

Likelihood ratios are preferable to sensitivity and specificity for bedside use for three reasons. They apply to individual results rather than to dichotomised categories, so a markedly elevated result and a marginally elevated result can be distinguished. They combine straightforwardly across independent findings. And they express directly the quantity a clinician actually wants to know.

Posttest probability is the result. It becomes the pretest probability for the next test, which is why sequential testing must be reasoned about as a sequence rather than as a set of independent verdicts.

2.3.3 Doing the arithmetic without a calculator

The formal calculation requires conversion to odds, multiplication, and conversion back. This is impractical in a corridor, and two approximations exist.

The first is the **Fagan nomogram**, a graphical instrument on which a line drawn from the pretest probability through the likelihood ratio intersects the posttest probability. It is accurate, requires no arithmetic, and exists in numerous pocket and application forms.

The second is a mental approximation adequate for most clinical purposes. For pretest probabilities below roughly 30 per cent, where most diagnostic questions live, a likelihood ratio of 2 adds approximately 15 percentage points to the probability, a ratio of 5 adds approximately 30 points, and a ratio of 10 adds approximately 45 points. The corresponding negative ratios subtract approximately the same amounts: 0.5 subtracts about 15 points, 0.2 subtracts about 30, and 0.1

subtracts about 45. These approximations degrade at the extremes and are unsuitable for formal work, but they are sufficient to distinguish a probability of 3 per cent from one of 40 per cent, which is usually the decision at hand.

2.3.4 The test and treatment thresholds

The reason to calculate probability is to make a decision, and decisions are governed by two thresholds, described formally by Pauker and Kassirer.

Imagine the probability of disease as a line running from 0 to 1. Two points divide it.

The treatment threshold is the probability above which treatment should be given without further testing, because the expected benefit of treating exceeds the expected harm of treating those who do not have the disease, and further testing would not change the decision.

The test threshold is the probability below which no test should be performed and the diagnosis should be abandoned, because the probability is so low that the harms of testing, including false positives and their cascades, exceed the benefit of the rare true positive found.

Testing is indicated only in the zone between the two thresholds. Above the treatment threshold, treat. Below the test threshold, stop. In between, test.

Where the thresholds sit depends on three factors, and reasoning about them explicitly resolves most disputes about whether a test is warranted.

- **Severity of the missed diagnosis.** The more catastrophic the miss, the lower both thresholds fall. This is why the test threshold for aortic dissection is far lower than for gastro-oesophageal reflux, and correctly so.
- **Risk and cost of treatment.** The more dangerous the treatment, the higher the treatment threshold rises. Anticoagulation in a patient with recent intracranial haemorrhage carries a much higher treatment threshold for suspected pulmonary embolism than anticoagulation in a healthy patient.
- **Risk and cost of the test itself.** The more harmful or inaccurate the test, the narrower the testing zone becomes. A test with substantial procedural risk has a much smaller window of legitimate use than a blood test.

This framework explains several things that otherwise appear inconsistent. It explains why two competent clinicians can reasonably disagree about whether to scan a patient: they may hold different estimates of pretest probability, or different valuations of the harms, and both are legitimate sources of disagreement. It also explains the single most common testing error in hospital practice, which is testing a patient whose probability was already above the treatment threshold. Ordering a confirmatory test in a patient you are going to treat regardless is not diligence. It is a delay with a false-negative risk attached.

2.3.5 A worked example

A 58-year-old man is admitted with pleuritic chest pain and mild dyspnoea, three days after a long flight. He has no leg swelling, no haemoptysis, no history of malignancy, a heart rate of 88, and no alternative diagnosis that is more likely.

Step one: pretest probability. Using a validated rule, this patient falls into an intermediate-probability category. In published cohorts, patients in comparable categories have a prevalence of pulmonary embolism of roughly 20 to 30 per cent. Take 25 per cent as the working estimate.

Step two: consider the thresholds. The missed diagnosis is potentially fatal, so the test threshold is low. The treatment is anticoagulation, which carries real bleeding risk, so the treatment threshold is meaningfully above zero but not extremely high, perhaps in the region of 50 to 60 per cent for empiric treatment without imaging. At 25 per cent, the patient sits squarely inside the testing zone. Testing is indicated.

Step three: choose the test and apply the likelihood ratio. A negative high-sensitivity D-dimer carries a negative likelihood ratio in the region of 0.1 in most published series. Applying the approximation: 25 per cent minus roughly 45 points would fall below zero, so the more careful calculation is needed, and it yields a posttest probability in the low single digits. That is below the test threshold for this diagnosis in most formulations, and the diagnosis can reasonably be abandoned.

Step four: consider the alternative result. Had the D-dimer been positive, the likelihood ratio for a positive result in this assay is close to 1.5 to 2, which is weak. It would raise the probability from 25 per cent to perhaps 35 to 40 per cent, which remains inside the testing zone and therefore mandates imaging. This is the correct and frequently misunderstood interpretation: a positive D-dimer is not a diagnosis and barely counts as evidence. It is an instruction to continue.

Step five: note what would change everything. Had this patient presented with syncope, hypotension, and right ventricular strain on the electrocardiogram, the pretest probability might have exceeded 60 per cent, placing him above the treatment threshold. In that circumstance, empiric anticoagulation before imaging is not an act of carelessness. It is the correct application of the framework.

2.3.6 Common quantitative errors

Five errors recur often enough to be worth naming explicitly.

Base rate neglect. The most consequential. A test with 95 per cent sensitivity and 95 per cent specificity, applied to a population with a disease prevalence of 1 per cent, produces roughly seventeen false positives for every true positive. Clinicians reliably underestimate this, and the practical consequence is a ward full of patients being investigated for findings that are almost certainly artefacts of the testing itself.

Conflating sensitivity with negative predictive value. A highly sensitive test rules out disease effectively only when the pretest probability is low to moderate. In a patient with a high pretest probability, a negative result on even a very sensitive test leaves a residual probability that may well remain above the test threshold.

Treating a numeric result as binary. A troponin at the ninety-ninth centile and a troponin twenty times that value carry radically different likelihood ratios. Reporting both as "positive" discards most of the information.

Assuming independence between tests. Likelihood ratios multiply only when the findings are conditionally independent. Many clinical findings are strongly correlated, and multiplying their ratios overstates the certainty, sometimes grossly.

Testing above the treatment threshold. Discussed above, and worth restating because it is the error most likely to be praised as thoroughness.

2.4 Diagnostic Error Taxonomy and the Anatomy of a Missed Diagnosis

2.4.1 Scale and definition

Diagnostic error is defined by the National Academy of Medicine as the failure to establish an accurate and timely explanation of the patient's health problem, or the failure to communicate that explanation to the patient. Three elements of that definition deserve attention. Accuracy is only one component; **timeliness** and **communication** are constitutive parts of the definition rather than aggravating factors. A correct diagnosis reached four days late is an error. A correct diagnosis never conveyed to the patient is an error.

Estimates of frequency vary with method. Autopsy series, which capture only fatal cases, have historically found major discrepancies between clinical and postmortem diagnoses in a substantial minority of deaths, with rates that have declined but not disappeared despite modern imaging. Studies of ambulatory and inpatient populations using record review suggest that a meaningful proportion of adults experience a diagnostic error at some point, and that diagnostic error contributes to a significant fraction of serious preventable harm in hospital. The precise figures are contested and readers should consult current primary sources, but the order of magnitude is not in dispute: this is the largest unaddressed category of preventable harm in medicine.

2.4.2 The three-part taxonomy

The most durable classification, developed by Graber and colleagues, divides diagnostic error by mechanism into three categories. The classification is useful precisely because each category implies a different remedy.

No-fault errors arise when the diagnosis could not reasonably have been made with the information available. Silent or atypical presentations, diseases masquerading convincingly as commoner conditions, and patients who provide inaccurate histories all fall here. These are irreducible in principle, though the boundary shifts as diagnostic technology improves. Genuine no-fault errors are less common than clinicians reviewing their own cases tend to conclude.

System errors arise from failures in the environment in which the diagnosis is made: a result that returns after discharge with no mechanism for follow-up, an imaging study reported but never viewed, a referral that is never scheduled, a specimen lost, an alert suppressed by alert fatigue, a handoff that omits the pending study. These are the most tractable of the three because they are amenable to engineering, and they are the natural target of the systems domain described in Chapter 1, section 1.2.2.

Cognitive errors arise from faulty knowledge, faulty data gathering, or faulty synthesis. This category attracts the most attention and is the least tractable, but it should be subdivided further because its subdivisions have different remedies. Faulty knowledge is a training problem. Faulty data gathering, meaning an incomplete history or examination, is a discipline problem. Faulty synthesis is the domain of the cognitive biases discussed in section 2.5.

Crucially, the categories are rarely exclusive. Most serious diagnostic errors, on careful review, involve elements of at least two, and typically a cognitive error that a system failure permitted to persist.

2.4.3 The anatomy of a miss

Missed diagnoses in hospital practice follow a recognisable sequence. The sequence matters more than the taxonomy, because it identifies the points at which interruption is possible.

Stage one: an early plausible label is applied. A patient with dyspnoea is labelled with a heart failure exacerbation in the emergency department, on the basis of a history of heart failure and a chest radiograph read as congestion. The label is not unreasonable; it is simply not verified.

Stage two: the label is transmitted rather than the data. The admission note records “admitted with heart failure exacerbation” rather than “admitted with dyspnoea, working diagnosis heart failure.” Every subsequent clinician inherits a conclusion rather than a question. This is the single most consequential step in the sequence and the one most amenable to individual correction, as discussed in Chapter 1, section 1.7.2.

Stage three: subsequent data are interpreted as consistent. The mildly elevated troponin is attributed to demand ischaemia in the setting of heart failure. The tachycardia is attributed to decompensation. The mild hypoxia is attributed to pulmonary oedema. Each interpretation is individually defensible. Collectively they constitute confirmation bias operating across a team.

Stage four: discordant data are explained away or not sought. The patient's failure to improve with diuresis on day two is attributed to inadequate dosing rather than to a wrong diagnosis. The leg asymmetry is not examined because no one is asking about it.

Stage five: the diagnostic question is never reopened. Handoffs transmit the plan rather than the reasoning. The weekend team inherits a diuresis protocol. No one reconstructs the original problem representation.

Stage six: the diagnosis is revealed by deterioration. The patient has a submassive pulmonary embolism, and it becomes apparent when they decompensate.

Reading this sequence, two features stand out. No individual step involves obvious incompetence. And the sequence is interruptible at every stage by the same single act: **restating the problem representation from the raw data rather than from the inherited label.**

2.4.4 Structural risk factors

Certain circumstances raise diagnostic error risk sufficiently that they warrant explicit heightened vigilance. The list is worth memorising.

- **Handoff and transitions.** The label crosses the boundary; the uncertainty does not.
- **The patient who does not improve as expected.** The most underused diagnostic signal in hospital medicine. Failure to respond to correct treatment is evidence against the diagnosis, and should be treated as such rather than as a dosing question.
- **The patient with an established diagnosis that explains everything.** Diagnostic overshadowing, in which new symptoms in a patient with a chronic condition, a psychiatric diagnosis, or a substance use disorder are attributed to the known problem. This is a major and documented source of disparity, discussed further in Chapter 19.
- **Atypical demographics.** The presentation that does not match the script's expected patient, including the young patient with a disease of older adults, the woman with a condition scripted as male, and the presentation altered by immunosuppression or age.
- **High census, night, and end of shift.** Discussed in Chapter 1, section 1.3.
- **The patient perceived as difficult.** Emotional response to a patient measurably degrades diagnostic performance, and the effect is largest in exactly the patients whose complaints are most likely to be dismissed.

2.4.5 Feedback: the missing loop

A structural feature of hospital medicine deserves particular emphasis. Diagnostic calibration requires feedback, and hospitalists receive very little of it.

The patient is discharged, and the outcome of the diagnosis is learned only if something goes wrong badly enough to return them. Correct diagnoses generate no feedback at all. Wrong diagnoses generate feedback only in the subset that deteriorate visibly and locally. The result is that a hospitalist's confidence is calibrated against a badly biased sample, and confidence rises with experience whether or not accuracy does.

Partial remedies exist and are worth institutional investment: structured review of readmissions within a defined window, morbidity and mortality conferences focused specifically on diagnostic process rather than management, routine feedback from pathology and radiology on discordant reads, and personal practices such as following a sample of discharged patients. None of these is complete. All are better than the default, which is no feedback at all.

2.5 Cognitive Debiasing Strategies: What Works and What Does Not

2.5.1 The honest state of the evidence

This section requires a caveat unusual in a clinical handbook. **The evidence that cognitive debiasing interventions improve diagnostic accuracy in practice is weak.**

The literature contains a large number of proposed strategies, a moderate number of studies demonstrating effects in artificial settings with written cases, and very few demonstrating durable improvement in real clinical outcomes. Enthusiasm has consistently outrun evidence. Readers should approach the recommendations that follow as reasoned practice rather than as established intervention, and should be sceptical of any curriculum that claims otherwise.

The reason for the disappointing results is instructive and connects back to section 2.1. If most diagnostic error arises from knowledge that is absent or poorly organised rather than from reasoning that is too fast, then interventions targeting the speed and style of reasoning are aimed at the wrong target.

2.5.2 Strategies with little or no demonstrated effect

Generic instruction to slow down and reflect. Repeatedly studied, repeatedly disappointing. Deliberation applied to a wrong hypothesis elaborates the error.

Teaching the catalogue of cognitive biases. Clinicians can learn to name anchoring, availability, confirmation bias, premature closure, and search satisfaction with high reliability, and this knowledge does not transfer to their own reasoning in the moment. Bias is recognised retrospectively in others and prospectively in almost no one. The catalogue remains valuable as a shared vocabulary for case discussion, which is a real benefit, but it is not an intervention.

Exhortation to consider the worst-case diagnosis. Without a structure specifying which worst cases and when, this degrades into either anxiety or ritual, and it drives overtesting without improving detection.

Confidence-based approaches. Asking clinicians to rate their confidence does not improve accuracy, because confidence and accuracy are poorly correlated, particularly at the extremes.

2.5.3 Strategies with a defensible basis

Several interventions have either supporting evidence or a mechanism specific enough to justify use.

Deliberate alternative generation. Rather than asking "am I confident?", asking "what else would produce exactly this picture, and what would distinguish it?" This directs cognition at hypothesis generation, which is where the failure actually occurs. It is the most defensible single recommendation in this section.

Diagnostic timeout at defined trigger points. A brief, structured reconsideration performed not routinely but at specified triggers: at handoff, when the patient fails to improve, before a procedure, and at discharge. Triggering matters, because untriggered timeouts become ritual and are performed without cognitive engagement.

Diagnostic checklists. General checklists prompting reconsideration have shown mixed results. Condition-specific checklists, listing the differential for a presenting syndrome, have performed better in several studies, and their mechanism is clear: they compensate for retrieval failure rather than attempting to alter reasoning style. A checklist for the causes of a raised anion gap acidosis works because it supplies a candidate the clinician possessed but did not retrieve.

Second opinions and structured consultation. Independent reconsideration by another clinician is among the more reliable interventions, provided the second clinician is given the raw data rather than the label. A consultant handed the conclusion will usually validate it. A consultant asked to interpret the presentation independently frequently will not.

Cognitive forcing at high-risk presentations. Rather than general debiasing, specific mandatory considerations attached to specific presentations. For example, a rule that every patient presenting with chest and back pain has dissection explicitly considered and documented. This is narrow, memorable, and addresses the presentations where misses are most catastrophic.

Environmental redesign. Reducing interruption, improving result follow-up systems, closing communication loops for pending studies, and displaying prior imaging and prior notes accessibly. These are systems interventions rather than cognitive ones, and they have the strongest evidence of anything in this section, which is itself the most important finding here.

Improving feedback. Discussed in section 2.4.5. Calibration cannot improve without it.

2.5.4 The practical synthesis

The realistic position for a practising hospitalist is this. You cannot reliably debias yourself in the moment through effort or awareness. You can build better scripts through deliberate exposure and case review. You can generate alternatives explicitly at defined trigger points. You can invite genuinely independent second opinions by transmitting data rather than conclusions. And you can work to change the environment so that the failures which do occur are caught by something other than your own vigilance.

That last point is worth stating plainly, because it runs against the professional instinct. The single most effective thing an individual clinician can do about diagnostic error is to stop relying on individual vigilance.

2.6 Evidence Appraisal at Speed: Guidelines, Systematic Reviews, and Their Failure Modes

2.6.1 The realistic constraint

A hospitalist deciding whether to anticoagulate at two in the morning has minutes, not hours. Formal critical appraisal as taught in evidence-based medicine courses is a valuable discipline and is not available at the point of decision. What is required is a set of rapid heuristics that identify, quickly, whether a given source can be trusted for this decision and what its specific weaknesses are likely to be.

The aim of this section is not to teach appraisal methodology in full, which is available elsewhere, but to identify the failure modes that most often mislead inpatient clinicians specifically.

2.6.2 Guidelines: how they fail

Clinical practice guidelines are the most-used evidence source in hospital medicine and the least critically examined. Six failure modes recur.

Recommendation strength is decoupled from evidence quality. A guideline may issue a strong recommendation on the basis of low-quality evidence, and frequently does. Under formal frameworks such as GRADE this is permissible in defined circumstances, but in practice a substantial proportion of strong recommendations in major cardiovascular and other guidelines rest on expert opinion or observational data rather than trial evidence. The practical habit is to read the evidence grade, not the recommendation grade, and to treat a strong recommendation on weak evidence as an opinion held firmly rather than as an established fact.

Population mismatch. Guidelines are derived from trials whose participants are systematically younger, less comorbid, less frail, more male in some fields and more female in others, and more adherent than the patients admitted to a general medical ward. Applying a recommendation derived from a trial population with a mean age of 62 and minimal comorbidity to an 89-year-old with five chronic conditions is an extrapolation, and should be recognised as one.

Failure to address competing risk. In an older patient with limited life expectancy, an intervention that prevents an outcome occurring on a five-year horizon may be irrelevant, because a competing cause of death intervenes first. Guidelines rarely model this, and the omission systematically overstates the benefit of preventive interventions in exactly the population most likely to be hospitalised.

Lag. The interval between the evidence and the guideline, and between the guideline and its revision, is frequently several years. A guideline published this year may reflect a literature search concluded three years ago.

Conflict of interest. Panel composition matters, and financial relationships between panel members and manufacturers of recommended interventions remain common despite reform efforts. This does not invalidate the recommendations, but it is a reason to look harder at recommendations that favour a proprietary intervention over a generic or non-pharmacological one.

Guidelines conflict with one another. Two specialty societies frequently issue contradictory recommendations on the same question, usually reflecting different valuations of the same evidence rather than different evidence. When this occurs, the disagreement itself is informative: it signals that the question is genuinely unsettled and that clinical judgement is legitimately in play.

A rapid appraisal sequence for a guideline takes about ninety seconds: check the publication date and the search cut-off; find the evidence grade for the specific recommendation rather than the overall document; check whether the trial populations resemble your patient; check the funding and panel disclosures; and check whether a competing society disagrees.

2.6.3 Systematic reviews and meta-analyses: how they fail

Systematic reviews sit at the top of most evidence hierarchies, which encourages uncritical acceptance. They have characteristic failure modes of their own.

Garbage in, garbage out. A meta-analysis of biased trials produces a precise estimate of a biased effect. The narrow confidence interval created by pooling conveys an impression of certainty that the underlying data do not support. Always look at the risk-of-bias assessment for the included studies before looking at the pooled estimate.

Clinical heterogeneity concealed by statistical pooling. Trials of different interventions in different populations with different comparators can be statistically poolable and clinically meaningless. A statistic quantifying heterogeneity does not detect the problem of pooling things that should not be combined; only reading the table of included studies does.

Publication bias. Trials with negative results are published less often, later, and in less visible venues. Funnel plot asymmetry and related tests detect this imperfectly and cannot detect it at all when the number of trials is small.

Dominance by a single large trial. A pooled estimate is sometimes driven almost entirely by one large study, with the remaining trials contributing negligible weight. In that circumstance the review is effectively a report on one trial, and should be read as such.

Composite outcomes. A significant effect on a composite of death, myocardial infarction, and revascularisation is frequently driven entirely by the least serious component. Always disaggregate.

Surrogate outcomes. An effect on a laboratory value, an imaging finding, or a physiological measure is not an effect on a patient-important outcome, and the history of medicine contains numerous instances where the two diverged in the harmful direction.

2.6.4 Reading a trial in five minutes

When a single trial is the relevant evidence, five questions extract most of what matters.

1. **Who was enrolled, and who was excluded?** Read the exclusion criteria before the results. This determines applicability and is where the trial population's dissimilarity from your patient becomes visible.
2. **What was the comparator?** A trial against placebo answers a different question from a trial against current standard care. Comparison against an inadequately dosed or outdated alternative is a common way to manufacture superiority.
3. **What was the primary outcome, and was it patient-important?** Check whether the reported outcome is the one that was pre-registered.
4. **What is the absolute effect?** Relative risk reduction is the number most often quoted and the least informative. Convert to absolute risk difference and number needed to treat, and apply the baseline risk of your actual patient rather than the trial's.
5. **What were the harms, and how were they ascertained?** Adverse events are systematically under-collected relative to efficacy outcomes, and a trial that reports harms only as investigator-attributed events has probably undercounted them.

2.6.5 When the evidence does not exist

A large proportion of decisions in hospital medicine are not addressed by any adequate evidence, and this is normal rather than exceptional. The appropriate response is not to locate a marginally relevant trial and over-apply it.

The appropriate response is to reason explicitly from mechanism, from the balance of plausible harms and benefits, from the patient's own values and goals, and from the reversibility of the decision. Preference should be given to the option that preserves future options. And the reasoning should be documented as reasoning, so that the next clinician understands that a judgement was made under uncertainty rather than that a standard was followed.

2.7 Diagnostic Stewardship: Ordering Less to Know More

2.7.1 The counterintuitive claim

Diagnostic stewardship is the practice of ordering the right test, for the right patient, at the right time, for a defined reason. Its central and initially counterintuitive claim is that **reducing test volume increases diagnostic accuracy.**

The claim follows directly from section 2.3. Testing at a pretest probability below the test threshold produces predominantly false positives. Each false positive generates further testing, and each further test carries its own false positive rate applied to an even lower-probability population. The result is a cascade that moves the clinician progressively further from the truth while generating an increasing volume of data. A patient with a great deal of information about them is not necessarily a patient who is better understood.

Stewardship therefore is not rationing. It is a precision intervention, and it should be argued and taught as one.

2.7.2 The core discipline

Every test order should be preceded by two questions, answered before the order is placed.

What is the question this test answers? If the question cannot be stated in a sentence, the test is not indicated.

What will I do differently for each possible result? If the answer is the same for every possible result, the test changes nothing and should not be ordered.

These two questions eliminate a substantial proportion of low-value inpatient testing on their own. They are also teachable, verifiable, and enforceable in a way that general exhortations to reduce utilisation are not. A trainee asked routinely to state the question and the contingent actions before ordering learns the discipline within weeks.

2.7.3 High-yield targets in inpatient practice

Several specific patterns account for a disproportionate share of low-value inpatient testing, and each has a well-described stewardship response. Institutional protocols vary, so the following should be adapted to local guidance.

Daily routine bloodwork. Repeat complete blood counts and chemistry panels on stable patients ordered as a standing daily series, rather than in response to a clinical question, contribute to iatrogenic anaemia, generate spurious findings requiring investigation, and disturb sleep. The stewardship response is to order laboratory tests as single events tied to a question rather than as recurring series, and to review standing orders daily.

Blood cultures. Cultures drawn in patients with a low pretest probability of bacteraemia generate contaminants at a rate that in some settings approaches or exceeds the rate of true positives. Each contaminant generates additional cultures, often unnecessary antimicrobial therapy, and occasionally a prolonged admission. The stewardship response is to define indications, to ensure adequate volume and technique, and in many institutions to restrict repeat culture sets in patients already on effective therapy.

Testing for *Clostridioides difficile*. This is the archetypal stewardship problem because the commonest assays detect colonisation as well as disease, and colonisation is prevalent among hospitalised patients. Testing a patient whose diarrhoea has an alternative explanation, most often laxatives or enteral feeding, produces positive results that represent colonisation and lead to treatment of a non-disease. The stewardship response is to test only patients with clinically significant unexplained diarrhoea who have not received laxatives recently, and to avoid tests of cure. Chapter 15 develops the clinical management.

Urine cultures. Asymptomatic bacteriuria is common, particularly in older adults and catheterised patients, and treating it produces harm without benefit in nearly all populations. Culturing urine in a patient without urinary symptoms, particularly a confused older patient in whom delirium has another explanation, is among the most common initiators of diagnostic error in hospital medicine. Chapter 18 addresses this in detail.

Broad serological and autoimmune panels. Ordering a large panel in a patient with a low pretest probability of connective tissue disease reliably produces a weakly positive result that requires explanation and generates referral, anxiety, and further testing.

Repeat imaging without a new question. Imaging repeated because time has passed rather than because a specific question has arisen produces incidental findings at a high rate.

Continuous telemetry and continuous oximetry without indication. These are diagnostic tests, though rarely thought of as such. They generate alarms at a rate that produces alarm fatigue, restrict mobility, disturb sleep, and thereby contribute directly to delirium and deconditioning.

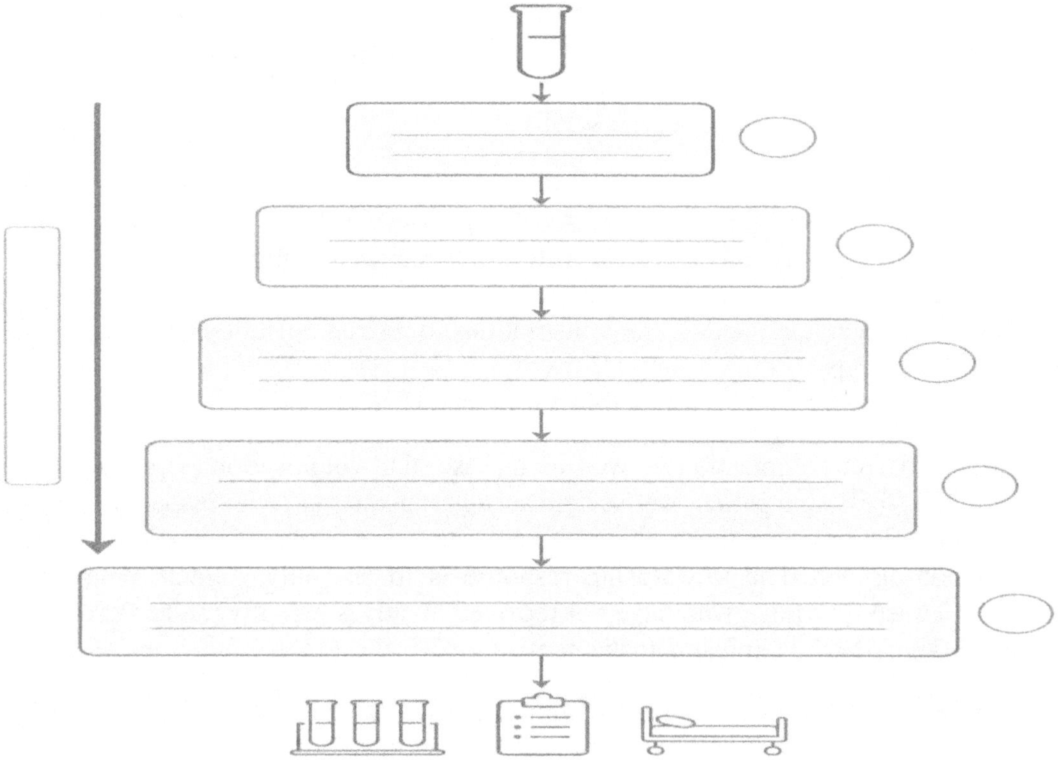

2.7.4 Stewardship in the diagnostic workup of the undifferentiated patient

A specific and difficult case deserves separate treatment: the patient in whom no diagnosis is apparent and the temptation is to test broadly.

The instinct to order widely in this situation is understandable and usually counterproductive, for the reasons set out above. The disciplined alternative has three components.

Return to the problem representation. Undifferentiated cases are frequently undifferentiated because the syndrome has been misnamed rather than because the diagnosis is rare. Reconstructing the representation from raw data, as described in section 2.2.3, resolves a meaningful proportion of these cases without any testing at all.

Test sequentially rather than in parallel, where time permits. Sequential testing preserves the Bayesian structure, since each result updates the probability for the next. Parallel broad testing destroys it, producing a set of results with no coherent interpretive framework.

Use time as a diagnostic instrument. Observation over twenty-four to forty-eight hours, with a defined plan for what would prompt escalation, is a legitimate and frequently superior diagnostic strategy. Many self-limiting conditions declare themselves as self-limiting, and many serious conditions declare themselves as serious. Time is the only test with no false positive rate.

The counterweight to all of this must be stated clearly. Stewardship applies to low-probability testing, not to the diagnostic evaluation of the acutely ill. In a patient who is deteriorating, in whom a time-critical diagnosis is plausible, the correct action is prompt and often broad investigation. The threshold framework in section 2.3.4 gives the reason: for catastrophic, time-sensitive, treatable diagnoses, the test threshold is very low, and testing at low probability is therefore appropriate. A clinician who invokes stewardship to justify not investigating a patient who is becoming unwell has misunderstood the principle entirely.

Chapter Summary

- Dual-process theory provides useful vocabulary but a misleading account of error. Intuitive reasoning is not systematically less accurate than analytic reasoning, and generic instruction to slow down does not reliably improve accuracy. Degraded working conditions, however, do reliably degrade diagnosis.
- Diagnostic knowledge is stored as **illness scripts** organised for clinical use. **Semantic qualifiers** convert raw data into the abstract form in which scripts are indexed, and qualifier density correlates with diagnostic accuracy.
- The **problem representation** is the central reasoning artefact. It should name the syndrome rather than the assumed cause, include informative negatives, and be explicitly revised when data change.
- A test **revises a probability**; it does not establish a diagnosis. Testing is indicated only between the **test threshold** and the **treatment threshold**. Testing a patient already above the treatment threshold is a delay with a false-negative risk attached.
- Diagnostic error divides into **no-fault**, **system**, and **cognitive** mechanisms, usually in combination. The characteristic anatomy of a miss is an early plausible label, transmitted as a conclusion rather than a question, followed by assimilation of all subsequent data.
- The evidence for **cognitive debiasing** is weak. Deliberate alternative generation, triggered timeouts, condition-specific checklists, genuinely independent second opinions, and environmental redesign have the strongest justification. Teaching the bias catalogue does not transfer.
- Guidelines fail through decoupled recommendation strength, population mismatch, competing risk, lag, and conflict of interest. Systematic reviews fail through pooled bias, concealed clinical heterogeneity, composite and surrogate outcomes, and single-trial dominance.
- **Diagnostic stewardship** increases accuracy by reducing testing below the test threshold. Two questions govern every order: what question does this answer, and what will I do differently for each result. Stewardship does not apply to the acutely deteriorating patient, in whom the test threshold is legitimately very low.

Review Questions

1. A patient with a pretest probability of pulmonary embolism of approximately 60 per cent has a negative D-dimer. State the approximate posttest probability, state whether the diagnosis can be excluded, and explain the reasoning error a clinician would be making if they excluded it.
2. Convert the following into a problem representation using semantic qualifiers, and state what the representation reveals that the raw narrative conceals: a 44-year-old woman with

two months of worsening breathlessness on exertion, occasional dizziness on standing, no chest pain, no cough, no fever, ankle swelling for three weeks, and a family history of sudden death in a sibling at 38.

3. Explain, using the threshold model, why two competent hospitalists might reasonably disagree about whether to obtain computed tomography in a patient with suspected aortic dissection, without either of them being wrong.
4. A guideline issues a strong recommendation for an intervention on the basis of low-quality evidence, in a population whose mean age is 61. Your patient is 88 with advanced frailty. Set out the specific appraisal steps you would take and the reasoning you would document.
5. Reconstruct the six-stage anatomy of a missed diagnosis for a patient admitted with a working diagnosis of alcohol withdrawal who is subsequently found to have a subdural haematoma, and identify the single act that would have interrupted the sequence at each stage.

CHAPTER 3: Transitions of Care: Admission, Handoff, Discharge

Learning Objectives

After studying this chapter, the reader should be able to:

1. Distinguish observation from inpatient status, explain the logic of time-based admission criteria, and describe the clinical and financial consequences of misclassification for the patient.
2. Perform a best possible medication history, identify the discrepancy types that most often cause harm, and explain why reconciliation is a diagnostic act rather than a clerical one.
3. Conduct a structured intra-hospital handoff using a validated framework, and analyse a handoff failure by identifying which element of the transfer was lost.
4. Write a discharge summary that functions as a clinical instrument, and state the elements whose omission most reliably causes downstream harm.
5. Apply readmission risk stratification appropriately, understanding both the utility and the substantial limitations of published prediction tools.
6. Reason systematically about post-acute disposition, including skilled nursing, inpatient rehabilitation, home-based services, and hospice.
7. Construct a defensible discharge plan for patients whose risk arises from housing instability, substance use disorder, or cognitive impairment.

Chapter Overview

Chapter 1 argued that hospital medicine purchases its advantages by severing longitudinal relationship, and that the specialty's quality apparatus exists to rebuild informationally what was given up relationally. Chapter 2 developed the reasoning discipline that produces a diagnosis. This chapter addresses what happens to that diagnosis, and to everything else known about the patient, when it crosses a boundary.

Transitions are where hospital medicine fails most often and most consequentially. The reason is structural rather than a matter of individual carelessness. At every transition, a large volume of tacit knowledge held in one clinician's head must be compressed into a written or spoken artefact, transmitted across a discontinuity, and reconstructed by someone who was not present for its acquisition. Compression is lossy. What is lost is systematically the same material each time: the uncertainty, the reasoning, the contingencies, and the things that were considered and rejected.

Three transitions structure the admission. **Entry**, where the patient crosses from the ambulatory or emergency environment into inpatient care and a status decision is made. **Internal handoff**, which occurs several times daily and dozens of times across a stay. **Exit**, where the patient leaves for home or a facility, and where the density of information that must transfer is greatest while the time available is smallest.

The chapter treats each in turn, then addresses the populations for whom the exit transition carries the highest risk. Readers outside the United States should note that section 3.1 and parts of section

3.6 describe payer structures specific to the American system; the underlying clinical logic generalises, but the administrative machinery does not, and local rules must be substituted.

3.1 The Admission Decision: Observation, Inpatient, and the Two-Midnight Logic

3.1.1 What the decision actually is

The admission decision is frequently mischaracterised as a clinical judgement about whether a patient needs to be in hospital. It is not. By the time a hospitalist is called, that judgement has usually been made by an emergency physician, and the patient is already occupying a bed.

The decision the hospitalist makes is different and narrower: **under what status is this hospital stay classified?** The two principal options in the American system are inpatient admission and observation, which is technically an outpatient service delivered in a hospital bed. The clinical care delivered is frequently identical. The consequences for the patient are not.

This is worth stating explicitly because the classification is often treated as an administrative annoyance to be delegated to utilisation review. It is not delegable, because its consequences are borne by the patient, and because the clinical documentation that justifies it can only be written by the clinician who examined them.

3.1.2 Consequences of the classification

Four consequences follow from the observation designation, and hospitalists should be able to explain all four to a patient.

Cost-sharing. Observation is billed under outpatient benefit structures, which typically involve different and sometimes higher out-of-pocket costs for the patient, including separate charges for services that would be bundled under inpatient status. Medications administered during an observation stay may not be covered in the way they would be for an inpatient.

Post-acute skilled nursing coverage. This is the consequence with the greatest clinical impact. Traditional Medicare has historically required a qualifying inpatient stay of a defined minimum duration before skilled nursing facility benefits are triggered. Time spent under observation does not count toward that requirement. A patient who spends three days in a hospital bed under observation status and then requires skilled nursing care may find that care entirely uncovered, and may face a bill of many thousands of dollars or, more commonly, a refusal of placement. Waivers and Medicare Advantage plan variations exist and have shifted over time, so current rules must be verified locally.

Notification requirements. Patients placed under observation for a defined duration must receive written and oral notice explaining the status and its financial implications. The obligation exists precisely because patients otherwise have no way of knowing that lying in a hospital bed for two days does not constitute admission.

Quality and readmission accounting. Observation stays are counted differently in readmission and mortality metrics, which creates a documented incentive for institutions to shift patients between categories. Clinicians should be aware that this incentive exists and should resist allowing it to influence the classification of an individual patient.

3.1.3 The two-midnight logic

The governing principle in the American system since 2013 has been time-based rather than severity-based. The general expectation is that inpatient admission is appropriate when the admitting clinician reasonably expects the patient to require medically necessary hospital care spanning at least two midnights. Stays expected to be shorter are generally appropriate for observation.

Three features of this rule are frequently misunderstood and matter practically.

It is an expectation standard, not an outcome standard. The relevant question is what the admitting clinician reasonably expected at the time of the decision, given the documented clinical circumstances. A patient admitted with a reasonable expectation of a three-day stay who improves rapidly and leaves the following morning was correctly admitted. The documentation must therefore capture the expectation and its basis, not merely the diagnosis.

Documentation is the entire substance of the justification. An expectation that is not recorded does not exist for review purposes. The admission note should state, in a sentence, why more than two midnights of hospital care are anticipated: the specific clinical instability, the planned interventions, the anticipated response, and what would need to occur before discharge is safe.

Exceptions exist. Certain procedures and circumstances permit inpatient admission regardless of expected duration, and case-by-case exceptions allow inpatient status for shorter stays where the clinical circumstances justify it, again provided the reasoning is documented.

Readers should verify the current version of these rules, which have been revised repeatedly since introduction and differ between traditional Medicare, Medicare Advantage plans, and commercial payers.

3.1.4 Practical approach

Several habits reduce both misclassification and its consequences.

Make the status decision explicitly and early, rather than allowing it to be assigned by default. A default assignment is usually observation, and converting later is administratively difficult and sometimes impossible.

Write the expectation into the admission note in clinical language. For example: "Anticipate at least two midnights given ongoing intravenous diuresis with a creatinine that has risen from baseline, requirement for daily electrolyte monitoring, and inability to ambulate safely at present."

Reassess status when the trajectory changes. A patient placed under observation who is clearly not going to leave within the expected window should have their status revisited that day, not on the third day. Mechanisms exist for conversion, and they are time-limited.

Tell the patient. A patient under observation who is planning on skilled nursing placement needs to know before the discharge planning process is complete, not on the day they are due to leave. This conversation is uncomfortable and it is a professional obligation.

Do not allow status to alter clinical care. The temptation to shorten a stay to fit a classification, or to order tests to justify one, is a form of the reasoning failure described in Chapter 2, section 2.7. The clinical question and the administrative question are separate, and the clinical one governs.

3.1.5 Systems outside the United States

For readers in systems without this classification, the underlying clinical decision remains and is usually framed as admission to a short-stay or ambulatory emergency care unit versus admission to a general ward. The relevant judgement is the same: whether the anticipated duration and intensity of required care justify a full inpatient pathway, and whether the patient can be safely managed with a defined short-interval reassessment instead. The clinical reasoning transfers; the financial consequences to the patient generally do not.

3.2 Medication Reconciliation as a Diagnostic Act

3.2.1 Reframing the task

Medication reconciliation is widely experienced as a clerical obligation: a list to be verified, a box to be ticked, a task delegable to whoever has time. This framing is both inaccurate and the direct cause of its poor performance.

Reconciliation is a diagnostic act, for two reasons.

First, **the medication list is a data source that frequently contains the diagnosis.** A patient admitted with confusion whose list includes a recently added anticholinergic, an opioid, and a benzodiazepine has an explanation for the confusion embedded in the list. A patient admitted with hyponatraemia on a thiazide has a probable cause. A patient with unexplained hypotension who has been continued on an antihypertensive during an acute illness has an iatrogenic explanation. Chapter 2 argued that diagnostic error arises most often because the correct hypothesis was never generated; the medication list is one of the richest available generators of hypotheses, and it is routinely skimmed.

Second, **the discrepancies themselves are clinically consequential at high rates.** Studies of admission medication histories consistently find that a majority of patients have at least one discrepancy between the recorded list and what they are actually taking, and that a meaningful minority of these discrepancies have potential for harm. Omission of a chronic medication is the commonest type and is frequently the most dangerous, particularly for antiepileptics, antiparkinsonian agents, immunosuppressants, antiretrovirals, anticoagulants, and drugs with withdrawal syndromes.

3.2.2 The best possible medication history

The reference standard is the **best possible medication history**, which is defined not by a single source but by systematic triangulation between several.

The available sources, each with characteristic failure modes:

- **The patient.** The only source that knows what is actually being taken, as distinct from what has been prescribed. Unreliable in delirium, cognitive impairment, and acute illness, and systematically inaccurate for medications the patient regards as unimportant, including inhalers, topical agents, eye drops, and injectables.

- **The family or carer.** Often the single most valuable source for older adults, and the source most often not contacted because they are not in the room at the time the history is taken.
- **The community pharmacy record.** Excellent for what has been dispensed. Blind to what has been dispensed and not taken, to samples, to over-the-counter agents, and to medications obtained elsewhere.
- **The primary care record.** Authoritative for intent. Frequently out of date, and typically does not reflect changes made by specialists or during other hospital admissions.
- **The prior discharge summary.** Useful and frequently the source of propagated error, since an incorrect list at one discharge is imported into the next admission and thereby laundered into apparent authority.
- **The medication containers.** The most underused source. Asking the family to bring in the bottles resolves a large proportion of ambiguity and reveals dosing that no record contains.
- **Prescription monitoring databases.** Essential for controlled substances and frequently the only reliable source for them.

The discipline is to use at least two independent sources for every patient and more for patients with polypharmacy, cognitive impairment, or high-risk medications, and to record which sources were used. A reconciliation that does not name its sources cannot be evaluated by the next clinician.

3.2.3 What to ask, and how

The interview technique substantially determines the yield. Several specific practices improve it.

Ask about categories the patient does not consider medications. Inhalers, eye drops, injectables, patches, creams, supplements, herbal preparations, over-the-counter analgesics, and sleep aids are routinely omitted from patient-reported lists because the patient does not classify them as medication. Each category should be asked about by name.

Ask about actual behaviour rather than the prescription. The useful question is not "are you taking the metformin?" but "how many times in the last week did you miss it?" The first invites a socially expected answer; the second normalises imperfect adherence and produces more accurate data. Adherence questions asked without judgement yield substantially better information, and adherence failures are themselves diagnostic: a patient admitted in heart failure who has not filled a diuretic prescription for six weeks has a different problem from one who has been taking it faithfully.

Ask why, not only what. A patient who cannot say why they take a medication is a patient at risk, and the answer frequently reveals a diagnosis absent from the record.

Ask about recent changes specifically. New medications, dose changes, and discontinuations in the preceding weeks carry disproportionate diagnostic weight for the presenting problem. This question should be asked of every patient and is often the single highest-yield question in the entire history.

Ask about non-prescribed and shared medications, including medications belonging to a family member, remaining supplies from previous illnesses, and substances obtained outside the medical system. This requires a non-judgemental framing to yield anything.

3.2.4 Reconciliation at every transition, not only admission

Reconciliation is required at three points, and the second is the one most often skipped.

On admission, to establish the true baseline.

On internal transfer, particularly transfer out of intensive care, where the risk is that medications started for a temporary indication become permanent. Stress ulcer prophylaxis, antipsychotics started for delirium, and analgesics escalated for procedures are the classic examples, and all three are regularly carried to discharge and then continued for years.

On discharge, where the task is not merely to produce a list but to reconcile three separate lists: what the patient took before admission, what they were taking in hospital, and what they should take now. Every difference between the first and third lists should be intentional, and every intentional difference should be explained in the discharge summary. An unexplained difference is indistinguishable from an error, and the receiving clinician will usually resolve the ambiguity by reverting to the preadmission regimen, which may be exactly the wrong action.

3.2.5 Deprescribing as part of reconciliation

Reconciliation is also the natural opportunity for deprescribing, and hospitalisation is one of the few moments when the whole regimen is visible to one clinician.

Candidate categories for review in every older inpatient include drugs with strong anticholinergic burden, sedative-hypnotics, long-term proton pump inhibitors without a persisting indication, medications prescribed to treat the side effects of other medications, and preventive medications whose benefit horizon exceeds the patient's likely remaining life expectancy, discussed further in Chapter 19.

Two cautions apply. Deprescribing initiated in hospital and not communicated clearly is frequently reversed on discharge, sometimes with harm. And withdrawal of certain agents, including beta-blockers, benzodiazepines, opioids, antidepressants, and corticosteroids, requires a taper and a plan rather than a cessation. The rule is that any medication stopped during admission requires an explicit statement in the discharge summary of what was stopped, why, and what should happen next.

3.3 Intra-Hospital Handoff: I-PASS, Structured Sign-Out, and Failure Analysis

3.3.1 The scale of the problem

A patient admitted for five days in a typical hospitalist service will be handed off between clinicians somewhere between ten and thirty times, counting evening cover, night cover, weekend cover, and service changes. Each handoff is a compression and reconstruction event of the kind described in the chapter overview.

The consequences are well documented. Handoff failure is among the most frequently identified contributing factors in serious adverse event analyses, and the mechanism is consistent: information that existed in one clinician's understanding did not exist in the next clinician's understanding at the moment a decision was required.

The material lost is not random. Handoffs reliably transmit the plan and reliably fail to transmit four things: **the reasoning behind the plan**, **the degree of diagnostic uncertainty**, **the contingencies for deterioration**, and **the alternatives that were considered and rejected**. This is precisely the material required to recognise that the plan is failing, which is why handoff failure characteristically presents as a delayed response to deterioration rather than as an overt error.

3.3.2 The I-PASS structure

The most rigorously evaluated handoff intervention is I-PASS, studied in a multicentre paediatric resident implementation and subsequently adapted widely. The published evaluation demonstrated a substantial reduction in medical errors and preventable adverse events following implementation, without lengthening handoff duration. It remains among the strongest pieces of evidence in the transitions literature.

The mnemonic structures the transfer as follows.

I: Illness severity. A single categorisation, typically stable, watcher, or unstable. This front-loads triage and tells the receiving clinician how to allocate attention across the list before any detail is transmitted.

P: Patient summary. A brief synopsis: the problem representation as developed in Chapter 2, section 2.2.3, the events of the admission to date, and the current working diagnosis with its confidence level.

A: Action list. What needs to be done, by whom, and by when. Tasks without an owner and a time are not transferred; they are mentioned.

S: Situation awareness and contingency planning. The most valuable element and the one most often omitted. This states what is expected to happen, what might go wrong, and what should be done if it does. The format is explicitly conditional: if the blood pressure falls below a stated threshold, do this; if the patient becomes more confused, consider that.

S: Synthesis by receiver. The receiving clinician summarises back what they have understood, and the sending clinician corrects it. This closes the communication loop and is the element most frequently dropped when the handoff is rushed, despite being the only element that verifies transmission actually occurred.

3.3.3 Conditions for effectiveness

Structure alone does not produce results. The published successes share several implementation features that are frequently absent when institutions adopt the mnemonic without the surrounding conditions.

A protected, predictable time and place. Handoffs conducted in a corridor, interrupted by pages, or performed piecemeal as clinicians happen to encounter one another lose their structure immediately.

A written document that accompanies the verbal transfer. Verbal handoff alone is unreliable for detail; written handoff alone is unreliable for emphasis and uncertainty. Both are required, and the written document must be updated rather than copied forward, or it will accumulate the same errors described in Chapter 1, section 1.7.2.

Explicit permission to interrupt and question. A handoff in which the receiver does not ask questions has usually failed, and hierarchy suppresses questions reliably.

Training and observation. The published interventions included direct observation with feedback. Institutions that distribute a mnemonic without observing its use generally see the structure decay within months.

3.3.4 Analysing a handoff failure

When a handoff-related adverse event is reviewed, the productive question is not whether a handoff occurred but **which element failed**. The five elements of the structure provide a ready diagnostic framework.

- If the receiving clinician did not prioritise the patient appropriately, the **illness severity** categorisation failed or was absent.
- If the receiving clinician acted on a diagnosis that was actually uncertain, the **patient summary** transmitted a conclusion rather than a working hypothesis. This is the failure described in Chapter 2, section 2.4.3, stage two.
- If a required task was not performed, the **action list** lacked an owner, a deadline, or both.
- If the receiving clinician responded slowly to a deterioration that the sending clinician had anticipated, the **contingency planning** failed. This is the commonest and most consequential failure.
- If the receiving clinician's understanding differed from the sending clinician's intent, the **synthesis** step was omitted.

This framework should be applied in morbidity and mortality review, and it converts a vague conclusion about communication into a specific and correctable finding.

3.3.5 The service-change handoff

One handoff deserves separate treatment because it is the highest-risk and least structured: the transfer of an entire patient list from one hospitalist to another at the end of a service block.

The risks are distinctive. The volume of information is large and must be transferred in a single session, which guarantees compression. The incoming clinician has no prior context for any patient. And crucially, the incoming clinician inherits diagnostic conclusions formed over several days by someone else, with all the anchoring risk that implies.

Three practices mitigate this.

Prioritise by uncertainty rather than by acuity alone. The stable patient with an unexplained finding deserves more handoff time than the sick patient with a clear diagnosis and a working plan.

State explicitly which diagnoses are secure and which are provisional. A single sentence per patient: "the heart failure is confirmed; the reason for the renal impairment is not established."

Treat service change as a scheduled opportunity for diagnostic reconsideration rather than only as a risk. The incoming clinician is the only person in the process with genuinely fresh eyes. Chapter 2, section 2.5.3, identified independent reconsideration as one of the few debiasing interventions with defensible support. Service change is the moment at which it is structurally available, and it is wasted if the incoming clinician's role is understood as passive receipt.

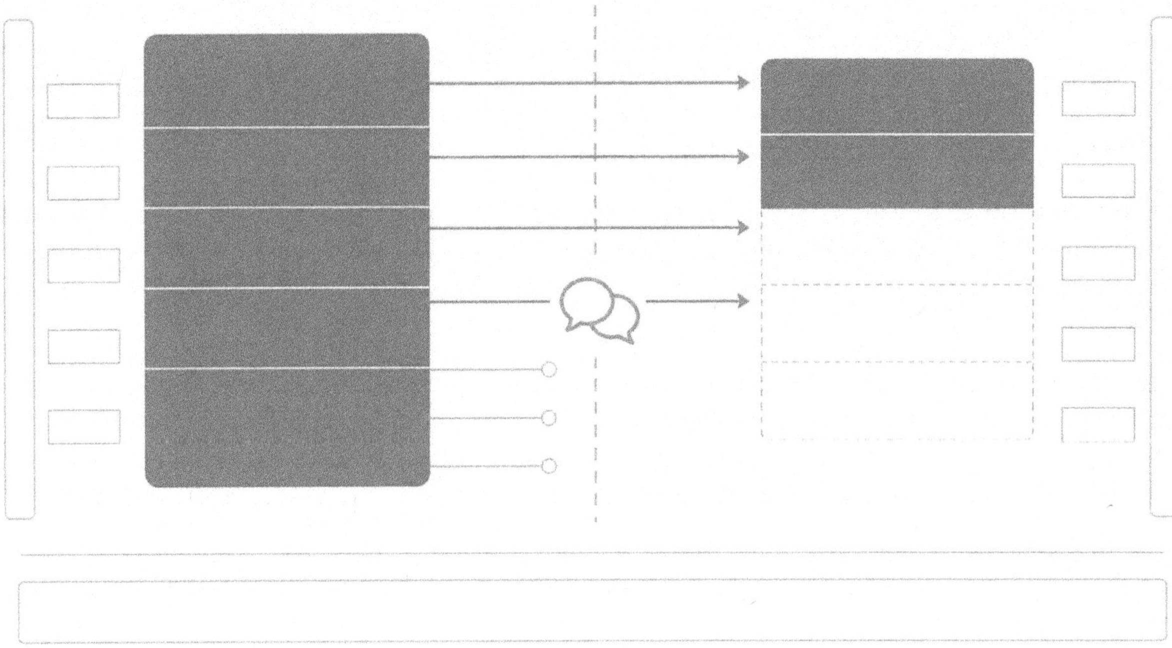

3.4 The Discharge Summary as a Clinical Instrument

3.4.1 What the document is for

The discharge summary is the only artefact that reliably crosses from the hospital to the outpatient world, and in most cases it is the sole record the next clinician will have of what occurred. Its quality determines whether the admission's diagnostic work survives.

The evidence on its performance is poor and has been consistently so. Studies of communication at discharge have repeatedly found that summaries reach the primary care clinician late or not at all, that they frequently omit key information including test results pending at discharge and the discharge medication rationale, and that primary care clinicians report having the summary available at a minority of first post-discharge visits.

Two consequences follow. The summary must be written on the assumption that it is the only source, and it must be completed at or before discharge rather than days later, because a summary that arrives after the first follow-up visit has failed regardless of its content.

3.4.2 The elements that matter most

Institutional templates typically mandate a long list of fields. In practice a small number of elements carry most of the clinical weight, and these are the ones most often written poorly.

The discharge diagnosis with an explicit confidence level. Not "pneumonia" but "community-acquired pneumonia, confirmed radiographically and clinically" or, when appropriate, "presumed aspiration pneumonitis; alternative of atypical infection not excluded." Chapter 2 argued that transmitting a conclusion rather than a hypothesis is the second stage in the anatomy of a missed diagnosis. The discharge summary is where that error is exported from the hospital into the community, where it may persist for years.

A brief hospital course organised as reasoning, not chronology. A day-by-day narrative is long and unusable. The useful form is problem-based and states what was thought, what was done, how the patient responded, and what that response implied. Three or four short paragraphs is usually sufficient.

Pending results at the time of discharge, with a named person responsible. This is among the most reliably harmful omissions in medicine. Cultures, biopsies, and imaging reported after discharge frequently reach no one. The summary must list each pending item and state explicitly who will review it. If the answer is the hospitalist, a mechanism must exist for them to do so.

Medication changes with reasons. Not the list alone but the differences from the preadmission regimen, each with a one-line rationale, as discussed in section 3.2.4. Include medications stopped and why, and any planned taper.

Follow-up with specificity. Not "follow up with primary care" but the interval, the purpose, and what should be assessed. "Primary care within seven days to repeat the basic metabolic panel and reassess volume status; if creatinine has risen further, the diuretic dose should be reduced."

Anticipatory guidance for the receiving clinician. What is expected to happen, what would represent deterioration, and what should be done if it occurs. This is the contingency planning element from section 3.3.2, applied to the outpatient setting, and it is almost universally absent.

Functional and cognitive status at discharge, compared with baseline. This determines the safety of the discharge environment and is essential information for the next clinician assessing decline.

What the patient and family were told, including the substance of any goals-of-care discussion. A patient discharged after a conversation about limitations on future intervention must not have that conversation lost.

3.4.3 Length, timing, and the audience problem

The summary has multiple audiences with conflicting needs: the primary care clinician, the receiving facility, the emergency clinician who will see the patient at three in the morning in two weeks, the patient themselves, and coders and auditors.

Two structural devices resolve most of the conflict. Place a **short synthesis at the top**, no more than a paragraph, containing the diagnosis, the confidence, the key changes, and the follow-up actions. Everything a clinician needs in an emergency should be readable in twenty seconds. Then allow the detail to follow for those who need it.

And **write for the patient as one of the audiences**, since open records legislation increasingly means they will read it. The considerations from Chapter 1, section 1.7.2, apply directly.

Timing is not negotiable. A summary completed at the time of discharge, even if slightly less polished, is worth considerably more than a perfect one completed four days later.

3.4.4 The patient-facing instructions are a separate document

The discharge summary is written for clinicians. The instructions given to the patient are a different artefact with different requirements, and treating them as an abbreviated version of the summary is a predictable source of failure.

Effective patient instructions share several features. They are written at a reading level substantially below that of the summary, since health literacy is frequently limited and is poorly predicted by education or articulacy. They are organised around actions rather than around diagnoses, because a patient does not need to understand the pathophysiology to execute the plan. They state a small number of things, since a list of fourteen instructions is functionally a list of none. And they include an explicit **return threshold**: the specific circumstances under which the patient should seek care again, stated concretely enough to be recognised. "Come back if you get worse" is not a threshold. "Come back if you gain more than two kilograms in three days, or if you cannot lie flat to sleep" is.

Two verification steps convert instructions from a document into a transfer of understanding. **Teach-back**, in which the patient explains the plan in their own words rather than confirming that they understood it, reliably reveals gaps that a confirmation question conceals. And **confirming the mechanics**, meaning asking how they will obtain the medication, how they will get to the appointment, and who will help them, which surfaces the failed assumptions described in section 3.7.1 while there is still time to address them.

A final point applies to both documents. The single most useful sentence a hospitalist can write for a patient and for the next clinician is an honest statement of what remains unresolved. A patient who leaves knowing that the cause of their symptom has not been established, and knowing what is being done about that, is safer than a patient who leaves believing the question was answered.

3.5 Post-Discharge Risk Stratification and Readmission Prediction

3.5.1 What readmission measures and what it does not

Readmission became a central quality metric because it is measurable, expensive, and intuitively connected to the quality of the index admission. Each of these justifications is partially valid and none is fully so, and hospitalists should understand the limitations because they shape how the metric should be used clinically.

Only a minority of readmissions are preventable. Structured reviews consistently find that the proportion judged preventable falls well below half, with estimates varying widely by method and reviewer. Many readmissions represent the natural history of advanced chronic disease in patients who are, correctly, being managed as long as possible.

Readmission is dominated by patient and social factors rather than by hospital performance. Housing, income, health literacy, social support, transport access, and insurance status predict readmission more powerfully than most measures of inpatient care quality. This is why unadjusted readmission rates systematically penalise institutions serving disadvantaged populations, a criticism that has driven successive adjustments to payment programmes.

Readmission is not always the wrong outcome. For some patients, a low threshold for return is the correct plan, and a readmission represents the system working. A metric that treats every return as a failure creates pressure to discourage appropriate returns, which is a documented and undesirable effect.

The clinical use of readmission risk is therefore not to avoid a penalty. It is to identify which patients require intensified transitional support, which is a genuinely useful application.

3.5.2 Prediction tools and their performance

Several validated instruments exist. The most widely used include the LACE index, which combines length of stay, acuity of admission, comorbidity, and emergency department utilisation; the HOSPITAL score, which incorporates haemoglobin, discharge from an oncology service, sodium, procedure during stay, index admission type, prior admissions, and length of stay; and the 8Ps assessment, which is a structured risk screen rather than a numeric score.

The honest summary of their performance is that **discrimination is modest.** Published values for area under the receiver operating characteristic curve for most general readmission models cluster in a range that indicates performance better than chance but well short of what would justify individual-level decision making in isolation. This is not a defect of the particular instruments; it reflects that readmission is driven substantially by factors outside the clinical record.

The practical implication is that these tools should be used to **triage the allocation of transitional care resources**, not to make binary judgements about individual patients. A high score should trigger intensified support. A low score should not reassure a clinician whose clinical judgement says otherwise.

3.5.3 Risk factors worth assessing directly

Independent of any score, several factors identify patients at elevated risk and, more usefully, point to specific interventions.

- **Prior admissions**, the single strongest predictor in nearly every model.
- **Polypharmacy and high-risk medications**, particularly anticoagulants, insulin, opioids, and diuretics.
- **Cognitive impairment**, which impairs the patient's ability to execute the discharge plan and is frequently undetected because it is not screened for.
- **Absence of a reliable carer**, or a carer who is themselves frail or unwell.
- **Housing instability**, addressed in section 3.7.
- **Substance use disorder**, addressed in section 3.7.
- **Depression**, which independently predicts readmission and is underdiagnosed in medical inpatients.
- **Low health literacy**, which is common, poorly correlated with education, and rarely assessed.
- **No established primary care relationship**, which makes follow-up nominal rather than real.
- **Discharge against medical advice** or a stay marked by conflict, which predicts poor follow-through independent of the clinical situation.

3.5.4 Interventions with evidence

The transitional care literature is one of the better-developed areas in health services research, and several structured programmes have demonstrated reductions in readmission.

The successful programmes share features that are more informative than the programme names. They involve **an identified individual responsible for the transition** rather than a distributed process. They include **contact within a short interval after discharge**, typically within two to three days, and typically by telephone at minimum. They involve **medication review after discharge**, in the patient's home where possible, because the discrepancies that matter emerge when the patient attempts to reconcile the hospital regimen with what is in their cupboard. They provide **coaching in self-management and in recognising deterioration** rather than only information. And they involve **early follow-up with a clinician who has the discharge information available**, which returns the analysis to section 3.4.

Single-component interventions perform poorly. A follow-up telephone call alone, a discharge information leaflet alone, or a scheduled appointment alone have generally not demonstrated meaningful effect. Bundles work; components do not.

The most useful conclusion for an individual hospitalist is that the elements they control directly are the summary's timeliness and quality, the accuracy of the medication reconciliation, the specificity of the follow-up instruction, and the honest identification of patients who need intensified support. These are necessary conditions for every successful programme, and none of them can be supplied by a transitional care team if the hospitalist has not done them.

3.6 Skilled Nursing, Rehabilitation, and Hospice-at-Discharge Decisions

3.6.1 Framing the disposition question

Post-acute disposition is often approached as a placement problem to be solved by case management. It is more usefully approached as a clinical question with three components: **what functional deficit exists, what is its expected trajectory, and what intensity of intervention will change that trajectory?**

Answering these requires information hospitalists frequently do not gather. Baseline function before the acute illness is the reference point against which everything is measured, and it must come from the patient or family rather than from the record. The question is specific: two weeks ago, could this person walk to the bathroom unassisted, prepare a meal, manage their own medications, and climb the stairs at home?

3.6.2 The principal options

The following describes the American post-acute landscape; the categories differ substantially elsewhere, though the underlying functional logic is transferable.

Home with no additional services. Appropriate when the patient has returned to or near baseline and has adequate support. The commonest error here is overestimating baseline because it was never established.

Home with home health services. Skilled nursing visits, physical or occupational therapy, and aide services delivered in the home. Appropriate for patients who can be safely at home but require ongoing skilled intervention, wound care, medication management, or therapy. Generally requires that the patient meet criteria related to difficulty leaving home. This is frequently the correct answer for patients who are reflexively referred to facilities.

Skilled nursing facility. Provides nursing care and therapy at lower intensity than inpatient rehabilitation, typically for patients who need daily skilled care but cannot tolerate or do not require intensive therapy. Coverage under traditional Medicare has historically depended on a qualifying inpatient stay, which returns to the status question in section 3.1.

Inpatient rehabilitation facility. Provides high-intensity multidisciplinary rehabilitation, conventionally characterised by an expectation of a substantial number of therapy hours daily and requiring that the patient be able to tolerate and benefit from that intensity, with physician oversight at a defined frequency. Appropriate for patients with significant functional deficit and genuine rehabilitation potential, classically after stroke, major trauma, amputation, or complex orthopaedic injury.

Long-term acute care hospital. For patients with prolonged, complex medical needs, most often prolonged mechanical ventilation or complex wound and infection management, who remain too unstable for skilled nursing but no longer require acute hospital resources.

Long-term custodial care. For patients whose functional deficit is permanent and who cannot be safely supported at home. This is generally not covered by acute medical insurance and is frequently the source of the most difficult family conversations of an admission.

Hospice, addressed in section 3.6.4.

3.6.3 Making the decision well

Several practices improve the quality of disposition decisions.

Involve therapy assessment early, ideally within the first day or two rather than as a discharge-day formality. Therapy assessment is a diagnostic test of function and should be ordered when the question arises, not when the bed is needed.

State the goal, not the destination. A referral that says "needs skilled nursing" transmits less than one that says "requires supervised ambulation and daily wound care for an anticipated two to three weeks with a goal of returning home independently." The second permits the receiving facility to plan and permits reassessment against a target.

Be explicit about trajectory. A patient improving daily and a patient who has plateaued require different dispositions even at identical function.

Address the family's expectations directly and early. Families frequently expect either full recovery or permanent placement, and the actual answer is usually neither. A conversation on day two is far easier than one on day six under discharge pressure.

Recognise the coverage constraint honestly. Placement is frequently determined by what is covered rather than by what is optimal, and pretending otherwise wastes days. Where the covered option is inadequate, that should be documented and escalated rather than silently accepted.

3.6.4 Hospice as a discharge decision

Hospice referral at discharge is among the most consequential decisions a hospitalist makes, and it is made too late far more often than too early.

Eligibility under most systems requires a prognosis of limited expected survival, conventionally six months or less if the disease follows its expected course, and a decision to pursue comfort-focused rather than disease-directed treatment for the terminal condition. Neither criterion requires that the patient be imminently dying, and both are widely misunderstood by patients, families, and clinicians.

The commonest errors are the following. Referring only when death is expected within days, which forfeits nearly all of the benefit. Presenting hospice as the abandonment of treatment rather than as a different and intensive form of treatment. Presenting it as a binary choice made once, when disenrollment is possible if circumstances change. And failing to recognise eligibility in non-cancer diagnoses, particularly advanced heart failure, chronic obstructive pulmonary disease, end-stage renal disease in patients declining or discontinuing dialysis, and advanced dementia, where prognostication is harder and referral is consequently delayed.

Prognostication is addressed in detail in Chapter 20, but one heuristic belongs here. The surprise question, asking oneself whether one would be surprised if this patient died within the next twelve months, is a crude instrument with modest predictive performance, and it is nonetheless useful as a trigger for further consideration rather than as a prediction in itself. A negative answer should prompt a goals-of-care conversation, not a hospice referral by itself.

The hospitalist's specific role is usually not to complete the hospice enrolment but to identify eligibility, to initiate the conversation honestly, and to ensure that the conversation is documented and transmitted. A patient who was told in hospital that their disease is terminal, and whose discharge summary does not record this, will encounter clinicians who do not know, and the conversation will have to occur again from the beginning.

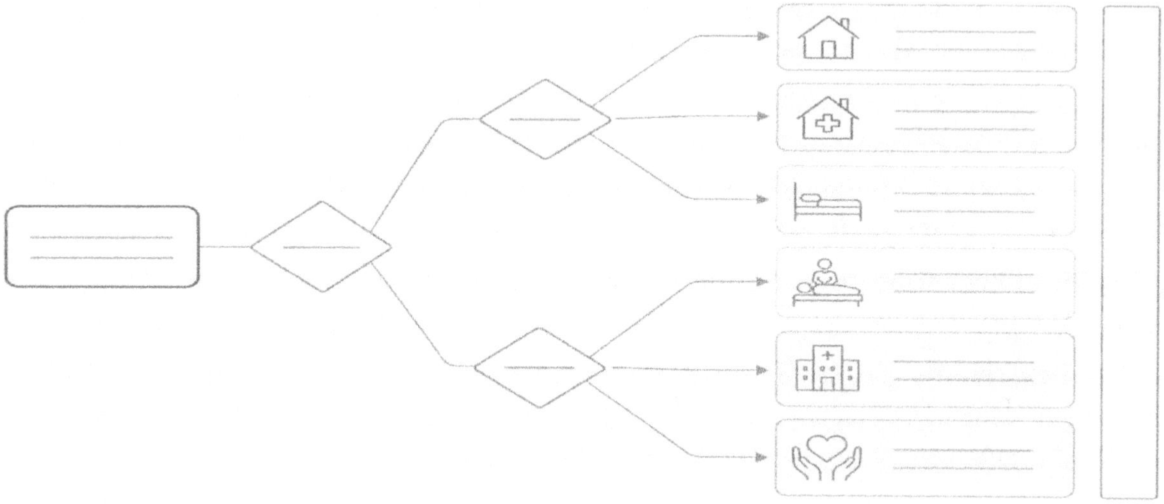

3.7 The High-Risk Discharge: Homelessness, Substance Use, Cognitive Impairment

3.7.1 The common structure

Three populations account for a disproportionate share of failed discharges, and although their circumstances differ, the failure has a common structure: **the discharge plan assumes capacities or resources the patient does not have.**

A plan requiring refrigerated medication assumes a refrigerator. A plan requiring twice-daily dosing assumes a stable environment in which to keep and take medication. A plan requiring attendance at a follow-up appointment assumes transport, a calendar, and an address at which a reminder can arrive. A plan requiring recognition of deterioration assumes intact cognition. When these assumptions fail, the discharge fails, and the failure is frequently attributed to the patient rather than to the plan.

The corrective discipline is to state the assumptions explicitly and test each one before discharge. This takes a few minutes and prevents a substantial proportion of avoidable returns.

3.7.2 Housing instability and homelessness

Patients experiencing homelessness have markedly elevated rates of readmission, of leaving before completing treatment, and of mortality following discharge, and the hospital admission frequently represents their only sustained contact with medical care.

Practical considerations for discharge planning:

- **Ask about housing directly and without assumption.** Housing status is frequently not recorded, and patients may not volunteer it. The question should be routine rather than reserved for those who appear unhoused.
- **Match the regimen to the environment.** Prefer once-daily dosing, avoid medications requiring refrigeration where alternatives exist, consider directly observed or long-acting formulations, and avoid regimens requiring careful titration against home monitoring.
- **Consider medical respite care** where it exists. Medical respite, also called recuperative care, provides a supervised environment for patients who are not sick enough for hospital but too unwell for the street or a shelter. Where available it substantially improves outcomes, and where unavailable its absence should be documented as an unmet need.
- **Do not discharge to the street at night or in extreme weather** without exhausting alternatives, and document the effort.
- **Provide medications in hand rather than a prescription** wherever the institution permits, since a prescription requiring a pharmacy visit, an address, and payment is frequently not filled.
- **Use the admission.** An inpatient stay is an opportunity for vaccination, screening, wound care, dental referral, and connection to services that may not recur for months.

3.7.3 Substance use disorder

Patients with substance use disorder experience high rates of premature discharge, readmission, and post-discharge mortality, and the period immediately following hospitalisation carries a markedly elevated overdose risk because tolerance falls during a period of abstinence in hospital.

Several practices are supported and are addressed clinically in Chapter 19.

Treat withdrawal adequately. Undertreated withdrawal is the single commonest reason patients with substance use disorder leave before completing treatment. The decision to leave is usually rational from the patient's perspective if the alternative is untreated symptoms.

Initiate medication for opioid use disorder during the admission rather than referring for it after discharge. Hospitalisation is a period of engagement, and initiation in hospital with a linked outpatient handover is associated with better retention than referral alone.

Provide overdose prevention supplies and education at discharge, including naloxone for the patient and any household member, with instruction. This is a low-cost intervention with a direct mechanism.

Manage pain adequately. Patients with substance use disorder frequently receive inadequate analgesia for genuine painful conditions, which drives conflict, premature discharge, and mistrust.

The considerations from Chapter 1, section 1.7.2, regarding documentation language apply with particular force here.

Plan for discharge against medical advice rather than treating it as a rupture. If a patient intends to leave, the correct action is to provide the best available partial plan: prescriptions, a return threshold, harm reduction supplies, and an explicit statement that they may return without judgement. Refusing to provide anything because the discharge is not sanctioned converts a partial outcome into a total one.

3.7.4 Cognitive impairment

Cognitive impairment is the most frequently undetected of the three risk factors, because it is not screened for routinely, because patients conceal it skilfully, and because a brief conversation with a socially intact patient does not reveal it.

Screen when the situation warrants it, which includes any patient over a certain age with a complex regimen, any patient whose history is internally inconsistent, any patient with an unexplained medication error at home, and any patient whose family expresses concern. Family concern is among the more reliable available signals.

Distinguish delirium from dementia from delirium superimposed on dementia, since the trajectory and the discharge implications differ entirely. Chapter 10 addresses the clinical distinction. A patient with unresolved delirium is not ready for a discharge plan requiring self-management, regardless of how well they appear during a morning conversation.

Assess whether the patient can execute the plan, not whether they understand it. Teach-back, in which the patient explains the plan in their own words, is the minimum standard and reveals a great deal. Asking whether they have questions reveals nothing.

Involve the person who will actually manage the medications. If that is a family member, they must be present for the discharge instruction, physically or by telephone. Instructions given only to a cognitively impaired patient have not been given.

Consider capacity explicitly where relevant. A patient who lacks capacity to consent to a discharge plan requires a surrogate decision maker, and the assessment should be documented rather than assumed. Chapter 20 addresses capacity assessment in detail.

Document baseline and discharge cognition. This is essential information for the next clinician, and it is almost never recorded in usable form.

Chapter Summary

- Transitions fail because compression is lossy, and what is lost is systematically the same material each time: uncertainty, reasoning, contingencies, and rejected alternatives.
- **Admission status** is a clinical documentation decision with direct financial and coverage consequences for the patient, particularly for subsequent skilled nursing coverage. The standard is the reasonable expectation at the time of admission, documented in clinical terms.
- **Medication reconciliation is a diagnostic act.** The list frequently contains the diagnosis, and the discipline of triangulating at least two independent sources, asking about behaviour

rather than prescriptions, and asking about recent changes yields more diagnostic information than most tests.

- **Handoff** transfers the plan reliably and the reasoning poorly. I-PASS provides a validated structure, and the two most frequently omitted elements, contingency planning and receiver synthesis, are the two that matter most.
- **The discharge summary** must be treated as the only artefact that reaches the next clinician. Timeliness outranks polish. Pending results with a named responsible person, medication changes with reasons, and specific follow-up instructions carry the greatest weight.
- **Readmission prediction tools** have modest discrimination and should allocate transitional resources rather than judge individual patients. Bundled transitional interventions work; single components do not.
- **Post-acute disposition** is a clinical question about functional deficit, trajectory, and required intensity, constrained but not determined by coverage. Hospice is referred too late far more often than too early, particularly in non-cancer diagnoses.
- **High-risk discharges fail because the plan assumes capacities the patient does not have.** Stating and testing those assumptions before discharge prevents a substantial share of avoidable returns.

Review Questions

1. A patient is placed under observation status and after two days requires skilled nursing placement. Explain the coverage consequence, the point at which the status decision should have been revisited, and what you would have documented on admission to support inpatient status.
2. Construct a best possible medication history plan for an 84-year-old admitted with recurrent falls who lives alone, has mild cognitive impairment, and attends three different specialists. Name the sources you would use, the specific questions you would ask, and the discrepancy types you would expect to find.
3. A patient deteriorates overnight and the covering clinician responds late. Using the five elements of a structured handoff, identify which element most likely failed and what specific sentence at handoff would have prevented the delay.
4. Write the top paragraph of a discharge summary for a patient discharged after an admission for heart failure in whom the precipitant was not established, the renal function worsened with diuresis, and a cardiac magnetic resonance study is pending. Include the elements that carry the greatest weight.
5. A patient experiencing homelessness with an infection requiring six weeks of intravenous antibiotics wishes to leave. Set out the discharge plan you would construct, including what you would change about the regimen, and state which assumptions in a conventional plan you are replacing.

CHAPTER 4: Patient Safety, Quality, and High-Reliability Practice

Learning Objectives

After studying this chapter, the reader should be able to:

1. Explain the systems account of harm, distinguish active failures from latent conditions, and describe the practical differences between the Safety-I and Safety-II perspectives.
2. Construct a measurement set for an improvement project using structure, process, outcome, and balancing measures, and interpret variation correctly using run and control chart logic.
3. Select an appropriate improvement methodology for a given problem, and identify the common failure modes of each.
4. Describe the evidence-based prevention of the principal categories of preventable inpatient harm, including where the evidence is weaker than commonly assumed.
5. Analyse a failure to rescue by identifying which link in the detection and response chain broke, and evaluate the evidence for rapid response systems honestly.
6. Conduct a disclosure conversation after harm, describe the second victim phenomenon and its management, and apply just culture reasoning to an individual case.
7. Identify the specific mechanisms by which the electronic health record both prevents and creates harm, and apply principles of effective clinical decision support.

Chapter Overview

The preceding three chapters described a specialty defined by a place, a reasoning discipline, and the transitions that reasoning must survive. This chapter addresses the environment in which all of it occurs, and the methods by which that environment can be changed.

The central claim of the patient safety movement is that harm in hospitals is predominantly a property of systems rather than of individuals, and that the traditional response to error, which is to identify the responsible person and improve their conduct, is both ineffective and counterproductive. This claim is now orthodoxy, and like most orthodoxies it has been simplified in transmission. Readers should hold it precisely: the claim is not that individuals bear no responsibility, nor that skill is irrelevant. It is that the same competent individual placed in a poorly designed system will produce predictable harm, and that redesigning the system produces larger and more durable improvement than exhorting the individual.

Chapter 1 identified the systems domain as one of the four in which hospitalists work, and observed that it is where the specialty generates much of its population-level value. This chapter supplies the methodology. It also, in sections 4.4 and 4.5, applies a discipline that recurs throughout this handbook: distinguishing what the evidence supports from what has become standard practice through repetition. Several widely mandated safety interventions have weaker support than their ubiquity suggests, and clinicians who do not know this cannot participate honestly in decisions about where to invest effort.

4.1 Systems Theory: Reason's Model, Latent Conditions, and Safety-II

4.1.1 The person approach and its failure

The traditional response to a harmful error is to locate the individual whose action was proximate to the harm, establish what they did wrong, and take measures directed at them: retraining, counselling, a policy reminder, discipline, or in serious cases removal.

This approach is intuitive, satisfying, and largely ineffective, for four reasons that are worth stating explicitly because the instinct behind it is strong and recurs even among people who have rejected it in principle.

It does not change the conditions that produced the error. The nurse who selected the wrong concentration from two similarly packaged vials stored adjacently will be replaced by another nurse facing the same two vials.

It relies on hindsight bias. After an outcome is known, the path leading to it appears obvious and the decision points appear clearer than they were at the time. Reviewers reliably overestimate how avoidable an error was and how much information was available to the person making it.

It suppresses the reporting on which improvement depends. If identifying the error results in personal consequence, errors are not reported, and the organisation loses its principal source of information about its own hazards. Near misses, which are the most valuable data because they are frequent and harmless, disappear first.

It misattributes the causal structure. The proximate action is the final element of a sequence that usually began long before and elsewhere.

4.1.2 Reason's model

James Reason's account, widely known through its illustration as layers of Swiss cheese, remains the most useful framework available for hospitalists.

The model holds that hazards are separated from patients by multiple layers of defence: protocols, checks, alarms, training, equipment design, staffing, supervision, and the vigilance of individuals. Each layer contains weaknesses, and the weaknesses are not static; they shift with circumstances. Harm occurs when the weaknesses in successive layers align, permitting a trajectory from hazard to patient.

The model distinguishes two categories of contribution.

Active failures are the unsafe acts of people in direct contact with the patient: the slip, the lapse, the mistake, the violation of protocol. They are proximate to the harm, easy to identify, and typically the focus of the person approach.

Latent conditions are the resident weaknesses built into the system long before the event, usually by decisions made far from the bedside and for reasons that had nothing to do with this patient. Understaffing, ambiguous protocols, similar drug packaging, poor equipment design, inadequate handoff structures, alarm configurations that produce fatigue, and production pressure are all latent conditions. They can lie dormant for years and combine with an active failure at a particular moment to produce harm.

The practical value of the distinction is directional. Active failures are numerous, individually unpredictable, and largely irreducible; humans in complex environments make errors at a stable base rate that training does not eliminate. Latent conditions are fewer, more predictable, and genuinely correctable. Effort spent on the second yields more than effort spent on the first.

A related concept from Vaughan's analysis of organisational disaster is **normalisation of deviance**: the process by which a departure from a standard, having been made repeatedly without visible harm, becomes the accepted local practice and ceases to be perceived as a departure at all. Hospitals are full of these. The hand hygiene step omitted when hurried, the identity check performed perfunctorily, the alarm limit widened to reduce noise, the double-check performed by a second person who signs without looking. Each was once a recognised shortcut and is now simply how the work is done. Recognising normalised deviance requires an outside perspective, which is why external observation and new staff are valuable sources of safety information and are routinely dismissed.

4.1.3 High reliability organising

Certain industries operate hazardous technologies with far lower failure rates than their complexity would predict. Weick and Sutcliffe characterised the organising principles that appear common to them, and these translate reasonably well to hospital settings.

Preoccupation with failure. Treating small anomalies as signals rather than noise, and actively seeking evidence of latent problems rather than waiting for events.

Reluctance to simplify. Resisting the convenient explanation that closes an investigation early. The finding that an error was caused by carelessness is a simplification that terminates inquiry.

Sensitivity to operations. Attention by leadership to how the work is actually performed at the point of care, as distinct from how policy describes it.

Commitment to resilience. Building the capacity to detect, contain, and recover from failures that will inevitably occur, rather than only attempting to prevent them.

Deference to expertise. During an evolving problem, decision authority migrating to the person with the most relevant knowledge regardless of their position in the hierarchy. This is the principle most frequently violated in medicine, where authority is strongly correlated with seniority rather than with proximity to the problem.

4.1.4 Safety-I and Safety-II

A more recent development, associated principally with Hollnagel, deserves attention because it changes what a hospitalist should look at.

Safety-I defines safety as the absence of adverse events and studies safety by studying failure. Incidents are investigated, causes identified, and defences added. This is the dominant model and it has produced real gains, but it has structural limitations: it studies a small and unrepresentative sample of events, it accumulates defences and thereby complexity, and it treats variability as a threat to be eliminated.

Safety-II defines safety as the capacity to succeed under varying conditions and studies safety by studying ordinary work. Its central observation is that things go right vastly more often than they go wrong, and that they go right largely because people adapt continuously to conditions that the formal system did not anticipate. On this account, human variability is the source of safety rather than a threat to it.

The most useful concept the perspective supplies is the distinction between **work-as-imagined** and **work-as-done**. Policies, protocols, and pathways describe work as imagined by those who designed them. What actually happens on the ward differs, always, because the designed process does not fit every circumstance and clinicians adapt to make it work. The gap is not a compliance problem. It is information about the design.

The practical consequence for a hospitalist attempting improvement is direct. Before changing a process, go and watch it being performed, and ask the people performing it what they do when the protocol does not fit. The workarounds are the map of the design's failures, and a change designed without knowing them will generate new workarounds within weeks.

The two perspectives are complements rather than rivals. Investigate harm; also study ordinary success.

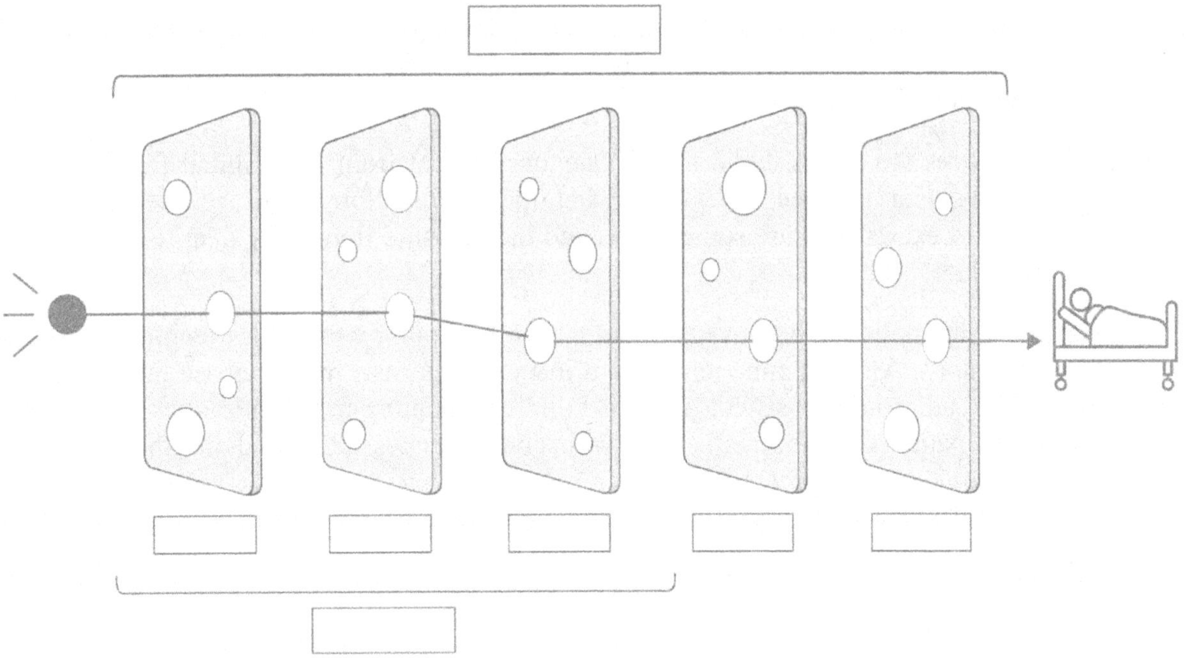

4.2 Measurement: Structure, Process, Outcome, and Balancing Measures

4.2.1 The Donabedian framework

Avedis Donabedian's classification remains the foundation of quality measurement and organises almost everything a hospitalist will encounter.

Structure refers to the attributes of the setting in which care occurs: staffing levels and skill mix, equipment availability, physical layout, information systems, and organisational arrangements. Structural measures are easy to collect and weakly connected to outcomes, since good structure permits good care without producing it.

Process refers to what is actually done: whether prophylaxis was prescribed, whether the medication was reconciled, whether the culture was drawn before antibiotics, whether the discharge summary was completed within the target interval. Process measures are the workhorse of improvement work because they are sensitive to change, attributable to specific actions, and require little risk adjustment. Their limitation is that they measure adherence rather than benefit, and a process measure is only as good as the evidence that the process improves outcomes.

Outcome refers to what happened to the patient: mortality, readmission, infection, functional status, symptom burden, experience of care. Outcomes are what matter, and they are the most difficult to use. They require risk adjustment, they occur infrequently enough that small units cannot detect change reliably, they are influenced heavily by factors outside the institution's control, and they are often delayed.

Balancing measures are the essential fourth category, absent from the original framework and added by improvement practice. They ask what the intervention might be breaking. Every improvement effort exerts pressure somewhere, and the pressure frequently manifests as harm in an unmeasured place.

Examples worth internalising, because they are real: a programme to reduce length of stay may increase readmissions. A programme to reduce urinary catheter use may increase falls in patients mobilising to the bathroom unassisted. A sepsis bundle mandating rapid antibiotics may increase antibiotic use in patients without infection, with consequences addressed in Chapter 18. An aggressive glycaemic control protocol may increase hypoglycaemia, addressed in Chapter 17. A project without balancing measures is not measuring its own harms, and therefore cannot know whether it produced net benefit.

4.2.2 Three purposes of measurement

A distinction drawn by Solberg, Mosser, and McDonald resolves a great deal of confusion, because the three purposes have incompatible requirements and are constantly conflated.

Measurement for improvement aims to guide change. It needs small samples, frequent collection, rapid feedback, and tolerance of imperfect data. Its standard is whether the data are good enough to decide what to do next.

Measurement for accountability aims to compare or judge. It needs complete data, careful risk adjustment, and standardised definitions, because a comparison drawn from imperfect data is unfair. It is slow and expensive, and it changes behaviour in ways discussed below.

Measurement for research aims to produce generalisable knowledge. It needs the most rigorous design of the three, including control of confounding and a defensible sampling frame.

The most common practical error is applying accountability standards to improvement work, which paralyses it. An improvement team that will not act until it has a fully adjusted, complete, validated dataset will not act. Twenty charts reviewed weekly is usually sufficient to guide a change.

The second most common error runs the other way: presenting improvement data as though it were accountability data, comparing units or clinicians on the basis of small, unadjusted samples. This produces unfair judgements and destroys the trust on which improvement depends.

4.2.3 Understanding variation

The single most consequential analytic skill in improvement work is distinguishing two kinds of variation, a distinction owed to Shewhart and popularised by Deming.

Common cause variation is the inherent, expected fluctuation of a stable process. A ward's fall rate will vary month to month even when nothing has changed. Reacting to common cause variation as though it were signal is called tampering, and it reliably makes processes worse while consuming enormous effort.

Special cause variation is variation arising from something outside the usual process: a genuine change, an unusual event, a new practice. This is signal and warrants investigation.

The instruments for distinguishing them are run charts and control charts, and hospitalists should be able to read both.

A **run chart** plots the measure over time against the median. Simple rules identify non-random patterns: a run of consecutive points on one side of the median, a trend of consecutive points moving in one direction, an unusual number of runs, and an astronomical single point. These rules are learnable in an afternoon and are sufficient for most improvement work.

A **control chart** adds statistically derived limits, conventionally at three standard deviations, and permits stronger inference about whether a process is stable and whether a change has occurred.

The practical importance is this. A hospitalist presented with a bar chart comparing this month's rate to last month's cannot tell whether anything happened. Two data points contain almost no information. The correct response to such a presentation is to ask for the time series, and this question, asked routinely, improves the quality of institutional decision making more than most interventions.

4.2.4 How measurement goes wrong

Four failure modes recur and should be recognised.

The denominator problem. Rates depend on who is counted, and definitional choices move rates substantially without any change in care. Infection rates depend on surveillance intensity; a unit that looks harder finds more.

Risk adjustment inadequacy. Adjustment models capture recorded comorbidity, not unrecorded severity, social circumstance, or frailty. Institutions serving sicker or poorer populations are systematically disadvantaged by imperfect adjustment, a point discussed in Chapter 3, section 3.5.1, in relation to readmission.

Gaming and the measure-target problem. When a measure becomes a target, it ceases to be a good measure, because effort shifts toward the measure rather than toward the underlying goal. Documentation changes, definitional reclassification, and patient selection are all easier than improving care. This is not usually conscious fraud; it is the predictable response of a system under pressure.

Measuring what is easy rather than what matters. Process measures proliferate because they are collectable. Outcomes that patients care about most, including function, symptom burden, and whether care aligned with their goals, are measured least often.

4.3 PDSA, Lean, and Six Sigma in the Inpatient Context

4.3.1 The Model for Improvement

The most widely used framework in healthcare improvement, developed by Langley and colleagues, poses three questions before any change is attempted.

What are we trying to accomplish? The answer is an aim statement, and its quality determines the project's fate. A good aim is specific, numerical, time-bound, and bounded to a defined population and location. "Reduce catheter-associated urinary tract infections on the two medical wards by fifty per cent within nine months" is an aim. "Improve catheter care" is a wish.

How will we know that a change is an improvement? The answer is the measurement set from section 4.2, including balancing measures.

What changes can we make that will result in improvement? The answer requires understanding the current process, which returns to the work-as-done principle from section 4.1.4. Process mapping, direct observation, and asking front-line staff what gets in their way generate better change ideas than a committee generates in a room.

A **driver diagram** is the standard tool for organising the answer: the aim on the left, primary drivers that must change to achieve it, secondary drivers beneath those, and specific change ideas at the right. Its value is that it makes the causal theory explicit and therefore falsifiable.

4.3.2 PDSA cycles and how they are misused

The Plan-Do-Study-Act cycle is a structure for testing a change on a small scale, learning from the result, and adapting before scaling.

Plan states the change, the prediction of what will happen, and how it will be measured. The prediction is not optional decoration; it is the element that makes the cycle a test rather than an implementation.

Do executes the test on a deliberately small scale. The canonical starting point is one clinician, one patient, one day.

Study compares the result to the prediction. The most valuable outcome is a failed prediction, because it means the underlying theory was wrong and has now been corrected.

Act adopts, adapts, or abandons the change, and specifies the next cycle.

Published analysis of PDSA use in healthcare, notably by Taylor and colleagues, has found that a large majority of reported applications do not meet the method's own criteria. The characteristic failures:

- **No prediction stated**, converting a test into an implementation with a form attached.
- **Starting at scale.** A change rolled out hospital-wide as a first cycle cannot be studied, cannot be reversed cheaply, and generates resistance.
- **A single cycle.** The method depends on iteration; one cycle is a pilot, not a learning system.
- **No data collected between cycles**, so adaptation is based on impression.
- **Retrospective labelling.** A change implemented by decision and later described in PDSA language, which is the most common form and produces no learning at all.

4.3.3 Lean

Lean, derived from manufacturing production systems, targets waste in processes and is most useful for problems of flow, delay, and duplication.

Its central concept is **value from the patient's perspective**: any step that does not contribute to what the patient needs is waste, however necessary it appears institutionally. Its canonical waste categories include waiting, unnecessary transport, unnecessary motion, overprocessing, inventory, defects requiring rework, and, importantly, underused human talent.

Value stream mapping, which traces every step from a defined start to a defined end and records the time consumed by each, reliably reveals that the great majority of elapsed time in hospital processes is waiting rather than doing. A discharge process that takes six hours typically contains twenty minutes of activity.

Lean fits inpatient problems including discharge delay, laboratory and imaging turnaround, operating theatre and procedure scheduling, supply availability, and admission flow. It fits diagnostic and therapeutic decision problems poorly, and applying manufacturing logic to clinical judgement is where Lean implementations generate the most staff resistance, usually justifiably.

The characteristic failure of Lean in healthcare is its adoption as a cost-reduction programme with the participatory elements removed. Lean depends on front-line staff identifying and solving problems; imposed from above as an efficiency exercise it produces the appearance of the method without its mechanism.

4.3.4 Six Sigma

Six Sigma targets defects and unwanted variation using a structured sequence conventionally abbreviated DMAIC: define, measure, analyse, improve, control. It is more statistically demanding than the alternatives and requires substantial data volume.

It fits high-volume, well-defined processes with a clear defect definition: laboratory specimen labelling errors, medication dispensing accuracy, appointment scheduling errors, billing accuracy. It fits low-volume, high-variability clinical problems poorly, because the statistical machinery has nothing to work with.

4.3.5 Choosing a method

The methods are not competitors and most institutions use elements of all three. A practical selection guide:

- **Problem of adherence to a known-good practice**, such as prophylaxis prescribing: Model for Improvement with iterative PDSA cycles.
- **Problem of delay, flow, or duplication**: Lean, beginning with a value stream map.
- **Problem of frequent defects in a high-volume standardised process**: Six Sigma.
- **Problem of a complex, poorly understood system with unclear causal structure**: begin with observation and process mapping before selecting any method.

Two cautions apply across all three. First, method selection matters far less than the quality of the underlying diagnosis of the problem, and projects fail most often because they addressed the wrong cause, not because they used the wrong framework. Second, sustainability is the unsolved problem in this field. Improvements decay when the project team disperses unless the change has been embedded in the default pathway, the order set, the staffing model, or the physical environment. A change that depends on remembering will not persist. The most durable improvements make the correct action the easy one.

4.4 Preventable Harm: Falls, Pressure Injury, Venous Thromboembolism, and Device Infections

This section treats four major categories of hospital-acquired harm. Throughout, the aim is to state both the accepted prevention practice and the actual strength of the evidence behind it, because several widely mandated interventions are supported less well than their ubiquity implies.

4.4.1 Falls

Falls are among the most frequent inpatient adverse events and among the least tractable, because the principal risk factors, meaning age, weakness, delirium, and the medications used to treat comorbid conditions, are not removable.

What is supported. Multifactorial assessment linked to individualised intervention has the best evidence, and the emphasis belongs on the linkage. Assessment alone changes nothing. Effective components include medication review with attention to sedatives, hypnotics, anticholinergics, and antihypertensives; treatment of delirium; assessment and correction of orthostatic hypotension; appropriate footwear; mobility aids within reach; timely toileting assistance, since a substantial share of falls occur en route to the bathroom; and adequate lighting and environmental arrangement.

What is weakly supported or unsupported. Bed and chair alarms as a standalone intervention have not demonstrated meaningful reduction in falls in controlled evaluation, and they contribute to alarm fatigue. Universal risk-scoring tools have modest discrimination and, used alone, do not reduce falls. Physical restraints increase harm, including injury and delirium, and should not be used for fall prevention. Bed rails are ambiguous; raised rails convert some falls into higher falls.

The balancing measure that matters. Fall prevention pursued through immobility produces deconditioning, delirium, thromboembolism, and pressure injury. The correct aim is fewer falls with preserved mobility, not fewer falls. A ward with no falls and no ambulating patients has traded one harm for several.

4.4.2 Pressure injury

Pressure injury is largely preventable, carries substantial morbidity, and is strongly associated with immobility, poor perfusion, moisture, malnutrition, and device contact.

What is supported. Systematic risk assessment on admission and at defined intervals, using a structured instrument as a prompt rather than as a prediction. Skin inspection at intervals, including under and around every device. Repositioning, though the optimal interval is less well established than commonly stated and should be individualised rather than fixed. Pressure-redistributing support surfaces for at-risk patients. Moisture management. Nutritional assessment and intervention where deficits exist. Early mobilisation, which is the intervention that addresses the underlying cause rather than its consequence.

Underrecognised. Device-related pressure injury, arising from oxygen tubing, nasogastric tubes, cervical collars, compression devices, catheters, and monitoring equipment, accounts for a substantial proportion of hospital-acquired injury and is frequently missed because inspection focuses on the sacrum and heels. Every device in contact with skin should be part of the inspection.

The hospitalist's specific contributions are attention to nutrition and perfusion, aggressive removal of unnecessary devices, and the prescription of mobility as an active order rather than an assumption.

4.4.3 Venous thromboembolism prophylaxis

This is the area where the gap between mandate and evidence is widest, and where a hospitalist most needs to reason rather than comply.

The established position. Hospitalised medical patients have elevated thromboembolic risk, and pharmacological prophylaxis reduces the incidence of venous thromboembolism in appropriately selected patients.

The complications. Trials of prophylaxis in medical inpatients have shown reductions in thromboembolic events with less consistent effects on mortality, and the absolute benefit in unselected medical inpatients is smaller than the near-universal prescribing pattern implies. Prophylaxis carries bleeding risk. Blanket prophylaxis for all medical inpatients therefore treats a large number of low-risk patients to prevent a small number of events, while causing bleeding in some.

The correct approach is individual risk assessment using a validated model, of which several exist for medical and surgical populations, combined with an explicit bleeding risk assessment, and a decision documented as a decision. Mechanical prophylaxis is appropriate where pharmacological prophylaxis is contraindicated, with the recognition that its evidence in medical patients is weaker still.

What hospitalists should resist is the conversion of prophylaxis into a compliance metric measured as the proportion of patients prescribed it, since that metric is optimised by prescribing for everyone including those who should not receive it. The appropriate process measure is the proportion of patients with a documented risk assessment and a decision consistent with it. Chapter 7 addresses perioperative prophylaxis and Chapter 14 addresses treatment.

4.4.4 Device-associated infection

Two categories dominate: central line-associated bloodstream infection and catheter-associated urinary tract infection. Both are among the clearest successes of the safety movement, and both have a shared underlying principle.

Central line infection. Insertion bundles combining hand hygiene, maximal sterile barriers, chlorhexidine skin antisepsis, avoidance of the femoral site where alternatives exist, and daily review of necessity have produced large and sustained reductions across many settings. Maintenance practices including hub disinfection and dressing integrity matter as much as insertion. The evidence for this bundle is among the strongest in the field.

Urinary catheter infection. The dominant risk factor is the presence and duration of the catheter. Interventions targeting insertion technique matter less than interventions targeting whether the catheter exists at all. Effective programmes restrict indications, require documented justification, prompt daily review, and empower nursing staff to remove catheters without a further order when criteria are no longer met. Chapter 18 addresses the distinction between catheter-associated infection and asymptomatic bacteriuria, which is essential because treating the latter is itself a common harm.

The shared principle, and the single most useful sentence in this section: *the most effective prevention for any device-associated harm is not having the device.* This applies to central lines, urinary catheters, peripheral cannulae, telemetry, supplemental oxygen, restraints, and continuous monitoring. Daily review of every device, with a default toward removal, prevents more harm than any bundle applied to devices that should not be present.

4.4.5 Other categories worth naming

Several further harms recur in inpatient practice and are addressed elsewhere in this handbook but belong on the hospitalist's mental list: hospital-acquired anaemia from diagnostic phlebotomy, discussed in Chapter 2, section 2.7.3; delirium, in Chapter 10; adverse drug events, in Chapters 3 and 19; hospital-acquired pneumonia and aspiration, in Chapter 18; deconditioning and functional decline, in Chapter 19; and hypoglycaemia from inpatient insulin protocols, in Chapter 17.

4.5 Rapid Response Systems and Failure to Rescue

4.5.1 The concept of failure to rescue

Failure to rescue, a concept introduced by Silber and colleagues, is among the most useful ideas in inpatient safety because it reframes what mortality differences between hospitals actually represent.

The observation is this. Hospitals differ relatively little in the rate at which complications occur. They differ substantially in the rate at which patients die once a complication has occurred. The difference in mortality between institutions is therefore driven less by complication prevention than by **the capacity to detect and respond to deterioration**.

This reframing has practical consequences. It directs attention away from the unattainable goal of preventing all complications and toward the attainable goal of ensuring that complications are recognised early and answered adequately. It also identifies where the failure occurs, which is almost never in the treatment itself. The treatment for most inpatient deterioration is well understood. The failure is in detection, escalation, and response.

4.5.2 The chain of rescue

Rescue depends on a sequence of links, each of which can break. Analysing a failure to rescue means identifying which one did.

Link one: monitoring. The deterioration must generate a detectable signal. Failures here include observations not taken at appropriate frequency, taken but not recorded, or a monitoring frequency set at admission and never revised as the patient's condition changed.

Link two: recognition. Someone must notice that the signal is abnormal. Failures include observations recorded but not reviewed, abnormal values normalised because the patient "always runs low", and single parameters assessed in isolation rather than as a pattern.

Link three: interpretation. The abnormality must be understood as significant. This is where the reasoning failures of Chapter 2 operate: a rising respiratory rate attributed to anxiety, a falling blood pressure attributed to sleep, a new confusion attributed to age.

Link four: escalation. The concern must reach someone able to act. This is the most frequently broken link and is discussed below.

Link five: response. The clinician who receives the call must attend, assess, and act with appropriate urgency.

Link six: treatment and disposition. The correct intervention must be delivered, and the decision about level of care must be made.

The empirical literature consistently identifies **link four, escalation, as the dominant failure point**, which is why it is sometimes called the afferent limb problem. A hospital may have an excellent response team and still fail patients if concerns do not reach it.

4.5.3 Early warning scores

Aggregate physiological scoring systems, which assign points to deviations in respiratory rate, oxygen saturation, blood pressure, heart rate, temperature, and consciousness level, are now widely implemented, with several national and institutional variants.

Their strengths are real. They convert subjective concern into a communicable number, they legitimise escalation by less senior staff, and they detect the pattern rather than the isolated parameter. Respiratory rate in particular is the earliest and most sensitive indicator of deterioration and is also the observation most often estimated rather than counted.

Their limitations should be understood equally. Discrimination is moderate rather than excellent. Scores perform less well in patients with chronic physiological derangement, in whom the baseline is already abnormal. They are insensitive to deterioration that is not primarily physiological, including neurological events and some haemorrhage. And a score threshold creates a binary where a trajectory is more informative: a patient whose score has risen steadily from one to four is often at greater risk than a patient stable at five.

The correct use is as a trigger for human assessment rather than as a substitute for it. A low score in a patient who a nurse thinks looks unwell should never override the nurse.

4.5.4 Rapid response systems: an honest reading of the evidence

Rapid response teams are now near-universal in developed health systems, and the evidence for them is more equivocal than their ubiquity suggests. Hospitalists should know this, because they are frequently asked to lead or resource these systems.

The largest cluster-randomised trial of a medical emergency team, conducted across Australian hospitals, did not demonstrate a reduction in the composite of cardiac arrest, unplanned intensive care admission, and unexpected death. Subsequent observational and before-and-after studies have frequently reported benefit, and meta-analyses have generally found reductions in cardiac arrest outside intensive care with less consistent effects on hospital mortality.

The most plausible reconciliation is that the effect depends heavily on implementation, and specifically on the afferent limb. A team that is not called cannot help. In the negative trial, activation rates were low relative to the theoretical need. Systems that achieve high activation rates, that have removed the social barriers to calling, and that treat calls as welcome rather than as a judgement on the calling clinician appear to do better.

The practical implications for a hospitalist:

- **The efferent limb is the easy part.** Resourcing a team is straightforward. Making it easy to call is the difficult and decisive work.
- **Measure activation rates as a process measure**, and treat a low rate as a problem rather than as evidence that the system is not needed.
- **Remove the hierarchy barrier explicitly.** Nurses and junior clinicians frequently do not call because of anticipated criticism, prior negative experience, or an expectation that they should first inform the primary team. Any system requiring a nurse to obtain permission before escalating has reintroduced the barrier it was designed to remove.

- **Never criticise a call that turns out to be unnecessary.** A single dismissive response propagates through a nursing unit within a shift and suppresses calls for months. This connects directly to Chapter 1, section 1.7.3.
- **Enable patient and family activation.** Programmes permitting families to call directly have been implemented in many institutions without the flood of inappropriate calls that was predicted, and families frequently detect subtle change that staff do not.

4.5.5 The hospitalist's role

Hospitalists occupy the pivotal position in this chain, as both the recipient of most escalations and, in many institutions, the responder.

Three behaviours matter most. **Go and look.** Deterioration cannot be assessed by telephone, and a substantial proportion of failures to rescue involve a clinician who managed a concerning call remotely. **Set explicit parameters at handoff**, as described in Chapter 3, section 3.3.2, so that the covering clinician's threshold is defined rather than improvised. And **document the ceiling of treatment where one exists**, because a substantial number of futile and distressing rapid response activations occur in patients for whom escalation was never appropriate and no one had recorded it. Chapter 20 addresses this directly.

4.6 Disclosure, the Second Victim, and Just Culture

4.6.1 Disclosure after harm

When a patient is harmed by their care, they are entitled to be told. This obligation is ethical before it is legal, and it rests on the same basis as informed consent: patients cannot make decisions about their care without accurate information about what has happened to them.

The practical barriers are substantial and familiar: fear of litigation, shame, uncertainty about whether an error actually occurred, uncertainty about who should speak, and institutional processes that delay disclosure while facts are established.

The evidence on litigation runs contrary to the intuition. Communication and resolution programmes, which combine prompt disclosure, investigation, explanation, apology where warranted, and proactive offer of compensation, have generally been associated with stable or reduced claims, reduced legal costs, and faster resolution in the institutions that have implemented them well. Patients frequently pursue litigation to obtain an explanation, and the explanation is cheaper than the litigation.

The structure of a disclosure conversation:

- **Do it promptly**, before the patient learns it elsewhere, which they usually will.
- **Have the right person present**, normally the responsible senior clinician, with institutional support available.
- **State the facts that are established**, plainly and without hedging.
- **Say clearly what is not yet known**, and commit to a defined process and timeline for finding out.

- **Apologise.** An expression of regret for what has happened is appropriate regardless of whether fault has been determined, and many jurisdictions have enacted protections for such expressions. Verify local law.
- **Explain what will be done**, both for this patient clinically and for the system to prevent recurrence.
- **Return.** A single conversation is not disclosure. The commitment to come back with findings is the element that most determines whether trust is retained.
- **Document the conversation** factually.

What to avoid: speculating about cause before it is known, attributing blame to a colleague or another service, minimising, and using the passive constructions that signal evasion.

4.6.2 The second victim

Wu's description of the clinician as a second victim named something previously unspoken: that the clinician involved in a harmful error experiences a predictable and severe reaction, and that this reaction is largely unsupported.

Scott and colleagues described a recognisable trajectory: an initial period of chaos and confusion; intrusive reflection with repeated replaying of the event; a period of anxiety about professional reputation and standing; a phase of seeking emotional first aid, frequently unsuccessfully; and finally one of three outcomes, described as dropping out, surviving, or thriving.

The consequences are real and measurable: depression, anxiety, post-traumatic symptoms, reduced job performance, attrition, and, in the most serious cases, suicide. Involvement in a serious adverse event is an established risk factor for physician suicide, and this fact belongs in any discussion of clinician wellbeing, alongside the material in Chapter 1, section 1.6.

What helps: rapid, non-judgemental peer support from a trained colleague within hours to days rather than weeks; explicit permission to step back from clinical duties if needed; clear information about the investigation process, since uncertainty about what will happen drives much of the distress; and inclusion in the improvement work that follows, which converts the experience into agency.

What harms: isolation, exclusion from the investigation, delayed or absent communication about outcome, and the implication that a strong clinician would not be affected.

For a hospitalist, the immediate practical obligation is toward colleagues. A colleague involved in a serious event should be contacted the same day by someone who does not ask them to explain what happened.

4.6.3 Just culture

Just culture is the framework that resolves the apparent conflict between a systems approach to harm and individual accountability. The systems approach is sometimes misread as holding that no one is ever accountable, which is neither true nor sustainable.

The framework, developed principally by Marx, distinguishes three categories of behaviour, each warranting a different response.

Human error is an inadvertent action: a slip, a lapse, a mistake. The appropriate response is to console the individual and to examine the system that permitted the error to reach the patient. Discipline for human error is both unjust and counterproductive.

At-risk behaviour is a behavioural choice that increases risk where the risk is not recognised or is mistakenly believed to be justified. This is the normalisation of deviance described in section 4.1.2. The appropriate response is to coach: to make the risk visible and to remove the incentives that made the shortcut attractive. Discipline is usually inappropriate, since the behaviour is typically widespread and locally normal.

Reckless behaviour is a conscious disregard of a substantial and unjustifiable risk. This is rare. The appropriate response is disciplinary, and applying it appropriately is what makes the framework credible; a system that never sanctions anything is not a just culture but an absent one.

The **substitution test** is the practical instrument for distinguishing these. Would three other clinicians of similar training and experience, in the same circumstances, with the same information and the same pressures, have acted similarly? If yes, the problem is systemic and the individual response should be support and system change. If no, examine whether the individual had adequate training, supervision, and support before considering accountability.

Two cautions. Just culture must be applied consistently across professions and seniority levels, and it frequently is not; nurses and junior staff are disciplined for behaviour that is tolerated in senior physicians, which destroys the framework's credibility faster than any other failure. And a just culture is demonstrated by what happens after a serious event, not by what is written in a policy document. Staff calibrate their reporting behaviour on observed outcomes, and they observe accurately.

4.7 The Electronic Health Record as Both Safety Instrument and Hazard

4.7.1 What it prevented

The electronic record eliminated several important categories of harm, and this should be stated before the criticism, because the counterfactual is frequently forgotten by clinicians who never worked without one.

Illegible handwriting no longer causes drug and dose errors. Orders no longer go missing. The record is available in more than one place simultaneously, which is the precondition for most of the transition work in Chapter 3. Allergy and interaction checking occurs automatically. Results are visible immediately rather than when a paper arrives. Dosing calculations are supported. Prior imaging and prior notes are retrievable rather than stored in a basement.

These were not trivial harms and their elimination was a genuine achievement.

4.7.2 What it created

The record also introduced new hazard categories, several of which were not anticipated.

Alert fatigue. Interruptive alerts fire at rates that make attention impossible, and clinician override rates for drug interaction alerts are extremely high in most published series, commonly exceeding ninety per cent. The predictable consequence is that the small proportion of alerts carrying serious information are overridden along with the rest. Alert burden is a patient safety hazard in its own right, and reducing the number of alerts is a safety intervention.

Wrong-patient errors. Multiple open records, similar names, and interface design permit orders to be placed on the wrong patient at a measurable rate. The retract-and-reorder metric, which detects orders cancelled and immediately reissued on a different patient, has been used to quantify this and reveals rates higher than clinicians assume.

Selection errors. Dropdown lists, autocomplete, and default values produce a category of error that did not previously exist: the adjacent-item selection, in which a plausible but wrong medication, dose, route, or frequency is chosen because it sat next to the intended one.

Note bloat and copy-forward. Automated import of results and copied prior text produces documents of great length and little content, with propagated errors that persist across an entire admission and beyond. Chapter 1, section 1.7.2, treats the professional obligation; the systems point here is that the feature makes the harmful behaviour the path of least resistance, which is a design failure rather than a discipline failure.

Loss of the narrative. The clinical reasoning that Chapter 2 identified as the most valuable content of any note is precisely the content that templates do not capture and that billing-driven structure crowds out.

Fragmented attention and interruption. Discussed in Chapter 1, section 1.3.2. The interface is itself an interruption generator.

Downtime vulnerability. Systems fail, and institutions that have not rehearsed downtime procedures discover during the failure that no one knows how to order a medication on paper.

Documentation burden and its contribution to burnout. Addressed in Chapter 1, section 1.6.

4.7.3 Effective clinical decision support

Decision support that works shares identifiable characteristics, commonly summarised as delivering the right information, to the right person, in the right format, through the right channel, at the right time in the workflow.

Design principles with support:

- **Deliver at the point of decision**, integrated into the order rather than appended afterward.
- **Be specific and actionable.** An alert that names the action to take is useful; one that states a concern is noise.
- **Prefer non-interruptive support** where the risk is moderate. Inline display, order set defaults, and passive indicators change behaviour without consuming attention.
- **Use defaults deliberately.** The default is the most powerful decision support instrument available and requires no attention at all. Setting the default dose, the default duration, the default monitoring frequency, and the default review interval correctly changes practice more reliably than any alert.
- **Tier by severity.** Reserve interruptive alerts for the small number of situations where the harm is severe and the alert is highly specific.

- **Monitor and prune.** Alerts should have override rates measured, and any alert overridden almost always should be reviewed for removal or redesign. Most institutions add alerts continuously and remove them never.

4.7.4 The hospitalist's role

Hospitalists are frequently the most intensive users of the inpatient record and are therefore positioned to influence its configuration, which is systems work of exactly the kind described in Chapter 1, section 1.2.2.

Practical contributions: participate in order set design, since order sets encode defaults and therefore practice; report usability hazards through the safety reporting system rather than developing a private workaround, because the workaround protects you and leaves the hazard for the next clinician; advocate for alert pruning with data; resist template expansion; and preserve a written assessment in every note regardless of what the template requires.

A closing observation connects this section to the whole chapter. The record is a **latent condition generator**. Its configuration decisions are made far from the bedside, often by people who will never use it clinically, and they lie dormant until they combine with an active failure at a particular moment. That is precisely Reason's description, and it means the record belongs in the same analytic frame as any other system component rather than being treated as a fixed feature of the environment.

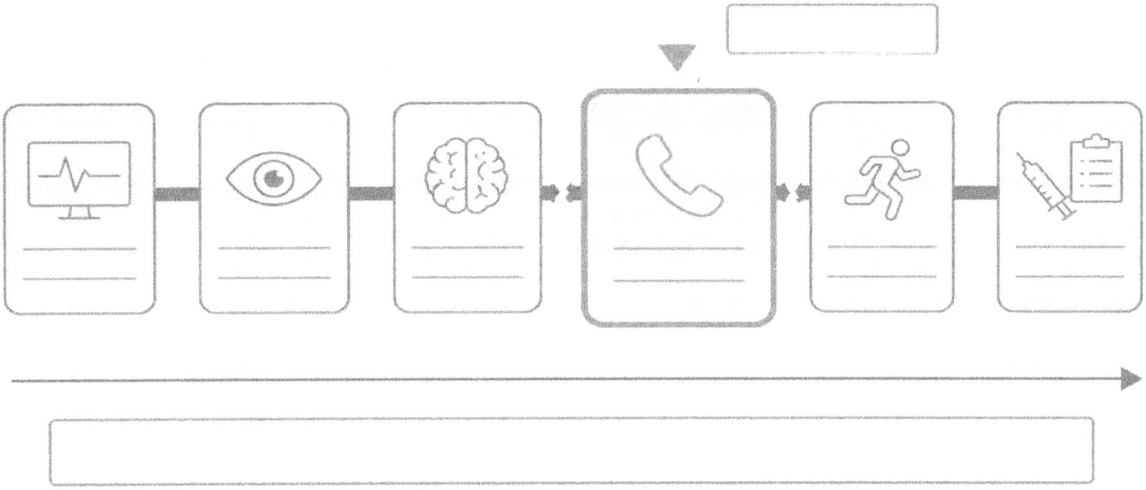

Chapter Summary

- Harm is predominantly a property of systems. **Active failures** are numerous, unpredictable, and largely irreducible; **latent conditions** are fewer, more predictable, and correctable, and are where effort yields most.
- **Normalisation of deviance** converts recognised shortcuts into invisible local practice. Detecting it requires an outside perspective.

- **Safety-II** directs attention to ordinary work and to the gap between work-as-imagined and work-as-done. Workarounds are a map of a design's failures and should be studied before any process is changed.
- Measurement requires **structure, process, outcome, and balancing measures**. Omitting balancing measures means the project cannot know whether it caused net benefit. Distinguish measurement for improvement from measurement for accountability, and never confuse the two.
- Distinguishing **common cause from special cause variation** is the central analytic skill. Two data points contain almost no information; ask for the time series.
- **PDSA fails most often through absence of a stated prediction, starting at scale, and single cycles.** Lean fits flow and delay problems; Six Sigma fits high-volume defect problems. Method selection matters less than correctly diagnosing the problem, and sustainability requires embedding the change in the default pathway.
- Among preventable harms, the evidence is strong for **central line bundles** and for **catheter avoidance**, moderate and multifactorial for **falls** and **pressure injury**, and weaker than the mandates imply for **blanket venous thromboembolism prophylaxis**. The most effective prevention for any device-associated harm is not having the device.
- **Failure to rescue** explains more of the mortality difference between hospitals than complication rates do. The **afferent limb** is the most frequently broken link, and criticising an unnecessary call suppresses future calls for months.
- **Disclosure** after harm is an ethical obligation, and communication and resolution programmes have generally been associated with stable or reduced claims. The **second victim** reaction is predictable, severe, and best answered with same-day peer contact.
- **Just culture** distinguishes human error, at-risk behaviour, and reckless behaviour, with the substitution test as the practical instrument. It is demonstrated by what happens after an event, not by policy text.
- The **electronic record** eliminated major harm categories and generated new ones. Defaults are the most powerful decision support instrument available and require no clinician attention at all.

Review Questions

1. A patient receives a tenfold insulin overdose because a nurse selected an adjacent item from a dropdown list during a busy night shift. Using Reason's framework, identify the active failure and at least four plausible latent conditions, and state which of these you would prioritise correcting and why.
2. You are designing a project to reduce urinary catheter days on two medical wards. Write an aim statement, and specify one structure, two process, one outcome, and two balancing measures.
3. A colleague presents a bar chart showing that falls rose from four last month to seven this month, and proposes hourly rounding across the hospital. Explain what is wrong with both the analysis and the proposed response, and state what you would ask for instead.
4. A rapid response system has been in place for two years with a low activation rate and no measurable change in cardiac arrests outside intensive care. Set out your diagnostic approach to this system and the three most likely explanations.

5. A junior colleague prescribed a medication to which the patient had a documented allergy; the allergy alert had fired and was overridden, as it is in the great majority of cases in your institution. Apply just culture reasoning, including the substitution test, and state what response you would recommend for the individual and for the system.

CHAPTER 5: Principles of Medical Consultation and Preoperative Assessment

Learning Objectives

After studying this chapter, the reader should be able to:

1. Establish the terms of a consultation, including the question, the urgency, and the boundaries of the consultant's role, and explain why each must be negotiated rather than assumed.
2. Assess functional capacity, describe the metabolic equivalent framework, and explain the substantial measurement problems with subjective assessment demonstrated by contemporary evidence.
3. Apply the principal global risk indices, state what each was derived to predict, and identify the populations in which each performs poorly.
4. Select preoperative investigations on the basis of whether the result will change management, and articulate why routine testing before low-risk surgery causes net harm.
5. Identify modifiable preoperative risk factors and describe the evidence for prehabilitation and targeted optimisation.
6. Communicate perioperative risk to surgeons, anaesthetists, and patients using formats that support understanding, and explain why the language of surgical clearance should be abandoned.

Chapter Overview

Part I established the specialty, its reasoning discipline, its transitions, and its systems methodology. Part II turns to the consultative role, in which the hospitalist advises rather than directs, and in which the value delivered depends as much on the structure of the relationship as on the clinical content.

Medical consultation is where hospitalists are most often ineffective, and the reasons are rarely clinical. The commonest failures are answering a question that was not asked, providing recommendations too numerous or too vague to be actioned, giving advice on matters outside the consultant's competence, and issuing a verdict when a quantification was wanted. Each of these is a failure of the consultation contract described in section 5.1, and each is preventable.

Preoperative assessment is the highest-volume consultative activity in most hospitalist practices and is the subject of the remainder of the chapter. Readers should approach it with a specific frame in mind. The purpose of preoperative assessment is **not** to decide whether the patient may have surgery. That decision belongs to the patient, informed by the surgeon regarding the benefit of the operation and by the consultant and anaesthetist regarding its risks. The consultant's purpose is to estimate risk accurately, to identify what can be modified, and to specify what should be done differently because of the patient's medical condition. Section 5.6 develops the implications of this frame, which are considerable.

Chapters 6, 7, and 8 develop the organ-specific and complication-specific material. This chapter establishes the method.

5.1 The Consultation Contract: Question, Urgency, and Boundaries

5.1.1 Why the contract must be explicit

A consultation is a transaction between two clinicians with different training, different information, and frequently different assumptions about what has been requested. When the terms are left implicit, the two parties proceed on divergent understandings, and the divergence is discovered only when the advice proves useless or, worse, when a task assumed to belong to one party belongs to neither.

Chapter 1, section 1.4, distinguished consultation from comanagement and identified diffusion of responsibility as the dominant failure of the latter. The equivalent failure in consultation is **question mismatch**: the consultant answers a general question when a specific one was asked, or a specific one when a general one was needed.

The classic articulation of effective consultation was published by Goldman and colleagues in 1983 as a set of commandments, subsequently re-examined and updated by Salerno and colleagues, whose survey work found that requesting physicians valued direct communication and specific, actionable advice far more than consultants assumed, and valued extensive differential diagnosis discussion far less. The principles below draw on that tradition and adapt it to contemporary hospitalist practice.

5.1.2 Establish the question

Determine what is actually being asked, and if it is not clear, ask.

Consultation requests are frequently written in a shorthand that conceals the real question. "Preop clearance" might mean any of the following: is this patient's heart failure adequately controlled; should the anticoagulant be stopped and when; is the anaemia significant enough to delay; does this patient need a cardiology opinion; or, occasionally, please share responsibility for a patient who worries me. Each requires a different response.

The remedy is a telephone call or a direct conversation, which takes ninety seconds and is the highest-yield action available in consultative medicine. It resolves the question, establishes urgency, reveals the underlying concern that the written request did not contain, and creates a relationship that makes the advice more likely to be taken.

When the request is genuinely open, meaning the requesting clinician wants a general medical assessment, that is a legitimate question and should be confirmed as such rather than assumed.

5.1.3 Establish urgency

Urgency should be established explicitly, in three broad categories: immediate, meaning the patient is unstable and the consultant should attend now; same-day, meaning a decision depends on the answer today; and routine, meaning the answer is needed before a scheduled event at a known time.

Consultants systematically underestimate urgency and requesting clinicians systematically fail to state it. The cost is borne by the patient in delayed operations and prolonged stays.

5.1.4 Establish boundaries

The scope of the consultant's role should be agreed at the outset, and this is the element most often omitted.

Specifically: will the consultant write orders, or only recommend? Will the consultant follow the patient daily, or provide a single assessment with availability for further questions? Who manages the medical problems that arise subsequently? Who communicates with the family about medical issues?

The answers vary legitimately between institutions and situations. What matters is that they are stated. A consultant who writes orders without agreement creates confusion and resentment; a consultant who declines to write orders in a comanagement relationship creates delay.

5.1.5 Doing the work

Several practices distinguish a useful consultation from an ornamental one.

Gather your own data. Review the record, take your own history, and examine the patient. Consultations produced from the chart alone are unreliable, and the value a consultant adds frequently derives from finding something the requesting team did not know. The murmur that was not documented, the medication the patient stopped taking, the functional decline the family reports, and the goals-of-care conversation that occurred at another institution are all found this way and only this way.

Be brief and specific. The single most common complaint about medical consultations is that they are long and do not say what to do. A five-page note with a comprehensive differential and no clear recommendation has failed. The useful structure is a short assessment paragraph followed by a small number of numbered, specific, actionable recommendations.

Limit the number of recommendations. Evidence on consultation adherence consistently indicates that a small number of clearly prioritised recommendations is followed more often than a long list. Where many issues exist, distinguish explicitly between what must happen before the operation, what should happen during the admission, and what can be deferred to outpatient follow-up.

Be specific about drugs and doses. "Optimise the diabetes regimen" is not actionable. "Hold the sodium-glucose cotransporter-2 inhibitor for three days before surgery; on the morning of surgery give half the usual basal insulin dose and no short-acting insulin; check capillary glucose hourly intraoperatively" is.

Provide contingency plans. State what should be done if the anticipated course does not occur. This is the same principle as the contingency element of handoff in Chapter 3, section 3.3.2, and it is equally neglected here.

Communicate verbally for anything important. A note is a record; it is not a reliable means of transmitting urgent information. Any recommendation that changes management materially should also be spoken.

Follow up. A single note with no subsequent contact is rarely sufficient. Following up demonstrates that the consultant is available, allows the recommendation to be adjusted as circumstances change, and catches the situation in which the advice was not followed for a reason the consultant should know about.

5.1.6 Respecting the boundaries of competence

Two boundary failures are worth naming because both damage relationships and both harm patients.

Advising outside your domain. A medical consultant should not opine on the technical conduct of the operation, the choice of anaesthetic technique, or whether the surgical indication is sound, unless specifically asked. These are matters of others' expertise, and unsolicited opinions on them reliably reduce the weight given to the consultant's legitimate advice.

Declining to engage with what is within your domain. The converse failure is a consultant who answers narrowly to avoid responsibility. A patient referred for assessment of cardiac risk who is found to have undiagnosed severe anaemia, uncontrolled diabetes, or unrecognised frailty should have all of it addressed. The question sets the minimum, not the maximum, and a consultant who noticed something important and did not mention it has failed regardless of what was asked.

The reconciling principle is that the consultant's expertise is medical, and everything medical is within scope, while everything outside medicine is not.

5.1.7 Teaching and disagreement

Two further situations recur.

Disagreement with the requesting team. When the consultant believes the plan is wrong, the disagreement should be raised directly and privately with the responsible clinician before it appears in the record, and it should be framed around the clinical stake rather than the error. Chapter 1, section 1.5.3, addresses escalation when direct discussion fails.

Teaching through the consultation. A consultation note is read by trainees and by clinicians outside your specialty, and a brief statement of the reasoning behind a recommendation is more valuable than the recommendation alone. This should be brief and should not become a lecture. The distinction is between explaining why anticoagulation is being bridged in this patient and reviewing the literature on bridging.

5.2 Functional Capacity Assessment and Its Measurement Problems

5.2.1 Why functional capacity matters

Functional capacity is the single most useful piece of information in preoperative risk assessment, and it is obtained by asking rather than by testing.

The reason it carries such weight is mechanistic. Surgery imposes a substantial physiological demand: increased oxygen consumption, catecholamine surge, fluid shifts, inflammatory activation, and, in the postoperative period, the metabolic cost of healing superimposed on immobility and pain. A patient who can meet an increased demand without symptoms has demonstrated reserve across the cardiac, pulmonary, and musculoskeletal systems simultaneously, which no single test does.

Functional capacity is conventionally expressed in **metabolic equivalents**, where one metabolic equivalent represents resting oxygen consumption. The traditional threshold of four metabolic equivalents corresponds approximately to climbing one to two flights of stairs, walking on level ground at a brisk pace, or performing heavy housework. Below this threshold, risk assessment has traditionally been intensified.

Approximate values worth knowing:

Activity	Approximate metabolic equivalents
Rest, sitting quietly	1
Eating, dressing, walking indoors	2
Walking on level ground at 3 to 5 km per hour	3 to 4
Climbing a flight of stairs, walking uphill	4 to 5
Heavy housework, scrubbing floors, moving furniture	5 to 6
Running a short distance, doubles tennis	6 to 8
Strenuous sport, swimming, singles tennis	above 10

5.2.2 The measurement problem

Here the chapter must complicate the standard teaching, because the evidence on how functional capacity is usually assessed is uncomfortable.

The Measurement of Exercise Tolerance before Surgery study, reported by Wijeysundera and colleagues, prospectively compared four methods of assessing functional capacity in patients undergoing major non-cardiac surgery: subjective clinical assessment by the responsible clinician, the Duke Activity Status Index questionnaire, cardiopulmonary exercise testing, and serum natriuretic peptide measurement.

The principal finding was that **subjective clinical assessment performed poorly.** Clinician estimation of whether a patient could achieve four metabolic equivalents showed weak agreement with objectively measured capacity and did not usefully predict postoperative myocardial injury or death. The structured questionnaire and the natriuretic peptide measurement both performed better than clinician impression.

This finding deserves to be taken seriously rather than absorbed as a footnote, because it undermines a step that appears in nearly every preoperative algorithm and is performed by nearly every consultant. The mechanism of the failure is instructive and connects to Chapter 2: clinicians ask a vague question, receive a socially conditioned answer, and convert it into a number by inference. A patient who says “I manage all right” has told the clinician almost nothing, and the clinician who records four metabolic equivalents has generated data rather than collected it.

5.2.3 Asking better

Several practices substantially improve the yield of functional assessment.

Ask about specific, recent, verifiable activities. Not "can you climb stairs?" but "when did you last climb the stairs at home, and did you have to stop?" The best questions have a location, a recent time, and an observable stopping point.

Ask what stops them. A patient limited by knee pain, by dizziness, by breathlessness, and by fatigue have four different problems with four different implications. A patient limited by osteoarthritis may have excellent cardiac reserve that is simply untestable by walking.

Ask a household member. Patients systematically overestimate their capacity, and the family observes what actually happens. This single question resolves a large proportion of ambiguous assessments.

Ask about change over time. A capacity of four metabolic equivalents that was eight metabolic equivalents six months ago is a very different finding from a stable four, and the trajectory frequently reveals an undiagnosed condition.

Consider a structured instrument. The Duke Activity Status Index is a brief validated questionnaire covering a defined list of activities, and it outperformed clinician impression in the study described above. Using it takes a few minutes and produces a reproducible number.

Distinguish "does not" from "cannot." A sedentary patient who never climbs stairs has not demonstrated incapacity. This is the commonest source of falsely low estimates, particularly in older adults and in patients whose environment does not require exertion.

5.2.4 Objective testing

Where functional capacity cannot be established by history and the answer would change management, objective assessment is available.

Cardiopulmonary exercise testing measures oxygen consumption directly during graded exercise and yields the anaerobic threshold and peak oxygen uptake. It is the reference standard, predicts postoperative outcome in several surgical populations, and is limited by availability, cost, and the requirement that the patient can exercise.

Simpler functional tests, including the six-minute walk test, the incremental shuttle walk test, gait speed, and timed chair stands, are practical, correlate imperfectly with formal testing, and have accumulating evidence particularly in older surgical populations. **Gait speed** in particular is quick, requires only a corridor and a stopwatch, and predicts postoperative morbidity and mortality in several cohorts.

Natriuretic peptides occupy an interesting position: not a functional test at all, but a biomarker that performed comparably to or better than functional assessment in predicting cardiac events. Their role is discussed further in section 5.4 and Chapter 6.

The practical synthesis: take a rigorous functional history using specific recent activities and a collateral source; use a structured instrument where feasible; and reserve objective testing for the patient in whom the history is genuinely uninterpretable and the result would alter the plan.

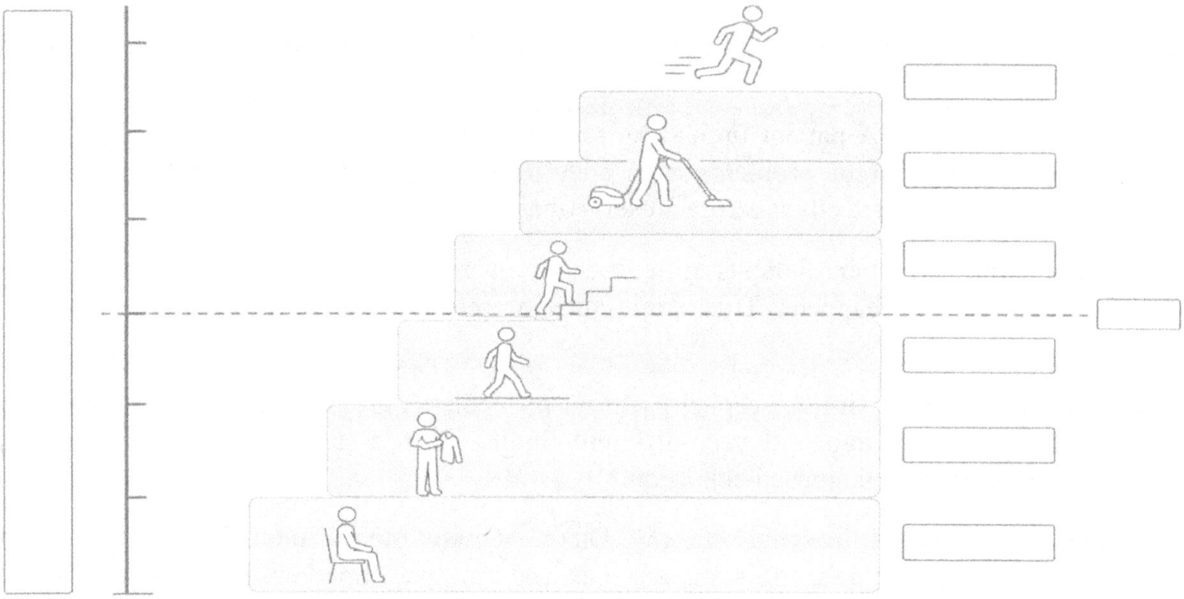

5.3 Global Risk Indices: RCRI, NSQIP MICA, Gupta, and Frailty Scores

5.3.1 What a risk index is and is not

A risk index converts a set of patient and procedure characteristics into an estimated probability of a specified outcome. Its value is that it anchors estimation to data rather than to impression, and Chapter 2, section 2.3.2, established why this matters: clinicians overestimate dramatic risks and underestimate common ones, and a validated model corrects both errors.

Three limitations apply to every index and should be stated before any of them are described.

Each predicts a specific outcome in a specific population. An index derived to predict cardiac events does not predict pulmonary complications, delirium, or functional decline, and using it as a general measure of operative risk is a category error.

Discrimination is moderate. Values for area under the receiver operating characteristic curve for the major perioperative indices generally fall in a range indicating useful but far from decisive performance. They stratify populations well and predict individuals imperfectly.

Derivation populations age. Perioperative care, surgical technique, and anaesthesia have changed substantially since several of these indices were derived, and event rates have generally fallen, which means older models tend to overestimate absolute risk even when their relative ordering remains valid.

5.3.2 The Revised Cardiac Risk Index

The Revised Cardiac Risk Index, published by Lee and colleagues in 1999, remains the most widely used perioperative cardiac risk instrument and is embedded in major guidelines.

It comprises six equally weighted predictors:

1. High-risk surgery, defined in the original derivation as intraperitoneal, intrathoracic, or suprainguinal vascular procedures
2. History of ischaemic heart disease
3. History of congestive heart failure
4. History of cerebrovascular disease
5. Diabetes mellitus requiring insulin
6. Preoperative serum creatinine above a defined threshold, conventionally 2.0 mg/dL or approximately 177 micromoles per litre

Risk of major cardiac complication rises with the number of factors present, and guidelines conventionally treat patients with none or one factor as low risk and those with two or more as elevated risk, with the elevated category triggering further consideration of functional capacity and, in selected cases, further testing.

Strengths. Simple, memorable, externally validated many times, and usable at the bedside without a calculator.

Limitations that matter clinically. It performs less well in vascular surgery specifically, which is a substantial limitation given that vascular patients carry high cardiac risk. It does not include age, which is counterintuitive but reflects the derivation. It uses coarse categories: any history of heart failure counts equally whether compensated or decompensated, and any ischaemic heart disease counts equally whether remote and revascularised or recent and symptomatic. And it does not capture the acute state of the patient, so a patient in current decompensation scores identically to the same patient when stable.

The practical rule is to use the index as a starting point and then to adjust explicitly for what it cannot see: current symptoms, recent change, valvular disease, arrhythmia, and pulmonary hypertension.

5.3.3 The NSQIP-derived calculators

Two instruments derived from the American College of Surgeons National Surgical Quality Improvement Program data are widely used.

The Gupta myocardial infarction or cardiac arrest calculator estimates the risk of perioperative myocardial infarction or cardiac arrest from five variables: age, functional status, serum creatinine elevation, American Society of Anesthesiologists physical status class, and the type of surgery. It was derived from a very large contemporary cohort and generally shows better discrimination for its specific outcome than the older index.

The ACS NSQIP Surgical Risk Calculator is broader, estimating the probability of multiple outcomes including death, serious complication, pneumonia, cardiac complication, surgical site infection, urinary tract infection, thromboembolism, renal failure, readmission, and discharge to a facility, from a larger variable set including the specific procedure code.

Strengths. Contemporary derivation, procedure-specific estimates, multiple outcomes, and output in a form suitable for discussion with a patient.

Limitations. They require a computer and the correct procedure code. They depend on variables recorded in a surgical database, which means they capture recorded comorbidity rather than severity or frailty. Functional status is entered as a coarse category, which returns the problem discussed in section 5.2.2. Calibration in populations dissimilar to the derivation cohort is variable, and several external validations have found systematic over- or underestimation in specific populations.

5.3.4 Frailty

Frailty deserves separate treatment because it predicts postoperative outcomes better than most conventional risk factors and better than chronological age, and because it is the variable most often absent from formal indices.

Frailty is a state of reduced physiological reserve across multiple systems, producing disproportionate vulnerability to stressors. Two conceptual models dominate.

The phenotype model, associated with Fried, defines frailty by the presence of a defined number of features among unintentional weight loss, self-reported exhaustion, weakness measured by grip strength, slow walking speed, and low physical activity.

The deficit accumulation model, associated with Rockwood, treats frailty as the proportion of a long list of possible deficits that an individual has accumulated, producing a continuous index.

For inpatient practice, several practical instruments exist.

- **The Clinical Frailty Scale** is a judgement-based nine-point ordinal scale assessed from history, requires no equipment, takes under a minute in experienced hands, and predicts outcomes across many settings. It has become the most widely used instrument in acute care.
- **Gait speed** alone, as noted in section 5.2.4, performs surprisingly well as a single-item marker.
- **Grip strength** is quick and requires only a dynamometer.
- **Modified frailty indices** derived from routinely collected comorbidity data can be calculated automatically from the record, which makes them attractive for institutional risk stratification even though they measure comorbidity accumulation more than frailty proper.

Why this matters for the consultant. Frailty predicts postoperative mortality, complications, delirium, prolonged stay, loss of independence, and discharge to a facility rather than home. Crucially, it predicts the outcomes patients care most about, which are frequently not death but the loss of the ability to live as they did before. A frail patient contemplating major surgery needs to know that the most likely adverse outcome is not dying on the table but never returning to independent living, and that information is available only if frailty has been assessed.

Assessment of frailty should therefore be part of every preoperative consultation in an older adult, and its result should appear explicitly in the note and in the risk discussion described in section 5.6.

5.3.5 Using indices well

Four practical rules.

Name which index you used and which outcome it predicts. A note stating "elevated perioperative risk" transmits nothing. A note stating "Revised Cardiac Risk Index of 2, corresponding to a major cardiac event risk of approximately 6 to 10 per cent in published cohorts, though contemporary rates are likely lower" transmits something usable.

Use a cardiac index for cardiac risk and something else for everything else. Pulmonary risk indices are addressed in Chapter 6; delirium risk in Chapter 10; and functional outcome is best predicted by frailty.

Adjust explicitly for what the index cannot see, and document the adjustment as a judgement rather than presenting it as an output.

Do not use an index to make the decision. The index informs the conversation described in section 5.6. It does not replace it.

5.4 Preoperative Testing: What to Order and When Nothing Is Right

5.4.1 The default should be nothing

Section 2.7 established the discipline: a test is indicated only when a question exists and the answer will change management. Preoperative testing is the single clearest application of that principle, and it is also where it is most widely violated.

The evidence on routine preoperative testing before low-risk surgery is unusually consistent. Multiple studies, including large analyses in cataract surgery, have found that routine preoperative investigation does not reduce perioperative complications, does not alter management in the great majority of cases, and generates abnormal results that lead to delay, further testing, and occasional harm without benefit. Major guideline bodies and Choosing Wisely recommendations across several specialties now advise against routine testing before low-risk procedures in asymptomatic patients.

The mechanism of harm is the cascade described in Chapter 2, section 2.7.1, and its cost is not only financial. A patient whose operation is delayed for six weeks to investigate an incidental finding has suffered a harm, and in oncological and symptomatic conditions the harm may be substantial.

The correct default position is therefore that **no preoperative test is indicated unless a specific question requires it**, and the burden of justification falls on ordering rather than on omitting.

5.4.2 When each test is actually indicated

The following describes the general position. Institutional and anaesthetic department requirements vary and should be followed where they exist, and readers should verify against current guidance.

Electrocardiogram. Reasonable in patients with known cardiovascular disease, significant arrhythmia, structural heart disease, or symptoms suggestive of these, undergoing surgery of at least intermediate risk. Not indicated routinely on the basis of age alone in asymptomatic patients undergoing low-risk surgery. Its principal value is as a baseline for comparison if postoperative ischaemia is suspected, which is a legitimate but limited indication.

Full blood count. Indicated where anaemia is suspected clinically, where the patient has a condition associated with anaemia, or where significant blood loss is anticipated. Detection of anaemia before major surgery is genuinely valuable, for reasons developed in section 5.5.

Renal function and electrolytes. Indicated in patients with known renal disease, heart failure, diabetes, or hypertension, in those taking diuretics, renin-angiotensin system agents, or nephrotoxic drugs, and where the result is required for drug dosing or for a risk index.

Coagulation studies. Not indicated routinely. A structured bleeding history, asking about prior surgical and dental bleeding, bruising, menorrhagia, family history, and anticoagulant or antiplatelet use, is a better screening instrument than the tests, which have poor performance for detecting clinically significant bleeding tendency in unselected patients. Indicated where the history is positive, in known liver disease, and in anticoagulated patients where a level is required.

Chest radiograph. Not indicated routinely, including on the basis of age or smoking history alone. Indicated where a new or unstable cardiopulmonary problem is suspected clinically.

Echocardiography. Not indicated routinely. Indicated for a new unexplained murmur with symptoms, suspected or known significant valvular disease without recent imaging, suspected heart failure of unclear cause, dyspnoea without explanation, and suspected pulmonary hypertension. Chapter 6 develops this.

Pulmonary function testing. Not indicated routinely, including in patients with known chronic obstructive pulmonary disease when the clinical status is established. Indicated principally for lung resection planning and for unexplained dyspnoea where the diagnosis will alter management.

Natriuretic peptides. An area of active change. Several guideline bodies, notably in Canada, now recommend preoperative measurement of B-type natriuretic peptide or its N-terminal fragment in defined higher-risk groups, on the basis that the result improves risk discrimination beyond clinical variables and identifies patients warranting postoperative troponin surveillance. Practice varies internationally and readers should verify current local guidance. Chapter 6 addresses postoperative troponin surveillance.

Pregnancy testing. Should be offered in accordance with local policy to patients of childbearing potential, with attention to consent and confidentiality.

Type and screen or crossmatch. Determined by anticipated blood loss and institutional protocol for the specific procedure.

5.4.3 The tests that produce most harm

Three ordering patterns cause disproportionate difficulty and are worth naming.

The panel ordered because it is available. Broad automated panels generate abnormal results at a rate governed by the number of analytes, and most such abnormalities are statistical rather than clinical.

Imaging ordered without a question. Incidental findings on preoperative computed tomography and echocardiography generate substantial downstream investigation, and the great majority prove insignificant.

Testing ordered to transfer responsibility. A test ordered so that the consultant can document having looked, rather than because the answer matters, is a defensive act that exposes the patient to the cascade without prospect of benefit.

5.4.4 When the answer is that no test is right

A specific and difficult situation deserves treatment: the patient in whom risk is clearly elevated, no test will change management, and the operation must proceed.

This occurs frequently. A frail patient with a hip fracture, severe aortic stenosis, and heart failure will not benefit from an echocardiogram that confirms what is known, will be harmed by a delay, and will not be a candidate for valve intervention before the fracture is fixed. The correct consultative action is not to order tests. It is to state the risk clearly, to specify what should be done differently intraoperatively and postoperatively, to ensure the anaesthetist has the information required, and to ensure the patient and family understand the situation.

Chapter 6 develops the cardiac specifics and Chapter 8 the postoperative management. The general principle belongs here: **the consultant's output is a plan, not a test.** A consultation that ends in an investigation has frequently deferred the work rather than done it.

5.4.5 What to do with an unexpected abnormal result

Having argued against unnecessary testing, the chapter must address the situation that unnecessary testing creates and that consultants face constantly: a result has come back abnormal, the operation is scheduled, and someone must decide what it means.

Four questions resolve most such situations.

Is this abnormality new? A creatinine of 140 micromoles per litre is alarming if it was 70 last month and unremarkable if it has been 140 for three years. Retrieving prior values is the first action and frequently the only one required. The commonest error in this situation is treating a value as an event when it is a baseline.

Is it clinically corroborated? An abnormal result in a patient with no corresponding symptom, sign, or risk factor is more likely to be a laboratory artefact, a statistical outlier, or a pre-analytic problem than a new disease. Repeating the test before acting on it is often the correct next step and is far cheaper than the alternative cascade.

Would knowing more change the perioperative plan? This is the same question as section 5.4.1, applied downstream. An incidental finding that will require outpatient investigation should be documented, communicated to the patient and the primary care clinician, and scheduled for after the operation. It should not delay the operation unless it changes perioperative management.

Does the delay cause more harm than the finding? For oncological, symptomatic, and time-sensitive surgery, delay is not a neutral act. The harm of a four-week postponement should be weighed explicitly against the expected benefit of the investigation, and the weighing should be documented as a judgement rather than resolved by default.

The consultant carries a specific responsibility here that is easy to evade. Incidental findings identified preoperatively are frequently lost, because the surgical team regards them as medical and the medical consultant regards their role as concluded once the operation is approved. The finding must be named explicitly in the note, communicated to the patient, and transmitted to whoever will follow it, with the same rigour applied to pending results in Chapter 3, section 3.4.2.

5.5 Prehabilitation and Modifiable Preoperative Risk

5.5.1 The window and what it is worth

Elective surgery provides something rare in medicine: a known date, a motivated patient, and an interval before a defined physiological stress. Prehabilitation is the deliberate use of that interval to improve the patient's capacity to withstand it.

The conceptual case is strong. Postoperative recovery is limited by physiological reserve, reserve is modifiable, and the preoperative period is when modification is possible. The empirical case is moderate and improving. Randomised trials and meta-analyses of multimodal prehabilitation, typically combining exercise, nutritional support, and psychological preparation, have generally shown improvements in preoperative functional capacity and postoperative functional recovery, with less consistent and more modest effects on complication rates and length of stay. Effects appear larger in higher-risk and more deconditioned patients, which is intuitive.

Readers should therefore present prehabilitation to patients honestly: as an intervention with good evidence for improving fitness and recovery of function, and weaker evidence for reducing complications.

The consultant's contribution is usually not to deliver the programme but to identify the modifiable factors and to trigger the relevant referral early enough to matter. **Timing is the binding constraint.** A patient seen three days before surgery cannot be optimised in any meaningful sense.

5.5.2 Anaemia

Preoperative anaemia is common, independently associated with postoperative morbidity and mortality, and frequently ignored until the day of surgery, at which point the only remaining option is transfusion, which carries its own risks and is itself associated with worse outcomes.

The correct approach, encompassed within patient blood management programmes, is to detect anaemia weeks before major surgery, to investigate its cause rather than treating it empirically, and to correct it where possible. Iron deficiency is the commonest treatable cause and is frequently present without anaemia, in which case it still warrants attention where significant blood loss is anticipated. Intravenous iron corrects deficiency substantially faster than oral iron and is the appropriate choice when the interval to surgery is short or oral iron is not tolerated or absorbed.

Two points are often missed. Anaemia in an older adult requires investigation for occult gastrointestinal blood loss in its own right, independent of the surgery, and the discovery may be more consequential than the operation. And correcting anaemia is not the same as transfusing; the aim is to avoid transfusion, not to achieve a threshold.

5.5.3 Smoking

Smoking cessation before surgery reduces pulmonary and wound complications, and the magnitude of benefit increases with the duration of abstinence before the operation. Cessation of several weeks, conventionally at least four, is associated with meaningful reduction in pulmonary complications, and longer intervals confer greater benefit.

Two practical points. There is no persuasive evidence that brief preoperative cessation increases complications, a concern that circulated for some years and should not be used to discourage quitting. And the preoperative period is among the most effective moments for cessation intervention in a smoker's life, because motivation is high and the connection between the behaviour and an imminent consequence is concrete. A consultant who offers pharmacological support and referral at this moment achieves cessation rates well above baseline, and the benefit extends far beyond the operation.

5.5.4 Alcohol

Hazardous alcohol use is associated with increased postoperative complications including infection, bleeding, and cardiopulmonary events, and with the risk of unrecognised withdrawal in the postoperative period, which is dangerous and frequently missed.

Preoperative abstinence of several weeks has been associated with reduced complications in trial evidence for heavy drinkers. Screening should be routine, and the consultant should specify a withdrawal management plan for the postoperative period where relevant, rather than assuming the surgical team will recognise it. Chapter 19 addresses withdrawal management.

5.5.5 Glycaemic control and diabetes

Poor preoperative glycaemic control is associated with increased surgical site infection and other complications. Where surgery is elective and glycaemic control is substantially outside target, delay for optimisation is reasonable, though the threshold at which delay produces net benefit is not well defined and the harm of delay must be weighed.

The consultant's more reliable contributions are practical and often neglected: specifying the perioperative medication plan in detail, including which agents to stop and when, how basal and prandial insulin should be adjusted on the day of surgery, and what glucose monitoring should occur. Newer agents have specific requirements, notably sodium-glucose cotransporter-2 inhibitors, which are associated with euglycaemic ketoacidosis perioperatively and require a defined period of withholding before surgery, and glucagon-like peptide-1 receptor agonists, which delay gastric emptying and have prompted specific anaesthetic guidance regarding fasting and aspiration risk. Both areas have evolved rapidly and current guidance should be verified. Chapter 7 develops perioperative diabetes management.

5.5.6 Nutrition

Malnutrition is common in surgical populations, particularly in oncological and gastrointestinal disease, and is independently associated with complications, impaired healing, and mortality.

Screening with a validated instrument should be routine before major surgery. Where significant malnutrition is identified, preoperative nutritional support for a period of weeks has evidence of benefit in reducing complications, and in some circumstances justifies delaying an operation. Perioperative carbohydrate loading and avoidance of prolonged fasting are components of enhanced recovery pathways with reasonable support.

5.5.7 Frailty, physical conditioning, and cognition

Exercise. Structured preoperative exercise programmes improve measured functional capacity reliably. Programmes combining aerobic and resistance training over a period of weeks are standard. Even brief programmes appear to produce measurable change in deconditioned patients.

Frailty. Identification, as discussed in section 5.3.4, should trigger comprehensive geriatric assessment where available, which has evidence for improving outcomes in older surgical patients. It should also trigger an explicit conversation about goals, since for some frail patients the correct answer is a less invasive procedure or no procedure at all.

Cognition and delirium risk. Preoperative cognitive assessment identifies patients at high risk of postoperative delirium, which is among the commonest and most consequential postoperative complications in older adults. Documented baseline cognition permits the postoperative change to be recognised. Multicomponent delirium prevention should be planned before the operation rather than initiated after it. Chapter 8 and Chapter 10 develop this.

Psychological preparation and expectation setting. Anxiety and unrealistic expectations are associated with worse reported outcomes, and structured preparation is a component of most prehabilitation programmes.

5.5.8 Medication optimisation

The consultant should produce an explicit, drug-by-drug perioperative medication plan rather than a general instruction. The categories requiring specific decisions include antiplatelet agents, anticoagulants, renin-angiotensin system agents, beta-blockers, diuretics, glucose-lowering agents, corticosteroids, immunosuppressants and biologics, psychotropic agents, opioids and agents for opioid use disorder, and hormone therapy. Chapters 6 and 7 address these in detail.

The plan should state, for each relevant medication, what to do before, on the day of, and after surgery, and who is responsible for restarting it. The final element is the one most often omitted and the one most often harmful: medications stopped before surgery and never restarted are a recognised source of preventable harm, and the restart plan belongs in the consultation note and in the discharge summary described in Chapter 3, section 3.4.2.

5.6 Communicating Risk to Surgeons, Anaesthetists, and Patients

5.6.1 Abandoning the language of clearance

The phrase "cleared for surgery" should not appear in a consultation note, and the reasoning is not pedantic.

Clearance implies three things that are all false. It implies that risk has been eliminated rather than estimated. It implies that the consultant has authority over whether the operation proceeds, which they do not. And it implies that responsibility has transferred, which creates a documented expectation that the consultant has underwritten the outcome.

What the consultant actually provides is an estimate of risk, an identification of what can be modified, and a set of specific recommendations for perioperative management. That is more useful than clearance and it is also accurate.

The replacement formulation is straightforward. State the estimated risk with its source, state what has been optimised and what remains, state the specific recommendations, and state explicitly that the decision to proceed rests with the patient and the surgical team weighing that risk against the benefit of the operation.

5.6.2 Communicating with the surgeon and anaesthetist

Three principles govern.

Give a number where one exists, and a qualifier where one does not. Surgeons and anaesthetists make decisions with these estimates, and "high risk" means different things to different people.

Separate the risk estimate from the recommendations. These are different products serving different purposes, and conflating them produces notes in which neither is findable.

Anticipate the anaesthetist's specific questions, which are frequently not the same as the surgeon's. The anaesthetist wants to know about airway, cardiovascular reserve, valvular disease, pulmonary hypertension, aspiration risk, positioning tolerance, anticoagulation, and the medications taken that morning. A consultation note that addresses these directly is far more useful than one organised as a general medical summary.

5.6.3 Communicating with patients

Risk communication to patients is a distinct skill with an evidence base, and several practices reliably improve understanding.

Use natural frequencies rather than percentages or relative risks. "About 4 out of every 100 people like you will have a serious heart complication" is understood far better than "your risk is 4 per cent" and immeasurably better than "your risk is doubled." Relative risk without absolute risk is the single most misleading format in common use.

Keep the denominator constant. Presenting one risk as out of 100 and another as out of 1,000 defeats comparison.

Give both the chance of the event and the chance of no event. Framing effects are real and presenting both sides reduces them.

Use a visual format for important decisions. Icon arrays, in which a grid of figures is shaded to represent the affected proportion, improve comprehension particularly in patients with lower numeracy, which is common and poorly predicted by education.

Present the outcomes the patient cares about, which are frequently not mortality. For an older patient, the probability of not returning to independent living, of needing a facility, of developing delirium, or of losing the ability to care for a spouse may matter far more than the probability of death, and these are the outcomes least often quantified.

Check understanding with teach-back, as described in Chapter 3, section 3.4.4.

Acknowledge uncertainty honestly. The estimates are population-derived and imprecise, and saying so does not undermine the discussion. It makes the subsequent advice more credible.

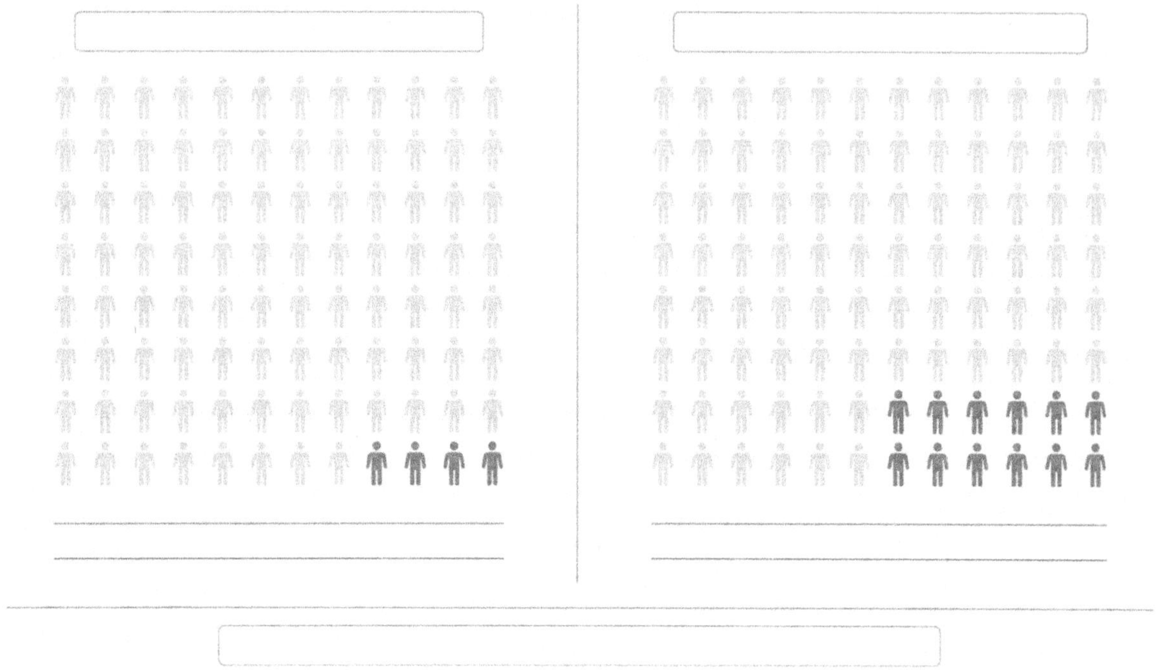

5.6.4 Documenting the consultation

The note should be structured so that each audience finds what it needs quickly.

A workable structure: a one-line statement of the question asked and who asked it; a brief assessment paragraph containing the problem representation and the risk estimate with its source; a short list of numbered, specific recommendations divided into preoperative, intraoperative or anaesthetic, and postoperative; an explicit medication plan including restart responsibility; a statement of what was discussed with the patient and what they understood; and a statement of availability and follow-up intention.

What should not appear: the word clearance; a comprehensive differential diagnosis; recommendations on surgical or anaesthetic technique that were not requested; and a recommendation list so long that its priorities are invisible.

5.6.5 When the consultant believes the operation should not proceed

Occasionally the consultant concludes that the risk is prohibitive or that the patient is unlikely to achieve an outcome they would regard as worthwhile.

This conclusion should be stated, clearly and without hedging, directly to the surgeon before it appears in the record, and the reasoning should be given. It should be framed as an assessment of risk and expected outcome rather than as a verdict on the indication, which remains the surgeon's domain.

The patient should be part of this conversation rather than its subject. A frail patient with a high probability of never returning home is entitled to know that, and frequently makes a different decision when told. Chapter 20 addresses the structure of these conversations, and the point that belongs here is that the preoperative consultation is one of the more common settings in which a goals-of-care conversation is indicated and one of the settings in which it is least often held.

Chapter Summary

- The **consultation contract** must be explicit: the question, the urgency, and the boundaries. A ninety-second conversation with the requesting clinician is the highest-yield action in consultative medicine.
- Effective consultations gather their own data, are brief and specific, limit and prioritise recommendations, specify drugs and doses, include contingencies, communicate verbally for anything important, and follow up.
- **Functional capacity** is the most useful single element of preoperative assessment, but subjective clinician estimation of it agrees poorly with objective measurement. Ask about specific, recent, verifiable activities, ask what stops the patient, ask a household member, and distinguish "does not" from "cannot."
- **Risk indices** predict specific outcomes in specific populations with moderate discrimination. The Revised Cardiac Risk Index is simple and validated but blind to acuity, severity, and age. NSQIP-derived calculators are contemporary and procedure-specific but depend on coarse functional and comorbidity inputs.
- **Frailty predicts postoperative outcomes better than chronological age**, and predicts the outcomes patients care most about, including loss of independence. It should be assessed in every older surgical patient.
- **The default for preoperative testing is nothing.** Routine investigation before low-risk surgery does not reduce complications and generates cascades. A structured bleeding history outperforms coagulation studies. The consultant's output is a plan, not a test.
- **Prehabilitation** has good evidence for improving fitness and functional recovery and weaker evidence for reducing complications. Anaemia, smoking, alcohol, glycaemic control, nutrition, conditioning, and cognition are the principal modifiable targets, and timing is the binding constraint.
- **Abandon the language of clearance.** Provide a risk estimate, an optimisation plan, and specific recommendations, and locate the decision with the patient and the surgical team.
- Communicate risk in **natural frequencies against a constant denominator**, use visual formats for important decisions, and quantify the outcomes the patient actually cares about.

Review Questions

1. A request reads "medical clearance for total hip arthroplasty." Set out the questions you would ask the requesting surgeon before seeing the patient, and explain what each would change about your assessment.
2. A 72-year-old man reports that he "gets around fine." Write the five specific questions you would ask to establish his functional capacity, and state what a positive or negative answer to each would imply.

3. A patient has a Revised Cardiac Risk Index of 1 but has developed orthopnoea over the past three weeks. Explain why the index is insufficient here, and state what you would do instead.
4. A colleague proposes routine electrocardiogram, chest radiograph, and coagulation studies for all patients over 65 before elective hernia repair. Construct the argument against, including the mechanism of harm and the evidence you would cite.
5. An 84-year-old woman with a Clinical Frailty Scale score of 6 is offered major abdominal surgery. Draft the risk communication you would deliver to her, using natural frequencies and specifying which outcomes you would quantify and why.

CHAPTER 6: Cardiac and Pulmonary Risk in Noncardiac Surgery

Learning Objectives

After studying this chapter, the reader should be able to:

1. Apply the stepwise perioperative cardiac evaluation algorithm, and identify the specific points at which it breaks down or rests on weak evidence.
2. Determine the appropriate interval between coronary stent placement and elective surgery, and construct an antiplatelet management plan that balances stent thrombosis against surgical bleeding.
3. State the findings of the POISE trial and their consequences for perioperative beta-blockade, and describe current practice regarding statins and renin-angiotensin system agents.
4. Assess and manage the patient with significant valvular disease, heart failure, or pulmonary hypertension undergoing noncardiac surgery.
5. Define myocardial injury after noncardiac surgery, describe its prognostic significance, and evaluate the arguments for and against routine troponin surveillance.
6. Apply pulmonary risk stratification, explain the physiology of perioperative atelectasis, and manage the patient with obstructive sleep apnoea.
7. Optimise and manage the perioperative course of patients with asthma and chronic obstructive pulmonary disease.

Chapter Overview

Chapter 5 established the method of preoperative consultation and argued that the consultant's product is a risk estimate and a management plan rather than a verdict. This chapter supplies the organ-specific content for the two systems that dominate perioperative morbidity and mortality.

Readers should approach the cardiac material with a particular caution in mind. Perioperative cardiology has an unusual evidential history. A substantial body of work that underpinned guideline recommendations for a decade, the DECREASE family of trials, was found to be scientifically unsound following investigation of its principal investigator, and guidelines on both sides of the Atlantic required revision as a result. Separately, the POISE trial produced a result that reversed prevailing practice, and the CARP trial showed that an intuitively appealing intervention conferred no benefit. The field is therefore one in which confident historical teaching has repeatedly proved wrong, and a degree of scepticism toward algorithmic certainty is warranted.

The pulmonary material has a different character. Postoperative pulmonary complications are at least as frequent as cardiac ones and contribute comparably to mortality and prolonged stay, yet they attract a fraction of the preoperative attention. Much of the useful intervention lies in intraoperative and immediate postoperative management rather than in preoperative testing, which means the consultant's contribution is largely a matter of communicating the right recommendations to the right people, as described in Chapter 5, section 5.6.2.

6.1 The Stepwise Cardiac Algorithm and Where It Breaks Down

6.1.1 The algorithm

Major guideline bodies present perioperative cardiac evaluation as a sequential algorithm. The versions differ in detail but share a structure, which is summarised here in the general form.

Step one: Is the surgery emergent? If the operation cannot be delayed without unacceptable harm, proceed. Perioperative surveillance and medical management are the only available interventions, and the assessment becomes a matter of anticipating and preparing for complications rather than preventing the operation.

Step two: Is there an acute coronary syndrome or other unstable cardiac condition? Acute coronary syndrome, decompensated heart failure, significant arrhythmia, and severe symptomatic valvular disease are conditions requiring evaluation and treatment in their own right, independent of the planned surgery. Elective surgery is deferred; urgent surgery proceeds with the condition managed concurrently.

Step three: Estimate the risk of a major adverse cardiac event. Using a validated index as described in Chapter 5, section 5.3, combined with the risk attaching to the specific procedure.

Step four: If the estimated risk is low, conventionally below one per cent, proceed to surgery without further cardiac testing. No further evaluation is indicated, and this step accounts for the majority of patients.

Step five: If the estimated risk is elevated, assess functional capacity. A patient with adequate functional capacity, conventionally four metabolic equivalents or more, proceeds to surgery without further testing regardless of the calculated risk.

Step six: If functional capacity is poor or unknown, ask whether further testing would change management. This is the pivotal question and it is frequently skipped.

Step seven: If testing would change management, perform pharmacological stress testing. If the result is abnormal, consider revascularisation or an alternative management strategy including a less invasive procedure, a modified anaesthetic plan, or no operation. **If testing would not change management**, proceed to surgery with medical optimisation and appropriate perioperative surveillance.

6.1.2 Where it breaks down

The algorithm is a reasonable organising structure and several of its joints are weaker than its presentation suggests. Hospitalists should know where.

The functional capacity step rests on unreliable measurement. Chapter 5, section 5.2.2, described the METS study finding that subjective clinician assessment of functional capacity agrees poorly with objective measurement and does not usefully predict postoperative myocardial injury or death. Step five is therefore a gate operated by an instrument that does not work reliably. This does not mean functional capacity is unimportant; it means it must be assessed rigorously rather than estimated, using specific recent activities, a structured instrument, or objective testing.

The "would it change management" question is usually answered wrongly. In practice, stress testing is ordered reflexively when functional capacity is poor, and the honest answer to step six is frequently that it would not change management, for the reason given below. Applying step six properly eliminates a large proportion of preoperative stress testing.

Prophylactic revascularisation before surgery does not improve outcomes. The Coronary Artery Revascularization Prophylaxis trial randomised patients with significant coronary disease undergoing major vascular surgery to preoperative revascularisation or medical management, and found no difference in mortality or perioperative myocardial infarction. This is the finding that hollows out step seven. If revascularisation performed because of a preoperative stress test does not improve outcomes, then the test that prompts it rarely changes management beneficially, and the chain from step six to step seven is broken in most patients.

The important exception is that revascularisation remains indicated where it would be indicated independent of the surgery, meaning for an acute coronary syndrome, for left main disease, or for symptoms refractory to medical therapy. The distinction is between revascularising because of the operation, which is not supported, and revascularising because the patient has an indication anyway, which is.

Revascularisation creates its own problem. A patient who receives a coronary stent before surgery now requires dual antiplatelet therapy and a delay of months, as described in section 6.2. The intervention intended to reduce perioperative risk has therefore either postponed the operation substantially or created a period of very high stent thrombosis risk. This consequence is frequently not considered before the stress test is ordered.

Part of the historical evidence base was unsound. The DECREASE trials, which reported large benefits from perioperative beta-blockade and other interventions and which heavily influenced guidelines in the 2000s, were the subject of institutional investigation concluding that the research was scientifically unsound. Recommendations resting on them were revised. Readers encountering older teaching or older guideline versions should be aware of this history, because a number of confident statements from that era have no remaining evidential support.

The algorithm is silent on the outcomes patients care about. It addresses cardiac events. It does not address delirium, functional decline, loss of independence, or the probability of returning home, which are frequently more important to the patient. Chapter 5, sections 5.3.4 and 5.6.3, addressed this.

6.1.3 A defensible practical approach

Given the above, the following approach is defensible and simpler than the formal algorithm.

Identify and treat unstable cardiac conditions on their own merits, independent of the planned operation.

Estimate risk formally, naming the index and the outcome, and combine it with an assessment of frailty.

Assess functional capacity rigorously rather than estimating it, using the methods in Chapter 5, section 5.2.3.

Order a stress test only when you can state, in advance, what an abnormal result will cause you to do differently, and when that action is one supported by evidence. In most patients the honest answer is that an abnormal result would lead to medical optimisation and surveillance, both of which can be instituted without the test.

Invest the effort saved in the things that do help: medication optimisation, volume status, anaemia correction, glycaemic management, delirium prevention, an explicit anaesthetic communication, and a plan for postoperative surveillance.

This last point deserves emphasis. The consultant's leverage in perioperative cardiac risk lies overwhelmingly in the postoperative period rather than in preoperative testing, and section 6.5 develops why.

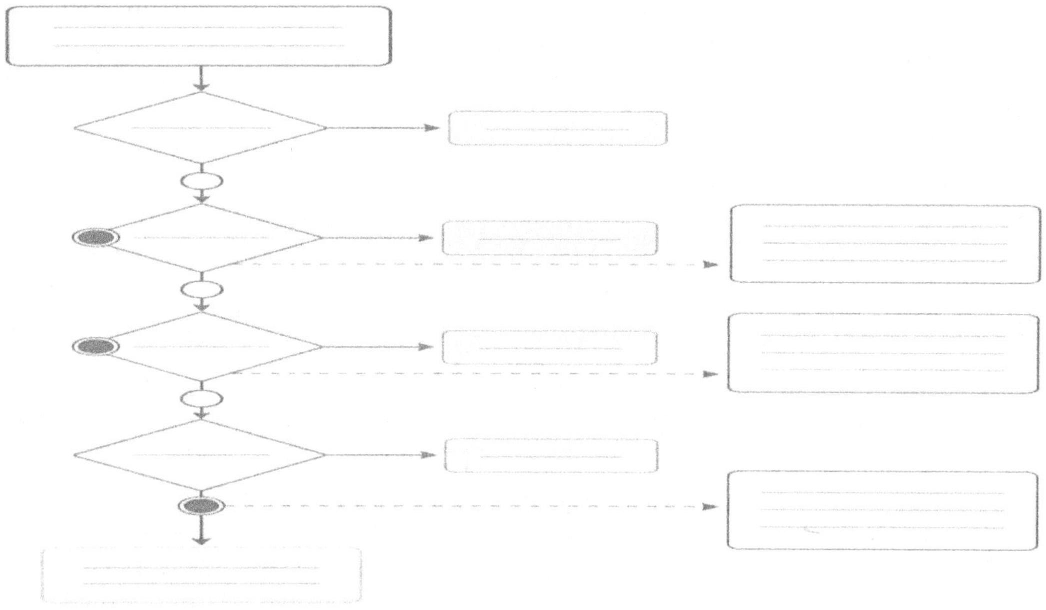

6.2 Coronary Stents, Dual Antiplatelet Therapy, and the Timing of Elective Surgery

6.2.1 The problem

A patient with a recently placed coronary stent presents a genuine dilemma with harm on both sides.

Stopping antiplatelet therapy risks stent thrombosis, which is a catastrophic event with a high mortality and a high rate of large myocardial infarction. Surgery compounds this risk independently, because the perioperative period is prothrombotic and proinflammatory.

Continuing antiplatelet therapy risks surgical bleeding, which varies enormously by procedure, from negligible in cataract or dermatological surgery to potentially fatal in intracranial or posterior chamber ocular surgery.

The risk of stent thrombosis is highest in the period immediately following implantation and declines with time as the stent endothelialises. The management question is therefore principally one of **timing**.

6.2.2 Recommended intervals for elective surgery

The following reflects the general position of major guidelines. Recommendations have changed as stent technology has improved and continue to evolve, so current guidance and the interventional cardiologist's specific advice should be sought.

Coronary intervention	Conventional minimum delay for elective noncardiac surgery
Balloon angioplasty without stent	At least 14 days
Bare metal stent	At least 30 days
Drug-eluting stent, elective surgery	Ideally at least 6 months
Drug-eluting stent, surgery that should not be delayed further	May be considered after 3 months, if the risk of further delay exceeds the risk of stent thrombosis
Stent placed for acute coronary syndrome	Longer intervals generally advised; individualised with cardiology

Contemporary drug-eluting stents have lower thrombosis rates than earlier generations, and the intervals have shortened accordingly over successive guideline versions. The direction of travel is toward shorter mandatory delays, and the specific stent type matters.

6.2.3 Managing antiplatelet therapy around the operation

Several principles apply.

Continue aspirin through surgery wherever the bleeding risk permits, particularly in patients with stents. This is standard practice for most procedures.

An important qualification arises from the POISE-2 trial, which randomised patients undergoing noncardiac surgery to aspirin or placebo and found no reduction in death or myocardial infarction with an increase in major bleeding. This result argues against initiating aspirin in patients not already taking it and against continuing it purely for cardiovascular prophylaxis in patients without a compelling indication. It does not apply straightforwardly to patients with recent coronary stents, who were largely excluded, and it should not be used to justify stopping aspirin in a patient with a stent.

Withhold the P2Y12 inhibitor for the shortest interval necessary, guided by the agent. Conventional preoperative intervals are approximately five to seven days for clopidogrel, five to seven days for ticagrelor, and seven days for prasugrel, though shorter intervals are increasingly used and local guidance should be followed.

Restart the P2Y12 inhibitor as soon as haemostasis permits, ideally within twenty-four to seventy-two hours. A loading dose may be appropriate and should be discussed with cardiology. This restart is among the most commonly forgotten steps in perioperative care and should be explicitly stated in the consultation note with a named responsible clinician, as described in Chapter 5, section 5.5.8.

Bridging with short-acting intravenous agents, such as a glycoprotein IIb/IIIa inhibitor or cangrelor, is used in some centres for very high-risk patients requiring interruption. The evidence base is limited, the protocols vary, and this should be a cardiology-directed decision rather than a hospitalist one.

Neuraxial anaesthesia has specific requirements regarding antiplatelet and anticoagulant timing because of the risk of spinal haematoma. These are the anaesthetist's domain, but the consultant should ensure the anaesthetist has complete and accurate information about every antithrombotic agent and its last dose.

6.2.4 Practical decision making

Three questions structure the decision.

Can the operation wait? If the indication is genuinely elective, waiting until the recommended interval has elapsed is almost always the correct answer, and the consultant should say so plainly. Much of the difficulty in this area arises from a reluctance to postpone an operation that has been scheduled.

If it cannot wait, what is the bleeding risk of this specific procedure? Procedures with low bleeding risk can generally proceed on full dual antiplatelet therapy. Procedures in closed spaces where bleeding is catastrophic require interruption regardless.

Who decides? This is a joint decision involving the surgeon, the anaesthetist, the interventional cardiologist, and the patient. The hospitalist's role is to convene it, to ensure the relevant information is in front of everyone, and to document the resulting plan explicitly. A perioperative antiplatelet plan agreed in a corridor and not written down will not be executed correctly.

6.2.5 The patient with a stent presenting for urgent surgery

When surgery cannot be delayed and the stent is recent, the plan should include the following elements, documented and communicated: continuation of aspirin if at all possible; the shortest feasible interruption of the P2Y12 inhibitor; availability of platelet transfusion and, where relevant, other haemostatic support; a defined restart plan with a named owner; postoperative troponin surveillance as described in section 6.5; and an explicit agreement with cardiology about what will happen if stent thrombosis occurs, including whether the patient would be a candidate for emergency catheterisation and how quickly that could be mobilised.

That last element is the one most often absent and the one that determines the outcome if the feared event occurs.

6.3 Perioperative Beta-Blockade, Statins, and the POISE Legacy

6.3.1 What POISE showed

The Perioperative Ischemic Evaluation trial randomised more than eight thousand patients undergoing noncardiac surgery to extended-release metoprolol, commenced two to four hours before the operation and continued for thirty days, or to placebo.

The results were internally consistent and consequential.

Beta-blockade reduced myocardial infarction. The mechanism is plausible: reduced heart rate reduces myocardial oxygen demand and lengthens diastolic filling time, which is exactly the physiology of demand ischaemia.

Beta-blockade increased death. All-cause mortality was higher in the treatment group.

Beta-blockade increased stroke, approximately doubling the rate, from a low baseline.

The mechanism of the harm was haemodynamic. Clinically significant hypotension and bradycardia were substantially more frequent in the treatment group, and the excess deaths and strokes were concentrated among patients experiencing these events. Sepsis and infection-related death were also more frequent, consistent with impaired haemodynamic response to a septic insult.

The interpretation that has endured is that the drug worked as intended physiologically and that the physiological effect, delivered at high dose in a fixed regimen to unselected patients starting on the day of surgery, caused net harm. A patient rendered hypotensive during an operation may avoid a myocardial infarction and sustain a stroke instead.

6.3.2 The DECREASE problem

The interpretation of POISE was complicated at the time by the DECREASE trials, which had reported large benefits from perioperative beta-blockade and which pulled meta-analytic estimates toward benefit. Following institutional investigation concluding that this body of work was scientifically unsound, subsequent analyses excluding it have found a picture consistent with POISE: a reduction in nonfatal myocardial infarction, an increase in stroke, and an increase in mortality or at best no mortality benefit.

The episode is worth remembering as a general lesson about evidence rather than only as a fact about beta-blockers. Chapter 2, section 2.6.3, addressed the failure modes of meta-analysis; the dominance of a pooled estimate by studies from a single group is one of them.

6.3.3 Current practice

Three positions follow, and they are stable across current guidelines.

Do not initiate beta-blockade on the day of surgery. This is the clearest and most important message from POISE. High-dose initiation immediately preoperatively is harmful.

Continue beta-blockers in patients already established on them. Abrupt withdrawal of chronic beta-blockade is associated with rebound tachycardia, ischaemia, and increased mortality. Chronic therapy should continue through the perioperative period, with attention to holding doses when the patient is hypotensive or bradycardic rather than administering them reflexively because they appear on the list.

If beta-blockade is being started for an independent indication, start it well in advance of surgery, at a low dose, and titrate to effect with monitoring of heart rate and blood pressure. Guidelines conventionally suggest an interval of at least several days and preferably longer, in order that tolerance and dosing are established before the physiological stress.

A practical corollary that applies on the ward: **the correct heart rate target is not the lowest achievable one.** Perioperative haemodynamic management aims to avoid both tachycardia and hypotension, and a patient with a heart rate of 50 and a mean arterial pressure of 55 is not being protected.

6.3.4 Statins

The position on statins is more favourable and less contested.

Continue statins in patients already taking them. This is a firm recommendation. Perioperative statin withdrawal is associated with worse outcomes, and there is no clinical reason to interrupt them for most surgery, including in patients who will be fasting, given the long duration of effect of most agents.

Initiation before surgery is supported by observational data and by mechanistic reasoning relating to plaque stabilisation and anti-inflammatory effects. The randomised evidence is weaker than the observational literature suggests, and several trials of perioperative initiation have not demonstrated benefit in their primary outcomes. Where a patient has an independent indication for a statin, meaning established atherosclerotic disease or a qualifying risk profile, initiating it preoperatively is reasonable and should be continued afterwards as a long-term therapy rather than as a perioperative intervention.

6.3.5 Renin-angiotensin system agents

Angiotensin converting enzyme inhibitors and angiotensin receptor blockers present a distinct problem. Continuing them through induction of anaesthesia is associated with increased intraoperative hypotension, sometimes refractory to conventional vasopressors, while withholding them risks postoperative hypertension and, in heart failure patients, loss of a disease-modifying therapy.

Observational and trial evidence has generally supported **withholding the morning dose before surgery**, particularly where the agent is prescribed for hypertension rather than for heart failure, and this has become common practice. The evidence is not uniform and practice varies.

Two practical points matter more than the specific decision. First, whichever course is chosen should be stated explicitly and communicated to the anaesthetist. Second, the agent must be **restarted** postoperatively once the patient is haemodynamically stable and renal function permits, and the restart must have a named owner. Chronic disease-modifying therapy silently discontinued during a surgical admission is a recognised and preventable harm.

6.3.6 Other agents in brief

Alpha-2 agonists. The POISE-2 trial also examined clonidine and found no reduction in death or myocardial infarction with increases in clinically important hypotension and nonfatal cardiac arrest. Routine perioperative clonidine is not recommended.

Calcium channel blockers, nitrates, and diuretics. Generally continued, with the usual attention to volume status and hypotension. Nitrates should not be started prophylactically.

Antiplatelet and anticoagulant agents are addressed in section 6.2 and in Chapter 7.

6.4 Valvular Disease, Heart Failure, and Pulmonary Hypertension

6.4.1 Aortic stenosis

Severe aortic stenosis is among the most important cardiac conditions in perioperative medicine because the physiology is unforgiving and because the management differs from most other cardiac disease.

The physiology. A fixed obstruction to left ventricular outflow means cardiac output cannot rise in response to vasodilation. The hypertrophied ventricle is stiff, dependent on atrial contribution to filling, and prone to subendocardial ischaemia. The consequence is that the patient tolerates hypotension, tachycardia, loss of sinus rhythm, and hypovolaemia poorly, and that a fall in systemic vascular resistance can produce a self-perpetuating spiral of hypotension, reduced coronary perfusion, and further ventricular dysfunction.

Assessment. Severity should be established by echocardiography if not already known and if the finding would alter management. Symptoms matter more than numbers: angina, syncope, and exertional dyspnoea in the presence of severe stenosis indicate a substantially worse prognosis and a different management pathway.

Management principles. For symptomatic severe aortic stenosis with elective surgery, valve intervention should generally be considered before the noncardiac operation, since the valve disease has an independent indication for treatment. Transcatheter approaches have made this feasible in many patients who previously would not have been surgical candidates, and have altered the calculus considerably.

Where surgery is urgent and cannot wait for valve intervention, it can proceed with careful attention to haemodynamics. The relevant instructions to the anaesthetic team are to maintain sinus rhythm, maintain preload, avoid tachycardia, avoid abrupt reductions in systemic vascular resistance, and treat hypotension promptly and with an appropriate agent. Invasive monitoring is frequently appropriate.

Balloon aortic valvuloplasty as a bridge has limited durability and a significant complication rate, and is reserved for selected circumstances rather than used routinely.

6.4.2 Mitral stenosis and regurgitant lesions

Mitral stenosis, now uncommon in many settings but persisting where rheumatic disease remains prevalent, is dominated by the requirement for adequate diastolic filling time. Tachycardia is poorly tolerated and atrial fibrillation with rapid ventricular response can precipitate pulmonary oedema. Rate control is the priority, together with attention to anticoagulation.

Regurgitant lesions, meaning aortic and mitral regurgitation, are generally better tolerated perioperatively than stenotic lesions, because afterload reduction improves forward flow. The principles are avoidance of bradycardia in aortic regurgitation, maintenance of a moderately reduced afterload, and attention to volume status. Severe regurgitation with ventricular dysfunction is nonetheless a significant risk factor and warrants echocardiographic assessment and cardiology involvement.

Prosthetic valves raise the question of anticoagulation interruption and bridging, which is addressed in Chapter 7. Mechanical mitral valves carry higher thrombotic risk than mechanical aortic valves and are managed more conservatively.

Endocarditis prophylaxis indications have narrowed considerably over successive guideline revisions and are now limited to defined high-risk cardiac conditions undergoing defined procedures, principally dental procedures involving manipulation of gingival tissue or the periapical region. Prophylaxis is not indicated for gastrointestinal or genitourinary procedures in the absence of established infection. Verify current local guidance.

6.4.3 Heart failure

Heart failure is among the strongest predictors of perioperative morbidity and mortality, and the distinction that matters most is between **compensated and decompensated** disease rather than between preserved and reduced ejection fraction.

Decompensated heart failure is a contraindication to elective surgery. A patient with orthopnoea, elevated venous pressure, worsening oedema, or a recent escalation of diuretic therapy should have the operation deferred and the decompensation treated. This is one of the clearest and least contested recommendations in perioperative medicine, and it is regularly overridden by scheduling pressure.

Assessment. Establish the current volume status clinically, establish the trajectory over recent weeks, review recent weights where available, and identify the precipitant of any recent deterioration. Echocardiography is indicated where the diagnosis is unclear, where there has been a change in clinical status, or where no recent study exists in a patient with significant disease. Routine repeat echocardiography in stable, well-characterised heart failure changes management rarely.

Optimisation. Achieve euvolaemia before the operation. Continue guideline-directed therapy with the specific exceptions discussed above regarding renin-angiotensin system agents on the morning of surgery, and noting that sodium-glucose cotransporter-2 inhibitors, now core heart failure therapy, require a defined preoperative withholding period because of euglycaemic ketoacidosis risk, as discussed in Chapter 5, section 5.5.5.

Perioperative principles. Patients with heart failure tolerate both hypovolaemia and fluid overload poorly, and the acceptable range is narrow. The anaesthetic and postoperative fluid plan should reflect this explicitly. Postoperative fluid administration is a common precipitant of decompensation, and a patient who received several litres of crystalloid intraoperatively will mobilise it on day two or three, which is when the pulmonary oedema appears.

6.4.4 Pulmonary hypertension

Pulmonary hypertension carries a high perioperative risk that is frequently underappreciated, with published series reporting substantial rates of morbidity and mortality even for procedures that would otherwise be considered low risk.

The physiology. The right ventricle is thin-walled and poorly adapted to acute increases in afterload. Anything that raises pulmonary vascular resistance, including hypoxia, hypercapnia, acidosis, pain, hypothermia, and certain anaesthetic manoeuvres, can precipitate right ventricular failure. Once the right ventricle fails, left ventricular filling falls, systemic pressure falls, right coronary perfusion falls, and the spiral is difficult to reverse.

Preoperative considerations. Establish the aetiology and severity, since pulmonary arterial hypertension differs substantially from pulmonary hypertension secondary to left heart disease or lung disease in both prognosis and management. Involve the specialist team managing the patient. Continue pulmonary vasodilator therapy without interruption; abrupt cessation of prostacyclin analogue infusions in particular can be fatal, and continuity of these infusions must be arranged explicitly rather than assumed.

Perioperative principles to communicate to the anaesthetic team. Avoid hypoxia and hypercapnia. Maintain sinus rhythm. Maintain systemic pressure and therefore right coronary perfusion. Consider regional rather than general anaesthesia where feasible. Anticipate that the postoperative period, particularly the first forty-eight hours, carries continuing risk and frequently warrants a higher level of monitored care than the procedure alone would suggest.

A specific caution. Patients with pulmonary hypertension undergoing minor procedures are the ones most likely to be harmed, precisely because the procedure appears trivial and the physiological risk is therefore not anticipated. The risk attaches to the patient rather than to the operation.

6.5 Postoperative Myocardial Injury: Detection and Meaning

6.5.1 The concept

Myocardial injury after noncardiac surgery, conventionally abbreviated MINS, describes myocardial injury of presumed ischaemic origin occurring within a defined period after an operation, detected by an elevated cardiac troponin, and prognostically important irrespective of whether it meets the formal criteria for myocardial infarction.

The concept emerged principally from the Vascular Events in Noncardiac Surgery Patients Cohort Evaluation studies, which measured troponin systematically in large numbers of patients after noncardiac surgery and correlated the results with outcomes. Three findings from that work reshaped the field.

Postoperative troponin elevation is common. A clinically meaningful proportion of patients over the age of 45 undergoing inpatient noncardiac surgery have a troponin elevation in the first days after operation.

It is strongly associated with mortality. Patients with postoperative troponin elevation have substantially higher thirty-day mortality than those without, and the risk rises with the magnitude of the elevation. The association is independent of whether the patient had symptoms.

Most of it is silent. The majority of patients with postoperative myocardial injury have no ischaemic symptoms at all. Chest pain is absent, obscured by analgesia, or attributed to the operation. This is the crucial practical point: an event with major prognostic significance is occurring in a substantial number of patients and is invisible unless it is looked for.

6.5.2 Mechanism and the type 1 versus type 2 distinction

Postoperative myocardial injury is heterogeneous, and the distinction between mechanisms matters for management.

Type 1 myocardial infarction results from acute atherothrombotic plaque rupture with thrombus formation. This is the classical mechanism and it does occur perioperatively, particularly in patients with unstable coronary disease and in the prothrombotic postoperative state.

Type 2 myocardial infarction and non-infarct injury result from a mismatch between myocardial oxygen supply and demand in the absence of acute plaque rupture. Perioperative contributors are numerous and frequently coexist: tachycardia, hypotension, anaemia, hypoxia, pain, catecholamine surge, sepsis, and hypovolaemia. This mechanism accounts for the majority of perioperative myocardial injury.

The distinction has direct management consequences. Type 1 injury may warrant antithrombotic intensification and consideration of coronary intervention. Type 2 injury is treated primarily by correcting the supply and demand imbalance: treating anaemia, controlling heart rate, correcting hypovolaemia and hypotension, managing pain, and treating infection. Reflexively applying an acute coronary syndrome pathway to a type 2 event may harm the patient, particularly through anticoagulation in a recently operated field.

Troponin elevation is not always ischaemic. Pulmonary embolism, sepsis, atrial fibrillation with rapid rates, renal failure, and myocarditis all raise troponin. The formal definition of myocardial injury after noncardiac surgery excludes elevations attributable to a clear non-ischaemic cause, and applying the label requires that judgement to be made rather than assumed.

6.5.3 The surveillance question

Whether to measure troponin routinely after noncardiac surgery in patients without symptoms is genuinely contested, and hospitalists should understand both positions because they will be asked.

The case for routine surveillance. The event is common, prognostically severe, and usually silent, so it will not be detected otherwise. Detection identifies a high-risk group who can be investigated for reversible contributors, managed medically, and followed more closely. The Canadian Cardiovascular Society guidelines recommend measurement of troponin daily for a defined period after surgery in patients meeting specified risk criteria, together with preoperative natriuretic peptide measurement to identify who should be screened. The MANAGE trial subsequently randomised patients with myocardial injury after noncardiac surgery to dabigatran or placebo and reported a reduction in major vascular complications, providing the first randomised evidence that the detected condition is treatable.

The case against routine surveillance. Detection of a marker does not by itself establish that acting on it improves outcomes, and much of the management triggered by a positive result consists of interventions of uncertain perioperative benefit. Screening generates investigation, anticoagulation and antiplatelet decisions in recently operated patients, prolonged stays, and patient anxiety. American guidance has historically been more cautious about routine screening in asymptomatic patients on the grounds that the actionability is unproven, though the position has softened as evidence has accumulated.

The practical position most hospitalists can defend: surveillance is reasonable and increasingly standard in patients at elevated risk undergoing surgery of at least intermediate risk, provided the institution has a defined pathway specifying what will be done with a positive result. Screening without a pathway generates harm through undirected investigation. If the answer to "what will I do differently?" is unclear, the reasoning in Chapter 2, section 2.7.2, applies here as it does everywhere.

6.5.4 Management of a detected elevation

A structured approach.

Establish whether this is ischaemic and, if so, which mechanism. Take a history for symptoms, obtain an electrocardiogram and compare it with the preoperative baseline, review the haemodynamic record for hypotension and tachycardia, check the haemoglobin, and consider pulmonary embolism, sepsis, and arrhythmia explicitly.

Correct the supply and demand imbalance, which is the highest-yield action in most cases: treat anaemia where significant, control heart rate, restore volume status and blood pressure, treat pain and hypoxia, and treat infection.

Consider antithrombotic therapy in the context of the surgical bleeding risk, in consultation with the surgical team. This decision requires an explicit weighing rather than a protocol, and the operating surgeon must be part of it.

Involve cardiology where the pattern suggests type 1 infarction, where there are dynamic electrocardiographic changes, where the patient is symptomatic or haemodynamically unstable, or where the elevation is large or rising steeply.

Reconsider the medication plan, including statin therapy and beta-blockade in patients with an established indication, noting the constraints in section 6.3.

Ensure the finding reaches the outpatient world. A patient with postoperative myocardial injury has been reclassified as having significant cardiovascular disease and warrants outpatient cardiovascular assessment and secondary prevention. This is precisely the sort of finding lost at discharge, and the requirements of Chapter 3, section 3.4.2, apply directly.

6.6 Pulmonary Risk Indices, Atelectasis Physiology, and Obstructive Sleep Apnoea

6.6.1 The scale of the problem

Postoperative pulmonary complications, encompassing atelectasis requiring intervention, pneumonia, respiratory failure, bronchospasm, and exacerbation of underlying lung disease, occur at rates comparable to or exceeding cardiac complications after major surgery, and carry comparable consequences for mortality, length of stay, and cost.

They receive substantially less preoperative attention, partly because there is no pulmonary equivalent of the coronary stress test to order, which is arguably an advantage rather than a deficiency, since it directs effort toward management rather than testing.

6.6.2 Risk factors

Patient factors with consistent evidence include advancing age, higher American Society of Anesthesiologists physical status class, functional dependence, chronic obstructive pulmonary disease, heart failure, current smoking, obstructive sleep apnoea, low serum albumin as a marker of nutritional status, anaemia, and recent respiratory infection.

Obesity, contrary to widespread assumption, is a weaker independent predictor of pulmonary complications than expected, though it interacts strongly with obstructive sleep apnoea and with positioning and mechanical factors.

Procedure factors are at least as important as patient factors and are frequently the dominant contributors: the surgical site, with upper abdominal, thoracic, and aortic procedures carrying the highest risk and the risk falling with increasing distance from the diaphragm; prolonged duration, conventionally beyond about three hours; emergency status; general rather than regional anaesthesia; and the use of long-acting neuromuscular blocking agents with inadequate reversal.

Risk indices exist, including the ARISCAT score, which combines age, preoperative oxygen saturation, recent respiratory infection, anaemia, surgical incision site, duration, and emergency status, and the NSQIP-derived calculators for postoperative respiratory failure and pneumonia. Their performance is comparable to cardiac indices, meaning useful for stratification and imperfect for individuals, and the same cautions from Chapter 5, section 5.3.1, apply.

6.6.3 The physiology of perioperative atelectasis

Understanding the mechanism explains why the interventions that work do work, and is worth the paragraph.

Functional residual capacity falls. Assuming the supine position reduces functional residual capacity substantially by cephalad displacement of the diaphragm and abdominal contents. General anaesthesia reduces it further through loss of inspiratory muscle tone and altered diaphragmatic configuration. The reduction begins within minutes of induction.

Closing capacity becomes relevant. Closing capacity, the lung volume at which small airways in dependent regions begin to close, rises with age and with lung disease. When functional residual capacity falls below closing capacity, dependent airways close during tidal breathing, and the alveoli they serve collapse. This is why age and obstructive disease amplify the effect: the two curves converge.

Three mechanisms of collapse operate. Compression atelectasis from the weight of the abdominal contents and the mediastinum on dependent lung. Absorption atelectasis, in which a region behind a closed airway has its gas absorbed into the blood, accelerated when the gas is a high concentration of oxygen because oxygen is absorbed far faster than nitrogen. And loss of surfactant function with prolonged low-volume ventilation.

The consequences. Collapsed but perfused lung produces shunt and hypoxaemia. Reduced clearance of secretions predisposes to infection. And reduced compliance increases the work of breathing at exactly the moment when pain, sedation, and abdominal splinting have reduced the patient's capacity to perform it.

Postoperatively the deficit persists. Functional residual capacity remains reduced for days after upper abdominal and thoracic surgery, and diaphragmatic dysfunction independent of pain contributes. This is why the risk period extends well beyond the operation and why postoperative management matters more than preoperative testing.

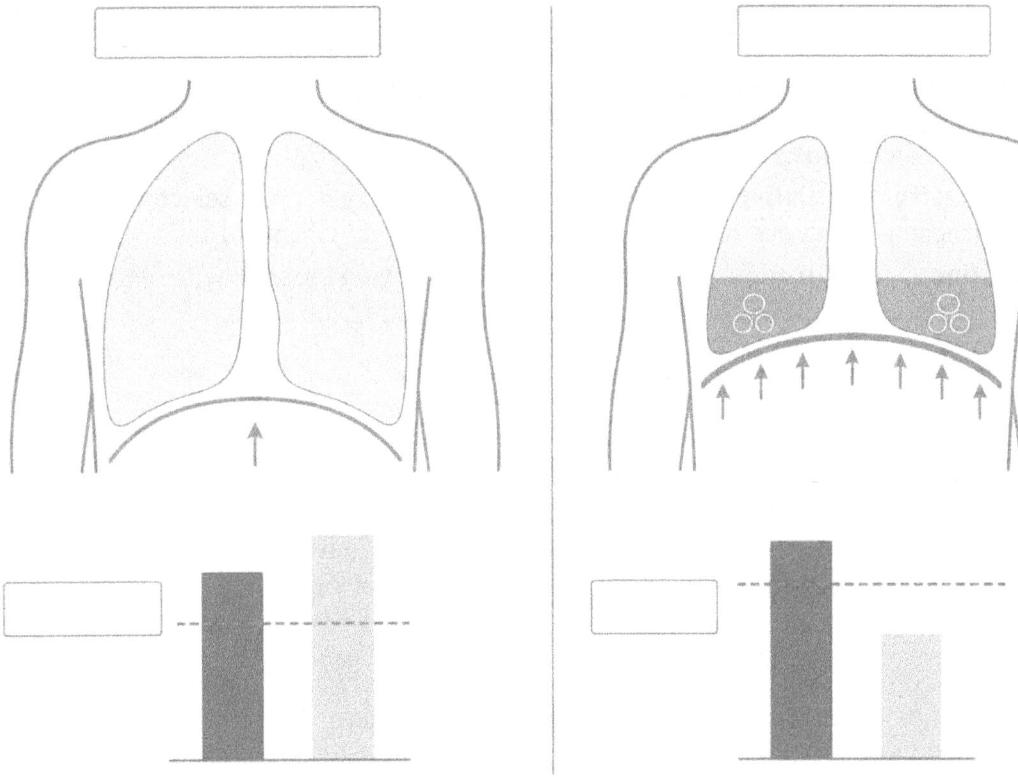

6.6.4 Interventions that reduce pulmonary complications

Intraoperative, meaning recommendations to communicate to the anaesthetic team rather than to implement directly. Lung-protective ventilation, combining lower tidal volumes calculated on predicted body weight with applied positive end-expiratory pressure and periodic recruitment manoeuvres, reduced postoperative pulmonary complications in randomised trials of abdominal surgery and is now widely adopted. Avoidance of excessive inspired oxygen concentration reduces absorption atelectasis. Complete reversal of neuromuscular blockade with objective monitoring reduces residual weakness and subsequent complications. Regional anaesthesia and regional analgesia, where feasible, reduce risk.

Postoperative, where the hospitalist has direct influence.

- **Early mobilisation** is the highest-yield intervention and the one most often deferred. Sitting out of bed and walking restore functional residual capacity mechanically.
- **Effective analgesia with opioid sparing.** Pain causes splinting, splinting causes atelectasis. Opioids cause hypoventilation and sedation, which also cause atelectasis. Multimodal and regional analgesia resolves the tension rather than trading one harm for the other, and is developed in Chapter 8.
- **Head-up positioning**, which is simple and consistently beneficial.
- **Lung expansion manoeuvres.** Incentive spirometry, deep breathing exercises, and positive expiratory pressure devices all aim at the same physiology. The evidence for incentive spirometry specifically as an isolated intervention is weak, and it is best regarded as one component of a programme that includes mobilisation and physiotherapy rather than as a substitute for them.
- **Oral care.** Structured oral hygiene reduces postoperative pneumonia in several studies, through reduction of the oropharyngeal bacterial load that is subsequently aspirated. It is cheap, safe, and consistently underused.
- **Noninvasive ventilation and high-flow nasal oxygen** for selected patients with established or threatened respiratory failure, addressed in Chapter 14.
- **Attention to aspiration risk**, including swallowing assessment where indicated, particularly in older adults and after procedures affecting the airway.

6.6.5 Obstructive sleep apnoea

Obstructive sleep apnoea is common, frequently undiagnosed, and associated with increased perioperative respiratory events, difficult airway management, and postoperative desaturation and arrhythmia. The interaction with opioids and sedatives is the central mechanism: agents that reduce pharyngeal tone and respiratory drive worsen an already compromised upper airway, and the effect is greatest during the rapid eye movement sleep rebound that occurs on the second and third postoperative nights.

Screening. The STOP-Bang questionnaire is the most widely used preoperative instrument, combining snoring, tiredness, observed apnoea, blood pressure, body mass index, age, neck circumference, and sex. It is highly sensitive and modestly specific, which is the correct trade-off for a screening tool intended to raise vigilance rather than to diagnose.

Preoperative management. Patients on established positive airway pressure therapy should be instructed to bring their device and to use it postoperatively, and this should be written explicitly in the orders rather than assumed. Patients screening positive without a diagnosis do not usually require formal sleep study before surgery unless the operation is elective, the interval permits, and the diagnosis would change perioperative management or the patient's long-term care.

Postoperative management. Minimise opioids and sedatives and use multimodal analgesia. Position the patient non-supine where feasible. Continue positive airway pressure therapy from the first postoperative night. Provide an appropriate level of monitoring, recognising that intermittent oximetry checks may miss significant events and that the risk period extends beyond the first night. Be cautious with supplemental oxygen without monitoring, since it can mask hypoventilation by maintaining saturation while carbon dioxide rises.

6.7 Perioperative Management of Asthma and Chronic Obstructive Pulmonary Disease

6.7.1 Asthma

The perioperative risk in asthma is dominated by **current control** rather than by the diagnosis itself. A patient with well-controlled asthma undergoing surgery has near-baseline risk; a patient with poorly controlled or recently exacerbated asthma has substantially elevated risk of intraoperative bronchospasm, laryngospasm, and postoperative respiratory complications.

Assessment focuses on control markers, not on the label. Ask about symptom frequency, night-time waking, rescue inhaler use, activity limitation, exacerbations in the preceding year, courses of oral corticosteroid, emergency attendance, and any previous intubation or critical care admission for asthma. Previous intubation for asthma is a marker of severe disease and should change the perioperative plan and the anaesthetist's preparation.

Timing. Elective surgery should be deferred during an exacerbation and for a period afterwards, since airway hyperreactivity persists beyond symptomatic recovery. A recent respiratory infection similarly increases risk and, for elective procedures, generally warrants postponement by a period of weeks.

Optimisation. Continue all inhaled therapy including the day of surgery. Ensure inhaler technique is adequate, which is frequently not the case and is checkable in a minute. Where control is inadequate and the operation is elective, escalate therapy and defer until control is achieved. A short course of oral corticosteroid before surgery is reasonable in patients with poor control and does not meaningfully impair wound healing at the doses and durations involved.

Perioperative specifics to communicate. Administer a bronchodilator before induction. Anticipate bronchospasm and have the plan for it agreed. Avoid known triggers, including certain drugs. In patients with aspirin-exacerbated respiratory disease, avoid aspirin and nonsteroidal anti-inflammatory agents, which is a significant constraint on multimodal analgesia and must be identified preoperatively rather than discovered afterwards. Patients on long-term systemic corticosteroids require consideration of perioperative supplementation, addressed in Chapter 7.

6.7.2 Chronic obstructive pulmonary disease

Chronic obstructive pulmonary disease is a consistent and important predictor of postoperative pulmonary complications, and the practical questions are what to assess and what can be improved.

No spirometric threshold contraindicates surgery. This point deserves emphasis because it is widely misunderstood. There is no forced expiratory volume value below which noncardiac surgery is prohibited. Spirometry does not add usefully to clinical assessment for risk stratification before non-thoracic surgery, and it should be reserved for lung resection planning and for cases where the diagnosis or the degree of reversibility is genuinely unclear and would change management.

What to assess instead: current symptom burden and its stability compared with baseline; exacerbation frequency, and specifically whether there has been one recently; current sputum volume, colour, and any change; oxygenation, including whether the patient uses long-term oxygen and whether they are a carbon dioxide retainer; functional capacity as in Chapter 5, section 5.2; and inhaler technique and adherence.

Optimisation. Treat any current exacerbation and defer elective surgery until recovery. Ensure the inhaled regimen is optimal and being taken correctly. Treat infection where present. Refer to pulmonary rehabilitation where the interval permits, since it improves functional capacity and is a component of prehabilitation as described in Chapter 5, section 5.5.7. Encourage and support smoking cessation, with the timing considerations from Chapter 5, section 5.5.3. Where sputum burden is significant, arrange chest physiotherapy preoperatively and ensure it continues postoperatively.

Perioperative principles. Regional anaesthesia and regional analgesia are preferable where feasible, since they avoid instrumentation of the airway and reduce systemic opioid requirement. Multimodal analgesia is important for the same reason. Bronchodilator therapy should continue throughout, including in the recovery area, and must be prescribed explicitly rather than assumed.

Oxygen therapy postoperatively requires specific care in patients with chronic hypercapnia. Uncontrolled high-flow oxygen in a carbon dioxide retainer can worsen hypercapnia through several mechanisms including reversal of hypoxic pulmonary vasoconstriction with increased dead space, the Haldane effect, and reduction of respiratory drive. Target saturation ranges should be specified in the orders for these patients rather than left to a default, and blood gas measurement should be used where hypercapnia is suspected. Chapter 14 develops this.

Noninvasive ventilation has a role in selected patients postoperatively, both therapeutically for hypercapnic respiratory failure and prophylactically in high-risk patients after major abdominal or thoracic surgery. The decision and the setting require respiratory or critical care input.

6.7.3 Two further points

The patient with undiagnosed obstructive disease. Preoperative assessment frequently uncovers a smoker with chronic productive cough and exertional limitation who has never been assessed. The correct response is to note it, optimise symptomatically for the operation, and ensure outpatient assessment is arranged afterwards, with the finding transmitted in the discharge summary. The operation is not usually the moment to complete the diagnostic workup, but the finding must not be lost.

Interstitial lung disease deserves brief mention because it is managed differently and carries high risk. These patients tolerate hypoxia poorly, may deteriorate acutely and unpredictably after surgery, and require specialist involvement. High inspired oxygen concentrations have been implicated in postoperative exacerbation in some series. Any patient with significant interstitial disease undergoing major surgery warrants respiratory specialist input rather than general perioperative management.

Chapter Summary

- The **stepwise cardiac algorithm** is a reasonable organising structure with weak joints. The functional capacity gate rests on unreliable measurement, the "would testing change management" question is usually answered wrongly, and prophylactic revascularisation before surgery does not improve outcomes, which breaks the link from stress test to action.
- **Order a stress test only when you can state in advance what an abnormal result will change**, and when that action is evidence-supported. Revascularise for an independent indication, not because of the operation.
- **Stent timing** governs antiplatelet management. Conventional minimum delays for elective surgery are 14 days after balloon angioplasty, 30 days after bare metal stent, and ideally 6 months after drug-eluting stent, with 3 months considered where further delay is harmful. Continue aspirin where bleeding risk permits, interrupt the P2Y12 inhibitor for the shortest feasible period, and name the person responsible for restarting it.
- **POISE** showed that beta-blockade started at high dose on the day of surgery reduces myocardial infarction while increasing death and stroke through hypotension and bradycardia. Do not initiate on the day of surgery; do continue chronic therapy; if starting for an independent indication, start early and titrate.
- **Continue statins.** Withhold the morning dose of renin-angiotensin system agents in most cases, and name the owner of the restart.
- **Severe aortic stenosis and pulmonary hypertension** are the valvular and vascular conditions least tolerant of perioperative haemodynamic disturbance, and the patient with pulmonary hypertension having a minor procedure is at particular risk precisely because the risk is not anticipated. **Decompensated heart failure is a contraindication to elective surgery.**
- **Myocardial injury after noncardiac surgery** is common, prognostically severe, and usually silent. Most is type 2, and the highest-yield management is correcting the supply and demand imbalance. Surveillance is reasonable in elevated-risk patients provided a defined response pathway exists.
- **Pulmonary complications** are at least as frequent as cardiac ones and receive far less attention. Procedure factors, particularly proximity to the diaphragm and duration, dominate. The physiology is a fall in functional residual capacity below closing capacity, and the interventions that work address that physiology: early mobilisation, opioid-sparing analgesia, head-up positioning, oral care, and lung-protective intraoperative ventilation.
- **Asthma risk is a function of current control, not of the diagnosis.** In chronic obstructive pulmonary disease, **no spirometric threshold contraindicates surgery**, and spirometry rarely adds to clinical assessment before non-thoracic operations.

Review Questions

1. A 68-year-old man with diabetes and prior stroke is scheduled for elective open aortic aneurysm repair. He cannot climb stairs because of knee osteoarthritis. Work through the stepwise algorithm, state where it breaks down for this patient, and state what you would actually do.
2. A patient received a drug-eluting stent seven weeks ago and now requires resection of a newly diagnosed colonic malignancy. Construct the antiplatelet and timing plan, state

who must be involved in the decision, and specify the five elements you would document.

3. A surgical resident proposes starting metoprolol on the morning of surgery in a patient with an elevated cardiac risk index who is not currently on a beta-blocker. Explain, with reference to trial evidence, why this is harmful and what you would recommend instead.
4. A troponin measured on the second postoperative day after hip fracture repair is elevated in an asymptomatic patient. Set out your diagnostic approach, the distinction you are trying to make, and the management that follows from each answer.
5. A patient with severe chronic obstructive pulmonary disease, chronic hypercapnia, and a recent exacerbation requires elective cholecystectomy. State what you would assess, what you would optimise, what you would communicate to the anaesthetist, and how you would write the postoperative oxygen orders.

CHAPTER 7: Perioperative Management of Complex Comorbidity

Learning Objectives

After studying this chapter, the reader should be able to:

1. Construct a perioperative glycaemic plan across the whole arc from the day before surgery to discharge, including specific handling of insulin, oral agents, and newer glucose-lowering drug classes.
2. Manage the patient with chronic kidney disease perioperatively, and appraise the contemporary evidence on contrast-associated kidney injury and its prevention.
3. Stratify operative risk in cirrhosis using validated instruments, and identify the circumstances in which the correct advice is not to operate.
4. Perform the risk-against-risk calculus governing anticoagulation interruption and bridging, and construct a specific interruption and resumption plan for warfarin and for direct oral anticoagulants.
5. Apply the principles of patient blood management, including preoperative anaemia correction, restrictive transfusion thresholds, and antifibrinolytic use.
6. Identify patients at risk of perioperative adrenal insufficiency and prescribe graded corticosteroid supplementation appropriate to the magnitude of surgery.
7. Manage antiplatelet, immunosuppressive, and biologic agents perioperatively, balancing disease flare against infection and impaired wound healing.

Chapter Overview

Chapters 5 and 6 established the method of preoperative consultation and the assessment of cardiac and pulmonary risk. This chapter addresses the comorbidities that most often complicate the perioperative course and that most often generate a request for medical input.

Two themes run through the chapter and are worth naming in advance.

The first is that **the drug plan is the deliverable.** In every section that follows, the consultant's most valuable output is a specific, drug-by-drug, timed instruction covering what happens before, on the day of, and after the operation, with a named owner for resumption. Chapter 5, section 5.5.8, made this point generally. This chapter supplies the content, and the recurring failure across all seven domains is the same: a medication stopped correctly and never restarted.

The second is that **several long-standing perioperative doctrines have been substantially revised by recent evidence**, and in each case the revision has been toward doing less. Bridging anticoagulation, high-dose corticosteroid stress regimens, liberal transfusion, and elaborate contrast nephropathy prophylaxis were all standard within recent memory and are now known to be unnecessary or harmful in most patients. Readers trained on older material should note where their practice may need updating, and readers trained recently should understand why senior colleagues may practise differently.

7.1 Diabetes and Hyperglycaemia: Insulin Strategies Across the Perioperative Arc

7.1.1 Why it matters and what the target is

Perioperative hyperglycaemia is associated with surgical site infection, delayed wound healing, prolonged stay, and mortality, and the association holds in patients without a prior diagnosis of diabetes as well as those with one. Surgery itself is hyperglycaemic: the catecholamine and cortisol response to tissue injury raises hepatic glucose output and induces insulin resistance, so a regimen adequate at home is frequently inadequate on the second postoperative day.

The target range in most guidance is approximately 6 to 10 millimoles per litre, roughly 110 to 180 milligrams per decilitre, with an acceptable upper extension to around 12 millimoles per litre in some settings. Two points about the target matter more than its precise boundaries.

Tight control is not the goal. Trials of intensive glycaemic control in critically ill and perioperative populations have demonstrated increased hypoglycaemia without consistent outcome benefit, and hypoglycaemia is itself associated with mortality. The aim is avoidance of both extremes.

Hypoglycaemia in the anaesthetised or sedated patient is undetectable clinically. This is the specific reason for caution intraoperatively and in the immediate recovery period, and it justifies a slightly higher target than would be accepted on the ward.

7.1.2 Preoperative assessment

Establish the type of diabetes, which determines everything that follows. **Type 1 diabetes requires basal insulin at all times**, and a patient with type 1 diabetes whose insulin is fully withheld while fasting will develop ketoacidosis. This is the single most important error to avoid in this section, and it is made regularly when a fasting patient's insulin is stopped by analogy with oral agents.

Establish the current regimen in full, including insulin types, doses, timing, pump use, and continuous glucose monitoring. Establish recent control, including a glycated haemoglobin measurement if not recent, and establish the frequency and awareness of hypoglycaemia, since impaired awareness changes the safety margin.

Where control is substantially outside target and the surgery is genuinely elective, deferral for optimisation is reasonable. The threshold at which delay produces net benefit is not well established, and various figures circulate without strong support. The defensible position is that the decision should weigh the magnitude of the derangement, the infection risk of the specific procedure, the achievable improvement in the available time, and the harm of delay, rather than applying a fixed cut-off.

Finally, **schedule the patient first on the operating list** where possible. This single logistical intervention shortens the fasting interval and prevents more perioperative glycaemic difficulty than most pharmacological adjustments.

7.1.3 Oral and non-insulin injectable agents

The general principle is that most non-insulin agents are withheld on the day of surgery, with two classes requiring longer and more specific handling.

Metformin. Withheld on the day of surgery in most protocols. The historical concern regarding lactic acidosis is now understood to be substantially overstated in patients with normal renal function, and some protocols permit continuation for short procedures with minimal fasting. Where renal impairment, significant contrast exposure, or a risk of perioperative acute kidney injury exists, withholding is appropriate, and it should not be resumed until renal function has been confirmed stable postoperatively.

Sulfonylureas and meglitinides. Withheld on the day of surgery because of hypoglycaemia risk during fasting. Sulfonylurea-induced hypoglycaemia can be prolonged, particularly with longer-acting agents and in renal impairment.

Dipeptidyl peptidase-4 inhibitors. Low hypoglycaemia risk and generally continued or withheld on the day according to local protocol; the decision is not consequential.

Sodium-glucose cotransporter-2 inhibitors. These require specific attention. They are associated with **euglycaemic diabetic ketoacidosis** in the perioperative period, in which ketoacidosis develops with glucose values that are normal or only mildly elevated, which delays recognition because the diagnosis is not considered. Regulatory and specialist guidance advises withholding these agents for a defined period before surgery, conventionally three to four days depending on the specific drug, and they should not be resumed until the patient is eating, euvolaemic, and not acidotic. Any perioperative patient on one of these agents who becomes unwell, nauseated, tachypnoeic, or acidotic should have ketones measured regardless of the glucose value. Chapter 17 addresses the management.

Glucagon-like peptide-1 receptor agonists. These delay gastric emptying, which raises concern about residual gastric contents and aspiration risk at induction. Initial anaesthetic guidance advised withholding daily agents on the day of surgery and weekly agents for a week beforehand. Subsequent multi-society guidance has moved toward a more individualised approach that weighs the risk of withholding against aspiration risk and incorporates gastric ultrasound and modified fasting in some pathways. This area has changed rapidly and current local anaesthetic department policy should be followed.

7.1.4 Insulin across the arc

The day before surgery. Continue the usual regimen. Some protocols reduce the evening basal dose modestly, commonly by around twenty per cent, in patients with tight control or a history of nocturnal hypoglycaemia.

The morning of surgery. Withhold short-acting and prandial insulin, since the patient is not eating. Continue basal insulin at a reduced dose, conventionally around sixty to eighty per cent of the usual dose, with the exact proportion depending on the agent, the degree of control, and the hypoglycaemia history. **Do not omit basal insulin entirely in type 1 diabetes.** Premixed preparations are generally withheld and replaced with a proportion of the basal component or with a variable rate intravenous infusion.

Intraoperatively and for prolonged fasting. A variable rate intravenous insulin infusion, with a substrate infusion providing glucose and appropriate potassium, is indicated for patients with type 1 diabetes undergoing anything other than a short procedure, for patients with poor preoperative control, for prolonged procedures, for those expected to miss more than one meal, and for emergency surgery. The infusion requires hourly glucose monitoring, defined adjustment rules, and attention to sodium and potassium.

The transition off the infusion is the most error-prone moment in this section. Subcutaneous basal insulin must be given before the infusion is stopped, with an overlap of a defined period, conventionally thirty to sixty minutes for rapid-acting analogues and longer for basal preparations. Stopping the infusion at the same moment the subcutaneous dose is given produces a gap in insulin coverage and, in type 1 diabetes, ketoacidosis. This transition should be written explicitly into the plan rather than left to the ward team to improvise.

Postoperatively. Resume a scheduled regimen as soon as the patient is eating. The evidence here is clear and frequently ignored: **basal-bolus regimens outperform sliding-scale correction alone** in hospitalised surgical patients, producing better control with comparable or lower hypoglycaemia. A correction scale is a supplement to a scheduled regimen, not a substitute for one. Chapter 17 develops inpatient glycaemic management in detail.

Anticipate that insulin requirements will be higher than baseline for several days because of surgical stress, corticosteroid administration where relevant, and reduced mobility, and will then fall as the stress response resolves and the patient begins eating normally. The fall is where hypoglycaemia occurs, and doses escalated on day two must be reviewed on day four.

Insulin pumps and continuous glucose monitors. Patients on pump therapy can generally continue basal delivery through short procedures with an agreed plan, and this requires prior discussion with the anaesthetist and the diabetes team rather than an improvised decision on the day. Continuous glucose monitors should not be relied upon for intraoperative or critical decisions, where capillary or blood gas measurement is preferred, and devices may need removal or shielding for certain imaging and diathermy.

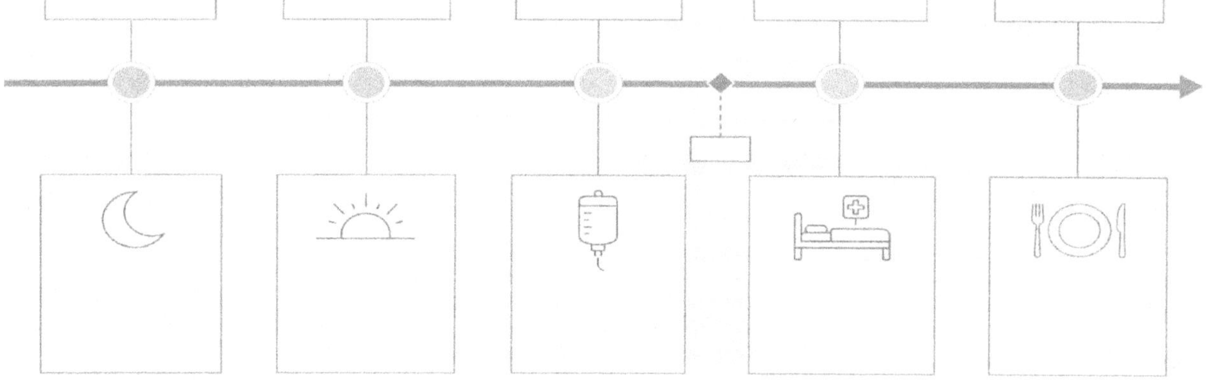

7.2 Chronic Kidney Disease and Contrast or Nephrotoxin Exposure

7.2.1 What chronic kidney disease changes

Chronic kidney disease alters perioperative management in several distinct ways, and listing them explicitly prevents the common error of treating it as a single risk factor rather than as a set of specific problems.

Drug handling. Dose adjustment is required for a long list of agents, including many antimicrobials, low molecular weight heparins, direct oral anticoagulants, opioids, and gabapentinoids. Morphine and codeine accumulate active metabolites in renal impairment and are poor choices; agents with less renally dependent clearance are preferred. Gabapentinoids accumulate and cause sedation and confusion, which is a frequent and avoidable cause of postoperative delirium.

Fluid and electrolyte handling. The margin between hypovolaemia and overload is narrow. Hyperkalaemia is a specific perioperative hazard, aggravated by tissue injury, transfusion of stored blood, acidosis, and drugs including renin-angiotensin system agents and potassium-sparing diuretics. A preoperative potassium should be checked in these patients and the threshold for delaying an elective procedure for significant hyperkalaemia is low.

Acid-base status. Metabolic acidosis reduces the buffering reserve available for the perioperative period.

Anaemia, which is common and multifactorial, and is addressed in section 7.5.

Platelet dysfunction. Uraemia impairs platelet function through mechanisms not reflected in the platelet count or conventional coagulation tests. Where clinically significant bleeding tendency exists, desmopressin has a role, as does correction of anaemia and, in some circumstances, dialysis.

Vascular access preservation. This is the item most often neglected by non-nephrologists and it has permanent consequences. In any patient with advanced chronic kidney disease who may require dialysis, the non-dominant arm veins should be preserved. Avoid venepuncture, cannulation, and peripherally inserted central catheters in that arm. Avoid subclavian venous catheters entirely where possible, since subclavian stenosis can render an entire arm unusable for fistula creation. In a patient with an existing fistula or graft, that arm must not be used for cannulation, venepuncture, or blood pressure measurement, and this should be written into the orders and signposted at the bedside.

7.2.2 The dialysis-dependent patient

Coordinate the operation with the dialysis schedule. Dialysis on the day before surgery is conventional, allowing correction of volume and electrolytes while avoiding the intravascular depletion, heparin exposure, and electrolyte shifts that follow immediately after a session.

Establish the dry weight and the residual urine output. Document the access type and location. Anticipate that potassium will rise postoperatively, particularly with tissue injury or transfusion, and plan the next dialysis session accordingly rather than waiting for a laboratory result to prompt it.

Peritoneal dialysis patients undergoing abdominal surgery require specific planning with nephrology, since the catheter and the peritoneum are directly involved.

7.2.3 Perioperative acute kidney injury

Acute kidney injury after surgery is common, associated with mortality and with progression to chronic kidney disease, and is substantially preventable. Chapter 16 develops the clinical management; the perioperative prevention points are as follows.

Avoid hypotension. Intraoperative and postoperative hypotension is among the strongest modifiable predictors of perioperative acute kidney injury, and the association is with both depth and duration. This is a matter for the anaesthetic team, and it is a legitimate item for the consultant to raise explicitly in a patient with pre-existing renal impairment.

Avoid nephrotoxins around the operation. Nonsteroidal anti-inflammatory drugs are the most commonly overlooked, and they are frequently prescribed as part of multimodal analgesia in exactly the patients who should not receive them. Aminoglycosides and vancomycin require dosing and monitoring attention. Renin-angiotensin system agents interact with intraoperative hypotension as discussed in Chapter 6, section 6.3.5.

Attend to volume. Both hypovolaemia and overload are harmful. Balanced crystalloids are preferred over high-chloride solutions, and hydroxyethyl starch preparations should not be used.

Avoid the assumption that a stable creatinine means stable function. Creatinine is insensitive to acute change and lags, particularly in patients with low muscle mass, in whom a normal value may conceal substantially reduced clearance.

7.2.4 Contrast-associated kidney injury: a revised picture

This topic requires specific treatment because the received teaching has been substantially revised and many clinicians still practise according to the older account.

The older account. Intravenous iodinated contrast was believed to cause acute kidney injury at a clinically significant rate, and elaborate prophylaxis was standard, including intravenous sodium bicarbonate, oral acetylcysteine, and prolonged hydration protocols, with contrast studies frequently avoided or delayed in patients with renal impairment.

What changed. Studies comparing patients receiving contrast with matched controls undergoing similar imaging without contrast found much smaller differences in renal outcomes than the uncontrolled literature had suggested, indicating that a substantial portion of the attributed injury reflected the underlying illness rather than the contrast. Randomised trials then examined the prophylactic interventions directly. The PRESERVE trial compared intravenous sodium bicarbonate with intravenous saline, and oral acetylcysteine with placebo, in patients with chronic kidney disease undergoing angiography, and found no benefit from either intervention on the primary outcome. The AMACING trial found no prophylaxis to be non-inferior to prophylactic hydration in high-risk patients.

The current position. The risk of contrast-associated kidney injury from modern low-osmolar and iso-osmolar agents is lower than previously believed, particularly for intravenous administration and in patients without severe renal impairment. Acetylcysteine and bicarbonate protocols are not supported. Intravenous isotonic fluid remains reasonable in patients with significant renal impairment receiving a substantial contrast load, particularly intra-arterially, though the magnitude of benefit is uncertain.

The clinical consequence that matters most is that a necessary contrast-enhanced study should not be withheld from a patient with renal impairment when the diagnostic information is important. Withholding a computed tomography study that would diagnose a treatable condition, in order to protect the kidneys from a risk that is smaller than believed, has caused substantial harm. The decision should be an explicit weighing of diagnostic value against renal risk, not a reflex.

Gadolinium carries a different concern, nephrogenic systemic fibrosis, which is associated with severe renal impairment. The risk with newer agent classes is very much lower than with the older agents that produced the original reports, and current guidance permits use in most patients with defined precautions. Verify current local radiology policy.

7.3 Cirrhosis, MELD, and the Decision Not to Operate

7.3.1 Why cirrhosis is different

Cirrhosis raises perioperative risk more steeply than almost any other chronic condition, and it does so through several simultaneous mechanisms rather than one.

Synthetic failure impairs production of coagulation factors, albumin, and complement. **Portal hypertension** produces varices, ascites, splenomegaly with thrombocytopenia, and a hyperdynamic circulation with low systemic vascular resistance that limits the response to further vasodilation. **Impaired drug metabolism** alters the handling of anaesthetic agents, sedatives, and analgesics. **Renal vulnerability** means that hypovolaemia, nephrotoxins, and sepsis precipitate hepatorenal physiology readily. **Encephalopathy risk** rises with sedation, opioids, gastrointestinal bleeding, infection, constipation, and electrolyte disturbance, all of which are common perioperatively. **Immune dysfunction** raises infection risk. And **sarcopenia and malnutrition** are near-universal in advanced disease and independently predict poor outcome.

Surgery adds hepatic ischaemia from anaesthesia-induced reductions in hepatic blood flow, which in a cirrhotic liver with already impaired reserve may precipitate decompensation.

7.3.2 Risk stratification

Three instruments are in common use.

The Child-Turcotte-Pugh classification grades severity using bilirubin, albumin, prothrombin time or international normalised ratio, ascites, and encephalopathy, producing classes A, B, and C. Older surgical series reported mortality for abdominal surgery rising steeply across the classes, with class C carrying prohibitive risk. The classification is simple and remains widely used, though it incorporates two subjective components and has coarse categories.

The Model for End-Stage Liver Disease, and its sodium-incorporating and updated variants, produces a continuous score from bilirubin, international normalised ratio, and creatinine, with sodium in later versions. It was derived for a different purpose, namely transplant allocation, but predicts postoperative mortality well. A widely cited derivation from Mayo Clinic data produced a postoperative mortality risk estimate incorporating the score, age, and physical status class, and the general relationship that emerged is that risk rises progressively with each point above a low threshold.

As broad orientation, scores below about 10 are associated with relatively acceptable operative risk, scores between about 10 and 15 with substantially elevated risk requiring careful weighing, and scores above about 15 with high risk for which elective surgery is usually inadvisable. These bands are approximate, vary with the operation, and should not be applied mechanically.

Newer procedure-specific instruments, including scores derived from large contemporary cohorts, offer better calibration than instruments repurposed from transplant allocation and incorporate the type of surgery explicitly. Where available, these are preferable, and readers should check for current validated options.

7.3.3 The operation matters as much as the score

Risk varies enormously by procedure in cirrhosis, more so than in most other conditions.

Highest risk procedures include open abdominal surgery, particularly hepatic resection, and cardiac surgery. Abdominal procedures disturb the portal circulation, are complicated by ascites and adhesions from prior decompensation, and carry high rates of wound complication and ascitic leak.

Intermediate risk includes many laparoscopic abdominal procedures, which are generally better tolerated than their open equivalents, and orthopaedic surgery.

Lower risk includes peripheral, superficial, and short procedures under regional or local anaesthesia.

The practical consequence is that the question is rarely whether the patient can have surgery in the abstract. It is whether this patient can have this operation, and whether a less invasive alternative exists.

7.3.4 When not to operate

Certain circumstances constitute contraindications to elective surgery, and the consultant should state them plainly.

- **Acute liver failure** or acute severe alcohol-associated hepatitis.
- **Child-Turcotte-Pugh class C disease**, or a very high Model for End-Stage Liver Disease score, for anything other than a life-saving procedure.
- **Acute decompensation**, including new or worsening ascites, encephalopathy, variceal bleeding, or spontaneous bacterial peritonitis, which should be treated and stabilised first.
- **Severe uncorrectable coagulopathy or profound thrombocytopenia** in the context of a high-bleeding-risk procedure.

- **Severe portal hypertension** with refractory ascites, where abdominal surgery carries very high rates of complication.

Chapter 5, section 5.6.5, addressed how to communicate this conclusion. The essential elements are to state it directly to the surgeon before it appears in the record, to give the reasoning, to include the patient in the conversation, and to identify whether a less invasive alternative or a palliative approach would serve the patient better.

7.3.5 Optimisation and perioperative management

Where surgery proceeds, several specific issues require attention.

Coagulopathy in cirrhosis is misunderstood. The prolonged international normalised ratio does not predict bleeding risk in cirrhosis, because the test measures only procoagulant factors while the disease reduces anticoagulant factors in parallel, producing a rebalanced but fragile haemostatic state. Patients with cirrhosis are at risk of both bleeding and thrombosis, including portal vein thrombosis and venous thromboembolism. The practical consequences are that **routine correction of the international normalised ratio with fresh frozen plasma before procedures is not indicated and causes volume overload and increased portal pressure**, and that thromboprophylaxis should not be withheld reflexively on the basis of a prolonged clotting time. Viscoelastic testing is used in some centres to guide product administration. Fibrinogen and platelet count carry more useful information than the international normalised ratio.

Ascites should be optimised preoperatively with diuretics and, where necessary, paracentesis with albumin replacement. Ascites raises the risk of wound dehiscence, hernia complications, and ascitic leak after abdominal surgery, and drainage plans should be agreed in advance.

Encephalopathy should be treated and its precipitants managed. Sedatives and opioids should be minimised and short-acting agents preferred. Constipation should be prevented actively, since it is a common and easily avoided postoperative precipitant.

Renal protection is critical. Avoid nonsteroidal anti-inflammatory drugs absolutely, avoid aminoglycosides, maintain volume, and treat infection promptly. Chapter 15 develops hepatorenal syndrome.

Nutrition should be assessed and supported, since sarcopenia predicts outcome independently and is potentially modifiable over a period of weeks.

Infection surveillance should be heightened, since cirrhotic patients present atypically and deteriorate rapidly. A low threshold for diagnostic paracentesis in any cirrhotic patient with ascites who becomes unwell postoperatively is appropriate.

7.4 Anticoagulation Interruption and Bridging: A Risk Against Risk Calculus

7.4.1 The structure of the decision

This is the classic perioperative problem in which both available actions cause harm, and the discipline is to quantify both rather than to default to one.

Interrupting anticoagulation exposes the patient to thromboembolism: stroke in atrial fibrillation, valve thrombosis and systemic embolism with mechanical valves, and recurrent venous thromboembolism.

Continuing or bridging anticoagulation exposes the patient to surgical bleeding, which ranges from trivial to fatal depending on the procedure.

The decision therefore requires two independent estimates: the patient's thromboembolic risk if anticoagulation is interrupted, and the bleeding risk of the specific procedure if it is not. These two axes generate the management plan.

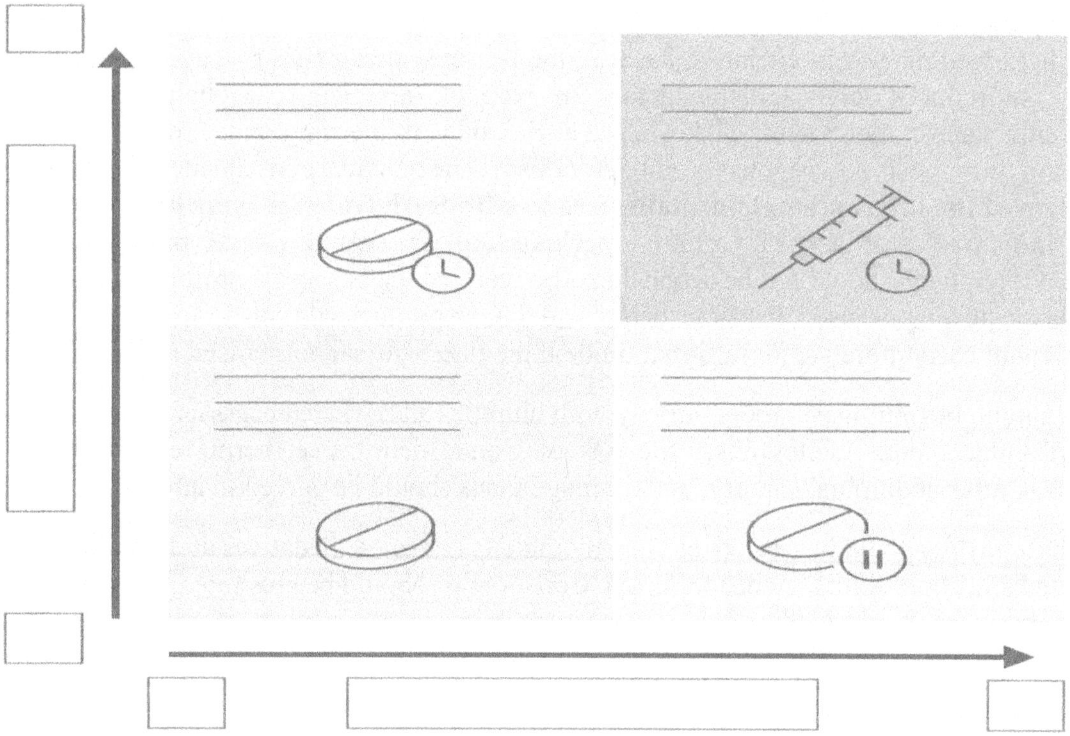

7.4.2 Estimating thromboembolic risk

Risk depends on the indication.

Atrial fibrillation. Stratified by a validated stroke risk score, with the highest-risk groups being those with very high scores and, particularly, those with a stroke or transient ischaemic attack within the preceding three months.

Mechanical heart valves. Risk depends on valve position, valve type, and additional factors. Mechanical mitral valves carry higher risk than mechanical aortic valves. Older valve designs carry higher risk than contemporary bileaflet valves. Additional atrial fibrillation, prior thromboembolism, or reduced ventricular function raise risk further.

Venous thromboembolism. Risk is dominated by recency. An event within the preceding three months represents the highest-risk category, and where possible elective surgery should be deferred beyond that window. Events between three and twelve months, and active malignancy or significant thrombophilia, constitute intermediate risk.

7.4.3 Estimating procedural bleeding risk

Procedures fall broadly into three groups, and the surgeon is the authority on which group applies.

Minimal bleeding risk, where anticoagulation can generally be continued: many dental procedures, cataract surgery, superficial dermatological procedures, and some endoscopic procedures without intervention.

Low to moderate bleeding risk, where interruption is appropriate but bleeding is manageable if it occurs.

High bleeding risk, including intracranial and spinal surgery, posterior chamber ocular surgery, major cardiac and vascular surgery, major abdominal and thoracic surgery, and any procedure in a closed space where haemostasis cannot be achieved by pressure. Neuraxial anaesthesia imposes its own timing requirements irrespective of the surgical bleeding risk.

7.4.4 Warfarin

Interruption. Warfarin is conventionally stopped approximately five days before surgery, allowing the international normalised ratio to fall. Measurement on the day before surgery permits administration of low-dose vitamin K if the value remains elevated.

Bridging. This is where practice has changed most.

The BRIDGE trial randomised patients with atrial fibrillation undergoing elective procedures to bridging with low molecular weight heparin or to no bridging. Forgoing bridging was non-inferior for arterial thromboembolism and produced significantly less major bleeding. The trial largely excluded patients at the very highest thromboembolic risk, so its result does not settle management for that group, but for the large majority of atrial fibrillation patients it established that bridging causes harm without benefit.

Subsequent evidence has extended similar reasoning to many patients with mechanical valves, though management there remains more conservative and more individualised.

The current position. Bridging should be reserved for a small population at genuinely high thromboembolic risk: mechanical mitral valves, older-generation mechanical valves, recent stroke or transient ischaemic attack, recent venous thromboembolism, and selected patients with severe thrombophilia. For most patients with atrial fibrillation and for many with contemporary mechanical aortic valves, bridging is not indicated.

Resumption. Warfarin is typically restarted within twenty-four hours of surgery once haemostasis is secure, recognising that therapeutic effect takes several days to re-establish, which is itself part of the risk calculation.

7.4.5 Direct oral anticoagulants

These are managed entirely differently from warfarin, and applying warfarin logic to them is a common error.

Do not bridge. Their rapid onset and offset make bridging unnecessary and harmful. Bridging a direct oral anticoagulant produces bleeding without benefit.

Interruption is based on the agent, renal function, and procedural bleeding risk. The PAUSE study evaluated a standardised interruption strategy without heparin bridging or perioperative coagulation testing, and found low rates of both bleeding and thromboembolism, providing a practical evidence-based schedule.

The general shape of that strategy is that factor Xa inhibitors are omitted for approximately one day before a low bleeding risk procedure and approximately two days before a high bleeding risk procedure, while dabigatran interruption is longer and is extended further in renal impairment because of its greater renal dependence. Precise intervals depend on the specific agent and creatinine clearance and must be taken from current guidance rather than memory.

Resumption is generally at approximately twenty-four hours after low bleeding risk procedures and forty-eight to seventy-two hours after high bleeding risk procedures. Because these agents achieve full anticoagulant effect within hours, resumption too early is a genuine bleeding hazard in a way that resumption of warfarin is not.

Routine preoperative coagulation testing is not required for these agents, and conventional tests do not reliably quantify their effect.

Reversal. Specific reversal agents exist for dabigatran and for the factor Xa inhibitors, and prothrombin complex concentrate is used where they are unavailable. Availability, cost, and local protocol vary substantially, and the consultant should know what is stocked in their institution before it is needed rather than discovering it during a haemorrhage.

7.4.6 Practical rules

Write the plan as a dated schedule, naming each day, each agent, each dose, and the person responsible for each step. A narrative instruction will not be executed reliably.

Confirm the procedural bleeding risk with the surgeon rather than assuming it. Surgeons and physicians frequently categorise the same operation differently.

Coordinate with the anaesthetist where neuraxial technique is contemplated, since the timing requirements are stricter than the surgical ones.

Name the person responsible for resumption, and state the criteria for it. Anticoagulation not restarted after discharge is a recognised and serious failure, and the discharge summary must carry the plan explicitly, as described in Chapter 3, section 3.4.2.

7.5 Anaemia, Transfusion Triggers, and Patient Blood Management

7.5.1 The three pillars

Patient blood management is a structured approach organised around three pillars, and the framing is useful because it directs attention away from the transfusion decision and toward the two interventions that precede it.

Pillar one: optimise the patient's own red cell mass. Detect and treat preoperative anaemia in advance of surgery.

Pillar two: minimise blood loss. Surgical technique, antifibrinolytics, cell salvage, management of anticoagulants and antiplatelets, and, on the ward, restraint in diagnostic phlebotomy.

Pillar three: optimise tolerance of anaemia. Restrictive transfusion thresholds, optimisation of oxygen delivery, and reduction of oxygen demand.

The single most important observation in this section is that **transfusion is the least good of the available options** and that the first two pillars are where outcomes are actually improved.

7.5.2 Preoperative anaemia

Preoperative anaemia is present in a substantial proportion of patients presenting for major surgery, is independently associated with postoperative morbidity, mortality, and prolonged stay, and is frequently detected only on the day of operation, when nothing can be done except transfuse.

Detection. Measure haemoglobin sufficiently far in advance of major surgery that correction is possible, conventionally several weeks. Chapter 5, section 5.5.2, addressed the timing constraint.

Investigation. Anaemia is a finding, not a diagnosis. Investigate the cause rather than treating empirically. Iron studies, including ferritin and transferrin saturation, are the first step, with the caveat that ferritin is an acute phase reactant and that a higher threshold applies in inflammatory states. Add vitamin B12, folate, renal function, and a reticulocyte count. In an older adult, iron deficiency anaemia requires investigation for occult gastrointestinal blood loss in its own right, and the finding may prove more consequential than the operation.

Treatment. Iron deficiency is the most common treatable cause. Intravenous iron corrects deficiency considerably faster than oral iron and is preferred where the interval to surgery is short, where oral iron is not tolerated, or where absorption is impaired by inflammation. Erythropoiesis-stimulating agents have a limited and specific role, principally in renal anaemia and in defined circumstances such as patients who decline transfusion, and carry thrombotic risk.

Iron deficiency without anaemia is also worth identifying before surgery with significant anticipated blood loss, since correcting it improves the reserve available.

7.5.3 Transfusion thresholds

The evidence supporting restrictive transfusion practice is among the more robust bodies of trial evidence in perioperative medicine, and it has consistently found that lower thresholds are non-inferior to higher ones across multiple populations.

The general position that has emerged:

A restrictive threshold of approximately 70 grams per litre is appropriate for most stable hospitalised patients without active bleeding or acute coronary syndrome.

A threshold of approximately 80 grams per litre is commonly applied in patients with pre-existing cardiovascular disease and in the postoperative surgical setting, including after orthopaedic surgery, where trial evidence specifically compared this threshold with a liberal one and found no difference in mortality or functional recovery.

Acute coronary syndrome is the population in which the picture is least settled. Trial evidence in patients with myocardial infarction and anaemia has been less clear-cut than in other populations, with some results favouring a more liberal approach on certain outcomes, and this remains an area of active discussion. Practice in this group should follow current cardiology guidance.

Active major haemorrhage is managed by a massive transfusion protocol rather than by a threshold, since the haemoglobin does not reflect the true deficit during ongoing bleeding. Chapter 17 addresses this.

Two operational rules follow from restrictive practice. **Transfuse a single unit and reassess** rather than prescribing two units by default; the practice reduces total transfusion substantially without harm. And **transfuse for a reason, not for a number**, meaning that a haemoglobin near the threshold in a comfortable, stable, asymptomatic patient does not itself require action.

7.5.4 Minimising blood loss

Tranexamic acid is one of the most cost-effective interventions in surgical medicine. It reduces bleeding and transfusion requirement across a wide range of surgical and traumatic settings, and large trials in trauma and obstetric haemorrhage have demonstrated mortality benefit when given early. Its use in elective surgery reduces bleeding and transfusion. Perioperative trial evidence has also examined the balance between reduced bleeding and thrombotic and seizure risk, and the general conclusion has been favourable, with attention required in patients with renal impairment, in whom dose adjustment applies, and with recognised dose-related seizure risk at high doses.

Cell salvage is appropriate for procedures with high anticipated blood loss and requires planning in advance.

Diagnostic phlebotomy is a significant and entirely avoidable cause of hospital-acquired anaemia, particularly in prolonged stays and in critical care. Chapter 2, section 2.7.3, addressed this. Ordering laboratory tests as single events tied to a question rather than as standing daily series is a patient blood management intervention as much as a stewardship one.

Anticoagulant and antiplatelet management is addressed in section 7.4 and in Chapter 6, section 6.2.

7.5.5 The patient who declines transfusion

Patients who decline blood products for religious or personal reasons require a specific plan established well before surgery, not discovered in theatre.

The essential elements: a clear, documented conversation establishing precisely which products and techniques are and are not acceptable, since positions vary between individuals and are not uniform; aggressive preoperative optimisation of haemoglobin, including intravenous iron and, where appropriate, erythropoiesis-stimulating agents; a surgical and anaesthetic plan that minimises blood loss, including antifibrinolytics and consideration of cell salvage where acceptable to the patient; involvement of any institutional bloodless medicine service; and, where the risk is substantial, an honest discussion of the consequences including the possibility of death from anaemia.

The patient's decision must be respected, and the consultant's role is to make refusal as safe as possible rather than to attempt to change it.

7.6 Adrenal Insufficiency and Perioperative Steroid Coverage

7.6.1 The physiology and the question

The adrenal response to surgical stress is a substantial increase in cortisol production, proportional to the magnitude of the operation and sustained for a period afterwards. A patient unable to mount this response may develop hypotension refractory to fluids and vasopressors, and in severe cases adrenal crisis.

Exogenous corticosteroid therapy suppresses the hypothalamic-pituitary-adrenal axis, and the degree and duration of suppression depend on dose, duration, and preparation. The perioperative question is therefore twofold: which patients are actually suppressed, and how much supplementation do they need.

Both parts of the question have been answered more conservatively over time. The historical practice of administering very large doses of hydrocortisone to any patient with recent corticosteroid exposure is now recognised as excessive and as carrying its own harms, including hyperglycaemia, impaired wound healing, and infection.

7.6.2 Who is at risk

The following is a widely used framework, and readers should recognise that the boundaries are approximate and that individual variation is considerable.

Almost certainly suppressed and requiring supplementation: patients with primary adrenal insufficiency or established secondary adrenal insufficiency, for whom this is not a matter of judgement; patients taking the equivalent of approximately 20 milligrams of prednisolone or more daily for three weeks or longer; and patients with clinical features of Cushing syndrome.

Almost certainly not suppressed: patients taking the equivalent of less than approximately 5 milligrams of prednisolone daily, for any duration; and patients who have received any dose for less than about three weeks.

Uncertain: the intermediate group, including doses between these thresholds, prolonged alternate-day therapy, and recent cessation of long-term therapy. Suppression may persist for months after stopping prolonged high-dose therapy.

Frequently overlooked routes. High-dose inhaled corticosteroids, potent topical preparations used over large areas, intra-articular injections, and intranasal preparations can all produce systemic suppression, and patients do not report them as steroids when asked about medications. Chapter 3, section 3.2.3, addressed this category of history-taking failure directly.

Testing. Where the situation is uncertain and time permits, an early morning cortisol measurement provides useful information, with very low values indicating insufficiency and clearly normal values making it unlikely. Intermediate values warrant dynamic testing with an adrenocorticotropic hormone stimulation test. Where testing is not feasible in the available time, covering empirically is reasonable, since the harm of unnecessary short-term supplementation is small.

7.6.3 Graded supplementation

The contemporary approach supplements in proportion to the surgical stress rather than administering a uniform high dose. The following reflects the general shape of current guidance; specific regimens vary and local endocrine protocols should be followed.

Continue the patient's usual daily corticosteroid dose throughout, converting to an intravenous equivalent while fasting. This is the foundation, and supplementation is additional to it rather than a replacement for it.

Minor procedures under local anaesthesia, including dental and superficial procedures, generally require the usual dose only, or a small single supplement.

Minor to moderate surgery generally warrants a modest supplement given at induction with a short continuation, in the region of 25 to 50 milligrams of hydrocortisone equivalent on the day, returning to the usual dose within a day.

Major surgery warrants a larger supplement, in the region of 100 milligrams of hydrocortisone in divided doses or by infusion over the first day, tapering over the following two to three days back to the usual dose as the patient recovers.

Three practical points. **Taper according to clinical progress rather than a fixed schedule**, extending supplementation if the patient develops complications, sepsis, or a return to theatre. **Anticipate hyperglycaemia** and adjust the diabetes plan accordingly, which connects directly to section 7.1. And **ensure the taper is completed and the usual dose resumed**, with the plan documented in the discharge summary, since a patient discharged on a supplementation dose that no one discontinues is a real occurrence.

7.6.4 Adrenal crisis

Every patient with established adrenal insufficiency undergoing surgery should have an explicit crisis plan, and every clinician managing them should recognise the presentation: hypotension disproportionate to the clinical situation and unresponsive to fluid and vasopressor, often with hyponatraemia, hyperkalaemia, hypoglycaemia, nausea, and abdominal pain.

Treatment is immediate intravenous hydrocortisone with fluid resuscitation, given on suspicion rather than after confirmation. Chapter 17 develops the management. The perioperative point is that the diagnosis is missed because it is not considered, and a patient known to have adrenal insufficiency should have this possibility flagged prominently in the handover and in the postoperative orders.

Etomidate deserves specific mention, since a single induction dose suppresses adrenal steroidogenesis for a period and should be used with awareness in patients with known or suspected insufficiency.

7.7 Antiplatelet, Immunosuppressive, and Biologic Agent Management

7.7.1 Antiplatelet agents outside the stent context

Chapter 6, section 6.2, addressed antiplatelet management in patients with coronary stents, which is the highest-stakes scenario. Several other situations recur.

Aspirin for primary prevention should generally be stopped before surgery and, in many cases, reconsidered entirely, since the balance of benefit and bleeding harm in primary prevention has shifted against routine use in recent guidance.

Aspirin for established atherosclerotic disease without recent stenting. The POISE-2 finding discussed in Chapter 6, section 6.2.3, argues against continuing it purely for perioperative cardiovascular protection. Decisions should weigh the specific indication, and continuation is appropriate for many patients with significant established disease undergoing procedures of low or moderate bleeding risk.

P2Y12 inhibitors for cerebrovascular or peripheral arterial disease. These are generally interrupted for procedures with meaningful bleeding risk, with the interval determined by the agent as described in Chapter 6, section 6.2.3, and resumed promptly.

Carotid and peripheral vascular surgery patients frequently have specific antiplatelet requirements determined by their vascular surgeon, and these should be confirmed rather than assumed.

7.7.2 Transplant immunosuppression

Solid organ transplant recipients undergoing unrelated surgery require particular care, and the governing principle is that **immunosuppression should not be interrupted**, since rejection is a more immediate and less recoverable harm than perioperative infection in most circumstances.

Practical elements: continue calcineurin inhibitors, antimetabolites, and corticosteroids without interruption, converting to intravenous equivalents while the patient is fasting, with dose conversion that differs by agent and requires pharmacy input. Monitor drug levels, since absorption, volume of distribution, and interactions all change perioperatively. Attend to nephrotoxicity, since calcineurin inhibitors are nephrotoxic and interact with perioperative hypotension and other nephrotoxins. Anticipate drug interactions, which are numerous and clinically significant, particularly with antimicrobials and antifungals. Provide corticosteroid supplementation per section 7.6. And **involve the transplant team early**, both for management advice and because they hold information about the graft that the surgical team does not.

7.7.3 Disease-modifying agents in rheumatic disease

This is a common and specific question, and reasonably clear guidance exists, principally from collaborative rheumatology and orthopaedic recommendations developed for elective joint arthroplasty and applied more broadly.

The competing considerations are that continuing immunosuppression raises infection and wound healing risk, while stopping it risks a disease flare that impairs rehabilitation and function, and flares are common and consequential.

The general shape of current recommendations:

Continue conventional synthetic agents through surgery, including methotrexate, leflunomide, hydroxychloroquine, sulfasalazine, and azathioprine. The evidence indicates that continuing methotrexate does not increase infection or wound complications and that stopping it precipitates flares. This represents a reversal of older practice and is worth stating explicitly.

Withhold biologic agents, timed to the dosing interval. The approach is to schedule surgery at the end of the dosing cycle for the specific agent, so that the trough coincides with the operation, rather than applying a uniform interval. Resumption is conventionally at approximately two weeks after surgery, once the wound shows evidence of healing and there is no sign of infection.

Withhold Janus kinase inhibitors for a short defined period before surgery, conventionally around three days, reflecting their short half-lives.

Rituximab requires longer planning because of its prolonged effect, with surgery ideally scheduled well into the dosing interval.

Severe systemic lupus erythematosus is handled differently, with continuation of therapy generally recommended because the risk of flare in severe organ-threatening disease outweighs the perioperative infection risk.

Corticosteroids in these patients raise the adrenal supplementation question in section 7.6, and long-term corticosteroid use is itself an independent risk factor for infection and wound complications.

7.7.4 Practical execution

Three points determine whether any of this is implemented correctly.

Write a dated schedule, agent by agent, covering the last dose before surgery and the planned resumption date and owner. This is the same instruction that closes section 7.4, and for the same reason.

Consult the prescribing specialist for biologics, transplant immunosuppression, and complex rheumatic regimens. These are not decisions a perioperative consultant should make unilaterally, and the specialist frequently has information about disease activity that changes the balance.

Ensure resumption actually happens. A biologic withheld before surgery and never restarted, because the rheumatologist assumed the hospital had restarted it and the hospital assumed the rheumatologist would, is a common and entirely preventable cause of disease flare weeks after an otherwise successful operation. The discharge summary must name the agent, the resumption date, the criteria, and the responsible clinician.

Chapter Summary

- **The drug plan is the deliverable.** Across every comorbidity in this chapter, the consultant's most valuable output is a dated, drug-by-drug schedule with a named owner for resumption. The recurring failure is a medication correctly stopped and never restarted.
- **Never fully withhold basal insulin in type 1 diabetes.** Withhold prandial insulin while fasting, reduce basal, and give subcutaneous basal insulin before stopping an intravenous

infusion with a defined overlap. Basal-bolus regimens outperform sliding-scale correction alone.

- **Sodium-glucose cotransporter-2 inhibitors** require several days of withholding and cause euglycaemic ketoacidosis, which is missed because the glucose is normal. Check ketones in any unwell perioperative patient taking one.
- In chronic kidney disease, **preserve the veins**, avoid subclavian access, avoid hypotension and nephrotoxins, and remember that nonsteroidal anti-inflammatory drugs are routinely prescribed to exactly the patients who should not have them.
- **Contrast-associated kidney injury has been substantially revised.** Acetylcysteine and bicarbonate protocols are not supported, and the risk from modern agents is lower than previously believed. A necessary contrast study should not be withheld from a patient with renal impairment when the diagnostic information matters.
- In cirrhosis, **the international normalised ratio does not predict bleeding**, routine plasma correction is not indicated, and thromboprophylaxis should not be withheld reflexively. Risk depends on the operation as much as on the score, and there are circumstances in which the correct advice is not to operate.
- **Bridging anticoagulation is harmful for most patients.** The BRIDGE trial established non-inferiority of no bridging in atrial fibrillation with less major bleeding. Reserve bridging for genuinely high thromboembolic risk. **Never bridge a direct oral anticoagulant.**
- **Patient blood management** places transfusion last. Detect and treat anaemia weeks in advance, minimise loss including diagnostic phlebotomy, use tranexamic acid, and transfuse restrictively, one unit at a time, for a reason rather than a number.
- **Perioperative corticosteroid supplementation should be graded to the magnitude of surgery**, added to the usual daily dose, and tapered by clinical progress. Historical high-dose regimens were excessive. Inhaled, topical, and injected preparations cause suppression and are not reported as steroids.
- **Continue methotrexate and other conventional synthetic agents** through surgery; **withhold biologics timed to the dosing cycle** and resume at around two weeks once healing is established; **do not interrupt transplant immunosuppression.**

Review Questions

1. A patient with type 1 diabetes on a basal-bolus regimen is scheduled for a four-hour bowel resection, second on the list. Write the complete glycaemic plan from the evening before to the second postoperative day, specifying each decision point.
2. A patient with an estimated glomerular filtration rate of 28 millilitres per minute requires urgent contrast-enhanced computed tomography for suspected mesenteric ischaemia. The surgical team wishes to avoid contrast because of renal risk. Set out your advice and the evidence supporting it.
3. A patient with cirrhosis has an international normalised ratio of 1.9 and a platelet count of 62 before an elective inguinal hernia repair. The surgeon requests correction with fresh frozen plasma. Explain why this is inappropriate and what you would recommend instead.

4. A 74-year-old with atrial fibrillation, a high stroke risk score, and no prior stroke is undergoing elective knee arthroplasty on apixaban. Construct the interruption and resumption schedule, and explain why bridging is not indicated.
5. A patient on 15 milligrams of prednisolone daily for eighteen months, plus adalimumab every two weeks and methotrexate weekly, requires elective hip arthroplasty. Set out your full perioperative plan for all three agents, including timing and resumption.

CHAPTER 8: Postoperative Complications: Recognition and Rescue

Learning Objectives

After studying this chapter, the reader should be able to:

1. Evaluate postoperative fever using a chronological framework, and explain why the traditional mnemonic and the attribution of fever to atelectasis are both unsupported.
2. Classify surgical site infection, recognise the features of a deep space collection and of necrotising infection, and describe evidence-based prevention.
3. Distinguish postoperative ileus from mechanical obstruction and from anastomotic leak, and recognise the early signs of leak before they become obvious.
4. Prevent, detect, and manage postoperative delirium, and describe what the evidence does and does not support regarding pharmacological approaches.
5. Apply venous thromboembolism prophylaxis appropriately after surgery, diagnose thromboembolism in the postoperative patient, and manage it when anticoagulation is hazardous.
6. Interpret the output and character of surgical drains and tubes, and apply the principle that every device requires an indication, an owner, and an exit criterion.
7. Construct a multimodal analgesic plan, practise opioid stewardship, and manage pain in the opioid-tolerant patient.

Chapter Overview

Chapters 5 through 7 concerned prediction and preparation. This chapter concerns what happens when preparation is insufficient, which is frequently.

Chapter 4, section 4.5, introduced the concept of failure to rescue: that hospitals differ less in the rate at which complications occur than in the rate at which patients die once a complication has occurred, and that the difference lies in detection, escalation, and response rather than in treatment. Postoperative care is the setting in which that concept applies most directly. Almost every complication in this chapter is treatable when recognised early and lethal when recognised late, and almost every failure follows the same shape: an abnormality attributed to the expected postoperative course until it is no longer possible to do so.

Three general principles run through the chapter.

The postoperative patient who is not progressing as expected has a complication until proven otherwise. Failure to progress is the single most useful signal available and the one most often explained away. Chapter 2, section 2.4.4, identified it as the most underused diagnostic signal in hospital medicine.

Tachycardia is the earliest and most reliable physiological sign of postoperative catastrophe, and it is routinely attributed to pain, anxiety, or fever. A persistently elevated heart rate in a postoperative patient deserves an explanation, not a rationalisation.

Go and look. The complications in this chapter are diagnosed at the bedside, by removing the dressing, examining the abdomen, inspecting the drain, and speaking to the patient. They are not diagnosed from the observation chart.

8.1 Postoperative Fever: A Chronological Approach

8.1.1 Two pieces of received teaching that are wrong

Most clinicians are taught a mnemonic for postoperative fever organised around the words wind, water, wound, walking, and wonder drugs, with each attributed to a particular postoperative day. It is memorable, it is widely taught, and as a diagnostic instrument it is poor.

Its two principal defects are worth stating.

The attribution of early fever to atelectasis is not supported by evidence. This is the most consequential error. Systematic examination of the literature has found no persuasive evidence that atelectasis causes fever. The association observed clinically arises because both atelectasis and fever are extremely common after surgery and both peak early, which is correlation rather than causation. The harm of the belief is specific and real: a genuine early fever gets attributed to atelectasis, incentive spirometry is prescribed, and the actual cause, which may be a developing necrotising soft tissue infection or an aspiration event, is not sought.

The day-based attributions are too rigid. Infections do not respect the schedule, and several important causes fall outside it entirely.

A chronological framework remains useful, because the differential genuinely does shift with time since operation. What must change is the content of each period and the recognition that the framework generates a prior, not a diagnosis.

8.1.2 The immediate period, within about 24 hours

Most fever in this window is not infection. Surgical tissue injury triggers release of inflammatory cytokines, including interleukin-6 and tumour necrosis factor, which act on the hypothalamus and produce fever proportional to the magnitude of the injury. This is a normal physiological response, it is self-limiting, and it requires no investigation in a patient who is otherwise well.

The important exceptions to look for:

- **Pre-existing infection**, present before the operation and not yet recognised or not yet controlled.
- **Malignant hyperthermia**, which is an anaesthetic emergency presenting with hyperthermia, rigidity, hypercapnia, and metabolic derangement, typically intraoperatively or in the immediate recovery period.
- **Transfusion reaction**, in patients who received blood products.
- **Drug reaction**, including neuroleptic malignant syndrome and serotonin syndrome where relevant agents were given.
- **Necrotising soft tissue infection**, which is rare but can begin within hours of surgery, particularly with group A streptococcal or clostridial organisms, and which is the reason

that an early fever with disproportionate wound pain requires inspection of the wound rather than reassurance.

8.1.3 The acute period, approximately days one to three

The differential broadens and infection becomes more likely, though a substantial proportion of fever in this window remains inflammatory.

Principal considerations: **pneumonia**, including aspiration, which is frequent after general anaesthesia and in patients with impaired swallowing or reduced consciousness; **urinary tract infection**, particularly with catheterisation, though with the caveats about asymptomatic bacteriuria in Chapter 18; **line-related infection**, including phlebitis at peripheral sites, which is frequently overlooked because peripheral cannulae are not inspected; **aspiration pneumonitis** as distinct from pneumonia; and **early necrotising infection**, as above.

Non-infectious causes in this window include venous thromboembolism, which can produce low-grade fever, and drug fever.

8.1.4 The subacute period, approximately days four to seven

This is the window in which the classic surgical infective complications appear, and in which the diagnostic effort should be most intense.

Surgical site infection typically declares itself in this period, addressed in section 8.2.

Anastomotic leak peaks in this window, addressed in section 8.3.5, and is the diagnosis that must not be missed.

Deep space collection or abscess may present here or later.

Catheter-related bloodstream infection, addressed in Chapter 18.

***Clostridioides difficile* infection**, particularly in patients who received perioperative antimicrobial prophylaxis.

Venous thromboembolism, which reaches a peak incidence around this period and later.

Drug fever, which characteristically appears after several days of a new agent, classically with beta-lactams and several other classes, and which is a diagnosis of exclusion but a real one. The patient with drug fever is often strikingly well despite a high temperature.

8.1.5 The delayed period, beyond about a week

Fever beginning or persisting beyond a week suggests a deep or contained process.

Principal considerations: **intra-abdominal or deep space abscess**; **anastomotic leak** presenting late or having been contained and then breaking down; **prosthetic or implant infection**; ***Clostridioides difficile***; **venous thromboembolism**; **drug fever**; and, in patients with prolonged stays, the accumulation of device-associated infections addressed in Chapter 4, section 4.4.4.

8.1.6 A practical approach

The following sequence is more useful than any mnemonic.

Establish whether the patient is well or unwell. This distinction, made at the bedside in thirty seconds, determines everything. A comfortable, mobile, eating patient with a temperature of 38.1 on the first postoperative day requires observation. A tachycardic, unwell, non-progressing patient with the same temperature on the fifth day requires urgent investigation regardless of how the fever is explained.

Take a history and examine, including the wound. Remove the dressing and look at it. Examine the abdomen. Inspect every line site, every drain, and both calves. Ask about swallowing, cough, urinary symptoms, and diarrhoea. This examination takes five minutes and answers most cases.

Review the medication list and the transfusion record. Chapter 3, section 3.2.1, made the case that the medication list frequently contains the diagnosis, and drug fever is a specific instance.

Review the operation. Know what was done, what was anastomosed, what was left in place, and what the surgeon was concerned about. This information is in the operation note and the surgeon's head, and the second source is usually better.

Investigate selectively rather than reflexively. The reflexive full septic screen, comprising blood cultures, urine culture, chest radiograph, and sputum culture on every febrile postoperative patient, is a poor use of testing and generates the cascades described in Chapter 2, section 2.7. Blood cultures are indicated where bacteraemia is plausible; urine culture where urinary symptoms or catheter-associated concern exists; and cross-sectional imaging where a deep collection or leak is suspected. In the well patient with early fever, the answer is frequently that no investigation is indicated at all.

Have a low threshold for cross-sectional imaging in the unwell patient after abdominal surgery. This is where diagnostic delay causes the most harm, and Chapter 7, section 7.2.4, addressed why renal concern should not prevent a necessary contrast study.

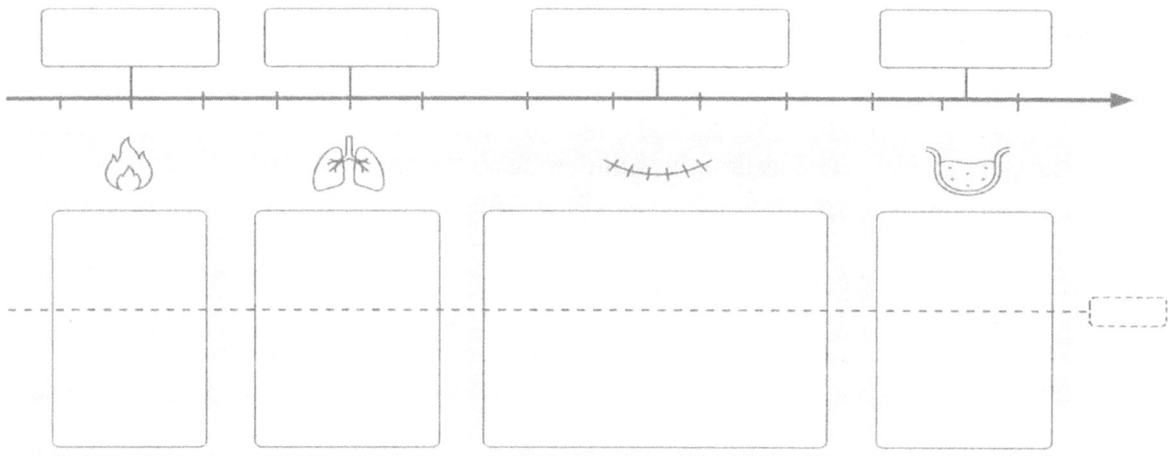

8.2 Surgical Site Infection and the Deep Space Collection

8.2.1 Classification

Surgical site infection is conventionally classified by depth, and the classification matters because management differs completely between categories.

Superficial incisional infection involves skin and subcutaneous tissue only.

Deep incisional infection involves fascia and muscle.

Organ or space infection involves any part of the anatomy opened or manipulated during the operation, including intra-abdominal abscess, empyema, and infection around an implant.

Surveillance definitions apply within a defined period after the operation, conventionally thirty days, extended to ninety days where an implant is placed. Practitioners should be aware that these definitions were designed for surveillance rather than for bedside diagnosis and are not always congruent with clinical judgement.

8.2.2 Prevention

Prevention is largely a matter of processes that occur before the hospitalist becomes involved, but several are within the consultant's influence and several represent common errors.

Antimicrobial prophylaxis timing. Prophylaxis should be administered so that adequate tissue concentrations are present at incision, conventionally within sixty minutes before incision for most agents and within one hundred and twenty minutes for agents requiring longer infusion. Administration after incision confers little benefit.

Redosing. For prolonged procedures or significant blood loss, intraoperative redosing at an interval based on the agent's half-life is required and is frequently omitted.

Weight-based dosing. Standard doses are inadequate in obesity, and underdosing is common.

Do not continue prophylaxis after wound closure. This is the recommendation most often violated. Current international guidance advises against continuing antimicrobial prophylaxis beyond the operation, including in the presence of a drain. Extended prophylaxis does not reduce infection and does cause resistance, *Clostridioides difficile*, and adverse drug events. A hospitalist consulted about a patient still receiving prophylactic antibiotics on the third postoperative day should raise it.

Normothermia during the operation reduces infection.

Glycaemic control, as addressed in Chapter 7, section 7.1.

Skin preparation with an alcohol-based chlorhexidine solution where not contraindicated, and **hair removal with clippers rather than razors**, or preferably not at all.

Smoking cessation, **nutritional optimisation**, and **anaemia correction**, as addressed in Chapter 5, section 5.5.

8.2.3 Recognising superficial and deep incisional infection

Superficial infection presents with local erythema, warmth, tenderness, induration, and discharge, typically in the subacute window. It is diagnosed clinically. The essential management is drainage: opening the wound where pus is present, which is the definitive treatment. Antibiotics alone will not resolve a collection, and this is the single most common error in wound management.

Distinguish infection from **normal postoperative inflammation**, which produces a narrow band of erythema at the incision without induration, systemic features, or discharge, and which is expected. Distinguish it also from **seroma**, **haematoma**, and **allergic contact dermatitis** from dressings or preparation solution, which is frequently misdiagnosed as cellulitis and presents with erythema in the exact distribution of the applied material.

Deep incisional infection produces more pain, more systemic disturbance, and frequently fascial involvement. It requires surgical assessment.

8.2.4 Necrotising soft tissue infection

This is the diagnosis that must not be missed, and it is missed regularly because the early appearance is unimpressive.

Features that should prompt immediate surgical involvement: pain markedly out of proportion to the visible findings; rapid progression over hours, particularly if the margin of erythema advances visibly; systemic toxicity disproportionate to the local appearance; skin changes including bullae, dusky discolouration, or anaesthesia of the overlying skin; crepitus; and a wound that drains thin, watery, malodorous fluid rather than frank pus.

Two practical points. Scoring systems intended to distinguish necrotising from non-necrotising infection have inadequate sensitivity to exclude the diagnosis and should not be used to reassure. And imaging should not delay surgical exploration when clinical suspicion is high; the diagnosis is made in theatre.

Management is emergency surgical debridement, broad-spectrum antimicrobial therapy including agents active against toxin production, and resuscitation. Chapter 18 develops the antimicrobial approach.

8.2.5 The deep space collection

Organ or space infection is the complication most likely to present as an unexplained failure to progress rather than as an obvious wound problem, and it is therefore the one requiring most active suspicion.

Presentation. Frequently non-specific. Persistent or recurrent fever. Tachycardia. Leucocytosis or a rising inflammatory marker. Ileus that does not resolve or recurs after resolving. Anorexia. New confusion, particularly in older adults. Diarrhoea, which can result from pelvic collection irritating the rectum and is often misattributed. Shoulder tip pain from subphrenic collection. And, most commonly, the patient who simply is not getting better and whose nurses report that something is wrong.

Diagnosis. Contrast-enhanced cross-sectional imaging is the investigation of choice. Ultrasound has a role in specific sites but is limited by bowel gas and by postoperative changes. Timing matters: imaging performed very early may be uninformative because a collection has not yet organised, and a negative early study in a patient who continues to deteriorate should be repeated rather than accepted.

Management. Source control is the priority and is achieved by percutaneous drainage where feasible or surgical drainage where not. Antimicrobial therapy is adjunctive. A collection that is not drained will not resolve on antibiotics, and prolonged antibiotic therapy in an undrained collection produces a partially treated, organism-selected abscess that is harder to manage subsequently.

The hospitalist's specific contribution in this situation is usually to be the person who insists that the failure to progress requires an explanation, and who arranges the imaging. Surgical teams under theatre commitments are frequently not at the bedside during the hours when the pattern becomes apparent, and the medical team is.

8.3 Ileus, Obstruction, and Anastomotic Leak

8.3.1 Normal postoperative gastrointestinal recovery

Motility does not return uniformly after abdominal surgery, and knowing the normal sequence prevents both premature alarm and delayed recognition.

Small bowel motility typically returns within several hours. Gastric emptying returns over approximately twenty-four to forty-eight hours. Colonic motility is slowest, typically returning over forty-eight to seventy-two hours, and the passage of flatus is therefore the conventional marker of recovery.

Postoperative ileus is the expected transient impairment of coordinated motility. It becomes **prolonged postoperative ileus**, and therefore a complication rather than an expected course, when it persists beyond the anticipated window, conventionally beyond about four days, or when it recurs after apparent resolution.

The physiology involves three overlapping mechanisms: a neurogenic phase mediated by sympathetic hyperactivity in response to surgical stimulation; an inflammatory phase driven by mediators released from the manipulated bowel wall, which is the dominant and most prolonged mechanism; and a pharmacological contribution from opioids acting on enteric mu receptors.

8.3.2 Preventing and managing ileus

The evidence-based measures are largely those bundled into enhanced recovery pathways, and the hospitalist can influence most of them.

Minimise opioids using the multimodal approach in section 8.7. This is the single most modifiable pharmacological contributor.

Avoid fluid overload. Excess intravenous crystalloid produces bowel wall oedema and demonstrably prolongs the return of function. Goal-directed rather than liberal fluid administration is standard in enhanced recovery protocols.

Mobilise early. The evidence that mobilisation itself accelerates motility is weaker than commonly assumed, but it addresses several other complications simultaneously and should be pursued regardless.

Feed early. Early oral intake after gastrointestinal surgery is safe in most circumstances and is associated with earlier return of function and shorter stay. Waiting for flatus before permitting oral intake is outdated practice in most enhanced recovery pathways.

Do not place a nasogastric tube routinely, discussed in section 8.6.3.

Correct electrolytes, particularly potassium and magnesium.

Consider a peripherally acting mu-opioid receptor antagonist where available and indicated, principally in bowel resection patients receiving opioids, where it has been shown to accelerate recovery of function.

Chewing gum has modest supporting evidence, is harmless, and is reasonable.

8.3.3 Distinguishing ileus from mechanical obstruction

This distinction matters because the management diverges.

Clinical features favouring mechanical obstruction: colicky rather than constant pain; high-pitched or hyperactive bowel sounds early, though this sign is unreliable; a period of normal bowel function followed by deterioration, which is the most useful clinical clue; and vomiting that is bilious or faeculent with abdominal distension proportionate to the level.

Clinical features favouring ileus: diffuse quiet abdomen, absent bowel sounds, gradual onset without an interval of normal function, and a temporal course consistent with the operation performed.

Imaging. Plain radiography is frequently equivocal and shows dilated loops in both conditions. Contrast-enhanced computed tomography is the investigation of choice and can identify a transition point, the level and cause of obstruction, and, critically, features of strangulation or a closed loop.

Early postoperative small bowel obstruction, occurring within the first weeks after abdominal surgery, is most often adhesive and frequently resolves with conservative management including nasogastric decompression and correction of fluids and electrolytes. The important exceptions requiring urgent operation are internal hernia, closed loop obstruction, and any features suggesting ischaemia: persistent tachycardia, localised tenderness, peritonism, rising lactate, acidosis, or leucocytosis with a left shift. Chapter 9 develops the assessment of acute abdominal pain.

8.3.4 The failure to progress as a diagnostic signal

Before addressing leak specifically, the general principle deserves separate statement because it is the organising idea of this chapter.

A patient who underwent an uncomplicated bowel operation and who, on the fourth or fifth day, has not passed flatus, is not eating, remains tachycardic, has a rising inflammatory marker, or simply seems unwell, has a complication. The most likely candidates are anastomotic leak and deep space collection. The management error is to interpret the picture as prolonged ileus, continue supportive care, and wait.

Prolonged ileus is a diagnosis of exclusion after leak has been considered and, where appropriate, investigated. Treating it as the default explanation is the mechanism by which most delayed leak diagnoses occur.

8.3.5 Anastomotic leak

Timing. Leaks characteristically declare between the fourth and eighth postoperative days, though they occur both earlier and considerably later, and late presentations after discharge are a recognised pattern.

Presentation is frequently subtle, and the classical picture of peritonitis is a late finding. The early signs, in approximate order of usefulness:

- **Tachycardia.** The earliest, most sensitive, and most consistently ignored sign. A persistent heart rate above about 100 in a postoperative bowel surgery patient requires an explanation and should not be attributed to pain without examining for alternatives.
- **New atrial fibrillation.** New arrhythmia after abdominal surgery is a recognised marker of intra-abdominal complication and should prompt evaluation for a septic source rather than being managed solely as a rhythm problem.
- **Failure to progress**, as above.
- **Ileus that fails to resolve or that recurs.**
- **A rising or non-falling inflammatory marker.** Serial C-reactive protein measurement after colorectal surgery has been studied specifically, and the pattern has a useful negative predictive value: a value that is falling appropriately by the third to fifth postoperative day makes leak unlikely, while a persistently elevated or rising value warrants investigation. This is one of the few situations in which a serial inflammatory marker earns its place.
- **Oliguria**, delirium, and unexplained hypotension, all of which reflect an evolving septic response.
- **Change in drain output**, discussed in section 8.6.2, including the appearance of enteric content or a rise in drain amylase.
- **The nursing report that the patient is not right**, which precedes the objective signs frequently enough to be treated as data.

Diagnosis. Contrast-enhanced computed tomography, with luminal contrast appropriate to the anastomosis, is the standard investigation. A negative study in a patient who continues to deteriorate does not exclude the diagnosis, and repeat imaging or surgical exploration should follow.

Management depends on the size of the leak, the degree of containment, and the patient's physiological state, and ranges from percutaneous drainage with antimicrobial therapy and bowel rest in a contained leak to urgent reoperation with diversion in a free leak with peritonitis. The decision is surgical. The hospitalist's contribution is early recognition, resuscitation, source control advocacy, and management of the septic physiology described in Chapter 18.

Risk factors worth noting because they raise the prior: low rectal anastomosis, emergency surgery, malnutrition, corticosteroid or biologic therapy, smoking, obesity, diabetes, intraoperative contamination, and anaemia or transfusion. Several were the subject of Chapter 7.

8.4 Postoperative Delirium and Neurocognitive Dysfunction

8.4.1 Scale and significance

Delirium is among the most common serious complications of surgery in older adults, with reported incidence varying widely by population and detection method and reaching high proportions after hip fracture repair and cardiac surgery.

It is not a benign or self-limiting inconvenience. Postoperative delirium is associated with increased mortality, longer stay, functional decline, institutionalisation, and persistent cognitive impairment. It is also distressing to patients, who frequently recall the experience, and to families.

Chapter 10 develops the pathophysiology, assessment, and management in detail. This section addresses the perioperative specifics.

8.4.2 Risk factors and prediction

Predisposing factors, present before the operation: advanced age; pre-existing cognitive impairment or dementia, which is the strongest single predictor and is frequently undiagnosed; frailty; sensory impairment, particularly uncorrected visual and hearing deficits; functional dependence; depression; alcohol use; polypharmacy, especially psychoactive agents; and prior delirium.

Precipitating factors, arising around the operation: the magnitude and duration of surgery; pain, particularly undertreated pain; medications including benzodiazepines, anticholinergics, and high opioid doses; sleep disruption; immobility and restraint; urinary catheters and other tethering devices; hypoxia; electrolyte disturbance; infection; anaemia; and constipation and urinary retention, which are unglamorous and common.

The relationship between the two categories is multiplicative rather than additive: a highly vulnerable patient develops delirium from a trivial precipitant, while a robust patient requires a major one.

Preoperative cognitive assessment should be routine in older surgical patients, both to identify risk and to establish the baseline against which postoperative change is measured. Chapter 5, section 5.5.7, made this point, and Chapter 3, section 3.7.4, addressed the general failure to document cognition.

8.4.3 Prevention

Multicomponent nonpharmacological prevention programmes have the strongest evidence in this area, with meta-analyses indicating meaningful reductions in incidence. The components are individually unremarkable and collectively effective.

- **Orientation and cognitive stimulation**, including visible clocks and calendars, and consistent staff where possible.
- **Sleep protection**, including clustering of overnight observations, reduction of noise and light, and avoidance of unnecessary nocturnal interventions. This requires institutional change rather than individual effort.
- **Early mobilisation** and avoidance of restraint.
- **Sensory optimisation**, ensuring glasses and hearing aids are available and used. This is trivially cheap and routinely omitted.
- **Hydration and nutrition.**
- **Adequate analgesia**, since undertreated pain is a potent precipitant. This is the point at which delirium prevention and opioid minimisation appear to conflict, and section 8.7 resolves the apparent conflict.
- **Avoidance of deliriogenic medications**, principally benzodiazepines and anticholinergics.
- **Removal of tethers**, including catheters, lines, and drains, as early as possible.
- **Bowel and bladder care**, including prevention of constipation and detection of urinary retention.

Anaesthetic factors. Trial evidence comparing regional with general anaesthesia for delirium prevention, particularly in hip fracture repair, has not demonstrated a clear advantage for regional technique, contrary to long-standing assumption. Evidence on processed electroencephalographic depth-of-anaesthesia monitoring has been mixed, with some trials suggesting benefit and others not. **Dexmedetomidine** has evidence for reducing delirium in some postoperative and critical care populations, and its use is an anaesthetic and intensive care decision.

Antipsychotics do not prevent delirium. Trials of prophylactic haloperidol and of atypical agents have not demonstrated reduced incidence, and they should not be used for this purpose.

8.4.4 Detection

Delirium is missed in a large proportion of cases, and the principal reason is that **hypoactive delirium is more common than hyperactive delirium and is quieter**. The withdrawn, drowsy, uncommunicative patient is not identified as delirious because they are not causing difficulty, and hypoactive delirium carries a worse prognosis than the hyperactive form.

Systematic screening with a validated instrument, applied at least daily in at-risk patients, is therefore necessary. Brief tools suitable for ward use include the 4AT and the Confusion Assessment Method, with an adapted version for intensive care settings. Screening should be performed by nursing staff as a routine observation rather than by a physician on suspicion.

Establish the baseline. Delirium is defined by acute change from baseline, and without a documented baseline the diagnosis cannot be made confidently. Family are the best source.

8.4.5 Management

Identify and treat precipitants. This is the treatment. Review medications, check for infection, hypoxia, electrolyte disturbance, pain, urinary retention, constipation, and alcohol or benzodiazepine withdrawal. New delirium in a postoperative patient should also prompt consideration of the surgical complications in sections 8.2, 8.3, and 8.5, since delirium may be the presenting feature of sepsis or of a leak.

Apply the nonpharmacological measures from section 8.4.3, which are as much treatment as prevention.

Pharmacological treatment is for severe agitation or distress that threatens safety, not for delirium itself. Antipsychotics have not been shown to shorten delirium duration or improve outcomes, and they carry risks including extrapyramidal effects, QT prolongation, and, in older adults with dementia, increased mortality. Where a drug is genuinely necessary because the patient is at risk of harm, the principle is the lowest effective dose of a single agent for the shortest possible period, with regular review for discontinuation.

Avoid benzodiazepines except for alcohol or sedative withdrawal, where they are the correct treatment, and for specific indications such as neuroleptic malignant syndrome.

Do not discharge a patient on an antipsychotic started for delirium without an explicit stopping plan communicated to the receiving clinician. This is a recognised source of long-term inappropriate prescribing, and it connects directly to Chapter 3, section 3.2.4.

8.4.6 Postoperative neurocognitive disorders

Beyond delirium, a broader spectrum of cognitive change is recognised after surgery, and the nomenclature has been revised to align with general psychiatric classification. The current framework distinguishes delirium occurring in the immediate period, delayed neurocognitive recovery within the first weeks, and postoperative neurocognitive disorder persisting beyond that, graded as mild or major.

Two practical points. The attribution of long-term cognitive decline specifically to anaesthesia has weakened considerably as studies have improved, and much of the observed decline reflects the underlying illness, the surgical insult, and pre-existing trajectory rather than the anaesthetic agent. And patients and families frequently ask about this, so hospitalists should be able to discuss it honestly: delirium is common and largely preventable, persistent cognitive change is less common, and the evidence implicating anaesthesia specifically is weaker than public perception suggests.

8.5 Venous Thromboembolism After Surgery: Prophylaxis, Diagnosis, and Treatment in the Bleeding Patient

8.5.1 Risk and prophylaxis

Surgery is a potent thrombotic stimulus, combining endothelial injury, immobility, and an acute phase prothrombotic state. Risk varies enormously by procedure and patient, and Chapter 4, section 4.4.3, argued against the blanket approach that a universal prophylaxis mandate encourages.

Risk stratification. Validated instruments exist for surgical populations, of which the Caprini score is the most widely used, combining patient factors, comorbidity, and the nature and duration of the procedure. As with all such instruments, discrimination is moderate and the value lies in structuring the assessment rather than in the precise output.

Highest-risk procedures include major orthopaedic surgery of the lower limb, major abdominal and pelvic surgery for malignancy, neurosurgery, major trauma, and spinal cord injury.

Pharmacological prophylaxis with low molecular weight heparin, or an alternative agent where indicated, is the mainstay. Timing relative to surgery and to neuraxial anaesthesia requires coordination with the anaesthetic team, and the intervals differ between agents and doses.

Mechanical prophylaxis with intermittent pneumatic compression is indicated where pharmacological prophylaxis is contraindicated by bleeding risk, and is used in combination in the highest-risk patients. Graduated compression stockings have a weaker evidence base and are contraindicated in significant peripheral arterial disease.

Extended prophylaxis beyond hospital discharge is indicated in defined populations, principally after major abdominal or pelvic surgery for cancer, where a period of approximately four weeks is conventional, and after major lower limb arthroplasty, where the duration is procedure-specific. Extended prophylaxis is frequently omitted at discharge, and the discharge summary must carry it explicitly with a named responsible clinician, as in Chapter 3, section 3.4.2.

Aspirin after arthroplasty has been used as an alternative to anticoagulant prophylaxis in some pathways. Trial evidence comparing aspirin with low molecular weight heparin after hip and knee arthroplasty has found aspirin inferior for symptomatic venous thromboembolism, and practice varies. Follow current orthopaedic guidance and local protocol.

The obligation to reassess. Prophylaxis prescribed on admission and never reviewed is a common failure. Bleeding risk changes, mobility changes, and the indication changes. A daily review of whether prophylaxis remains appropriate is the correct standard.

8.5.2 Diagnosis in the postoperative patient

Diagnosis is harder after surgery than in other settings, for three reasons that must be understood.

D-dimer is uninterpretable. It is elevated in essentially all postoperative patients as part of the normal response to tissue injury. A negative result retains some value in excluding disease if the pretest probability is genuinely low, but a positive result carries no information whatsoever. Applying the outpatient diagnostic algorithm from Chapter 2, section 2.3.5, to a postoperative patient is a specific and common error.

Clinical decision rules perform poorly, having been derived and validated in populations that largely excluded recent surgery.

The clinical picture is confounded. Leg swelling after lower limb surgery, dyspnoea after abdominal surgery, tachycardia after any surgery, and chest pain after thoracic surgery all have several explanations.

The practical consequence is to proceed directly to imaging when the diagnosis is suspected: compression ultrasound for suspected deep vein thrombosis, and computed tomographic pulmonary angiography for suspected pulmonary embolism, with ventilation-perfusion imaging as an alternative where contrast is contraindicated. The threshold for imaging should be lower than in other settings precisely because the clinical assessment is less reliable.

Consider the diagnosis in atypical presentations, including unexplained tachycardia, unexplained hypoxia, new atrial fibrillation, syncope, and unexplained fever. Chapter 14 develops the assessment and severity stratification of pulmonary embolism.

8.5.3 Treatment when anticoagulation is hazardous

This is the genuinely difficult scenario: a confirmed thromboembolism in a patient in whom full anticoagulation risks catastrophic bleeding, typically within days of major surgery, after neurosurgery, or with an active bleeding source.

The decision requires the same structure as Chapter 7, section 7.4: two independent estimates, of thrombotic consequence and of bleeding consequence, made explicitly rather than by default.

Assess the thrombotic stakes. A distal calf vein thrombosis in a mobile patient carries very different consequences from a large proximal thrombus or a pulmonary embolism with right ventricular strain. Not every thrombus requires immediate full anticoagulation.

Assess the bleeding stakes with the surgeon. The surgeon knows whether the operative field can tolerate anticoagulation, and this judgement cannot be made from the medical side alone.

Options along the spectrum:

- **Full therapeutic anticoagulation**, appropriate for most patients once an interval has elapsed and haemostasis is secure. The interval is shorter than clinicians often assume for most operations.
- **Delayed initiation**, with close surveillance and serial imaging, appropriate for a distal thrombus or a small subsegmental embolism where the immediate risk is low.
- **Reduced-intensity anticoagulation** as a temporising measure, though evidence for this is limited and it should be a documented deliberate choice rather than a drift.
- **Serial ultrasound surveillance** for isolated distal thrombosis, with treatment if propagation occurs.
- **Retrievable inferior vena cava filter**, for the specific circumstance of proximal deep vein thrombosis or pulmonary embolism with an absolute contraindication to anticoagulation. This warrants particular care: trial evidence has not demonstrated benefit from adding a filter to anticoagulation, filters carry complications including thrombosis, migration, and perforation, and retrieval rates in practice are poor. A filter placed must have a documented retrieval plan with a named owner and a date. An unretrieved filter is a lifelong complication generator.
- **Reperfusion therapy** for haemodynamically significant pulmonary embolism, where the calculus changes entirely because the alternative is death. Catheter-directed approaches may be preferable to systemic thrombolysis in the recently operated patient, and this requires urgent multidisciplinary input. Chapter 14 develops the decision.

Document the reasoning. This is a situation in which a decision under uncertainty is made and in which the next clinician must understand what was weighed. Chapter 2, section 2.6.5, addressed documentation of reasoning where evidence is absent.

8.6 Drains, Tubes, and the Physiology of Surgical Hardware

8.6.1 The governing principle

Chapter 4, section 4.4.4, stated it: the most effective prevention for any device-associated harm is not having the device. Applied to surgical hardware, the principle generates a simple daily discipline.

Every device on a postoperative patient must have three things: a stated indication, a named owner, and an exit criterion. If any of the three is missing, that is the finding, and the device should be questioned. A drain whose purpose no one can articulate, a catheter no one has reviewed, and a nasogastric tube placed on the first day and forgotten are all common and all harmful.

The hospitalist is frequently the person best placed to conduct this review, because they see the patient daily and are not the person who placed the device.

8.6.2 Surgical drains

Purposes. Drains are placed either **therapeutically**, to evacuate an existing collection, or **prophylactically**, to detect or evacuate an anticipated one. The evidence for the two purposes differs sharply.

Therapeutic drainage of an established collection is sound. Prophylactic drainage has been examined in several surgical fields and has frequently been found not to reduce complications, and in some settings to increase them, by providing a route for infection, causing tissue erosion, prolonging stay, and reducing mobility. Enhanced recovery pathways in several specialties have moved away from routine prophylactic drainage. The consequence for the hospitalist is that a prophylactic drain is a candidate for removal earlier than tradition suggests, and the question should be asked of the surgical team rather than assumed.

Monitoring output and character. This is where hospitalists add real value, because the change in drain fluid frequently precedes the clinical deterioration.

- **Volume trend.** A sudden increase, or a sudden decrease where output had been high, both warrant attention. The second is easily missed and may mean the drain has blocked or become displaced, not that the problem has resolved.
- **Blood.** Frank blood, or a fall in haemoglobin with serosanguinous output, suggests surgical bleeding.
- **Enteric content or faeculent material.** Anastomotic leak until proven otherwise.
- **Bile.** Biliary leak. Drain fluid bilirubin markedly exceeding serum bilirubin confirms it.
- **Amylase-rich fluid.** Pancreatic leak or fistula after pancreatic or upper gastrointestinal surgery. Drain fluid amylase measured on a defined postoperative day is standard practice after pancreatic resection and should be checked rather than assumed normal.
- **Milky fluid.** Chyle leak, confirmed by drain triglyceride content, and requiring specific nutritional management.
- **Clear fluid with high creatinine.** Urine leak, after urological or pelvic surgery.
- **Turbid or purulent fluid**, with or without odour, suggesting infection.

The general instruction is that **any change in the character of drain output requires the surgical team to be informed and the fluid to be tested rather than described.** Sending drain fluid for biochemistry costs almost nothing and answers the question definitively in several of the categories above.

8.6.3 Nasogastric tubes

Routine nasogastric decompression after abdominal surgery is not indicated. Meta-analyses have consistently found that routine placement delays return of bowel function, increases pulmonary complications, and increases patient discomfort without reducing anastomotic leak or other complications. It persists as practice in many settings through tradition.

Legitimate indications include established mechanical obstruction, symptomatic gastric distension with vomiting, and specific operations where the surgeon has a defined reason. A tube placed for one of these should have a defined criterion for removal.

A nasogastric tube is also a tether that impairs mobility, a source of discomfort that increases analgesic requirement, a contributor to sinusitis and aspiration, and a cause of nasal pressure injury, which is device-related pressure injury of the kind discussed in Chapter 4, section 4.4.2.

8.6.4 Chest drains

Hospitalists encounter chest drains after thoracic surgery and in medical contexts including pneumothorax and effusion.

The underwater seal system performs three functions: it permits air and fluid to leave the pleural space while preventing return; it provides a visual indication of pleural pressure through the movement of fluid in the water seal chamber, conventionally called swinging; and, where suction is applied, it regulates the level of suction independent of the wall source.

What to observe. Swinging with respiration indicates the drain is patent and communicating with the pleural space; loss of swinging means either the lung has re-expanded fully or the drain is blocked or displaced, and these must be distinguished. Bubbling in the water seal chamber during expiration or coughing indicates an air leak; continuous bubbling through the respiratory cycle suggests a large leak or a system leak, which should be excluded by checking connections. Output volume and character follow the same principles as section 8.6.2.

Practical cautions. Keep the system below the level of the patient. Do not clamp a bubbling drain, since this risks tension pneumothorax. Milking or stripping drains is generally discouraged because of the high negative pressures generated. And a drain that has stopped functioning should be assessed rather than removed on the assumption that it is no longer needed.

8.6.5 Other hardware

Urinary catheters should be removed at the earliest opportunity, for the reasons in Chapter 4, section 4.4.4, with attention to the risk of retention after pelvic surgery or neuraxial anaesthesia, which requires a defined post-removal monitoring plan rather than an assumption.

Central and peripheral vascular access should be reviewed daily for continued need and for site complications.

Epidural and regional catheters carry specific considerations, including timing relative to anticoagulation, monitoring for haematoma with any new neurological deficit or unexpected motor block, and infection surveillance. New back pain or lower limb weakness in a patient with an epidural catheter is an emergency requiring immediate imaging and anaesthetic involvement, and this must not be attributed to the block wearing off unevenly.

Implants and prostheses create a permanent susceptibility to infection, and any patient with an implant who develops bacteraemia requires specific consideration of seeding. Chapter 18 develops prosthetic infection.

8.7 Postoperative Pain, Opioid Stewardship, and Multimodal Analgesia

8.7.1 Why undertreated pain is a complication

Pain is not merely an experience to be minimised for comfort, though that alone would justify treating it. Undertreated postoperative pain has specific physiological consequences that appear elsewhere in this chapter.

It causes **splinting and reduced ventilation**, producing the atelectasis physiology described in Chapter 6, section 6.6.3. It causes **immobility**, contributing to thromboembolism, deconditioning, and pressure injury. It is a potent **precipitant of delirium**, as in section 8.4.2. It produces a **sustained catecholamine response** with tachycardia, hypertension, and increased myocardial oxygen demand, contributing to the type 2 injury described in Chapter 6, section 6.5.2. And severe acute postoperative pain is a risk factor for **chronic postsurgical pain**, which affects a meaningful minority of patients after several common operations and is difficult to treat once established.

The apparent tension between adequate analgesia and opioid minimisation is therefore false. Both are achieved by the same strategy, which is to use several agents with different mechanisms so that the opioid requirement falls without the analgesia failing.

8.7.2 The multimodal structure

Paracetamol should be prescribed regularly rather than as required for almost all postoperative patients, with dose adjustment for low body weight and hepatic impairment. It is the foundation and is frequently omitted or prescribed only as needed, which wastes its opioid-sparing effect.

Nonsteroidal anti-inflammatory drugs provide substantial opioid sparing and are underused because of contraindication anxiety. They are genuinely contraindicated or hazardous in significant renal impairment, active gastrointestinal bleeding risk, hypovolaemia, heart failure, and known aspirin-exacerbated respiratory disease. A long-standing concern regarding an association with anastomotic leak after colorectal surgery has produced variable practice and remains unresolved, and local surgical preference should be followed for those patients. Outside these situations, and particularly for short courses in patients with normal renal function, they are valuable.

Regional and neuraxial techniques provide the most effective analgesia for many operations with the least systemic drug exposure, and include epidural analgesia, peripheral nerve blocks, catheter techniques, and fascial plane blocks. Their availability depends on the anaesthetic service, and the consultant's role is to advocate for them in patients for whom systemic opioids are particularly hazardous, including those with obstructive sleep apnoea, significant respiratory disease, frailty, or opioid tolerance.

Local anaesthetic infiltration by the surgeon, wound catheters, and intravenous lidocaine infusion in selected settings.

Ketamine at low dose has an established opioid-sparing role, particularly in opioid-tolerant patients and after major surgery, and is generally an anaesthetic-directed intervention.

Dexamethasone, given as a single perioperative dose, provides analgesic benefit in addition to its antiemetic effect, with attention to glycaemic consequences as in Chapter 7, section 7.1.

Gabapentinoids deserve specific comment because practice is changing. Routine perioperative gabapentin and pregabalin were widely adopted on the basis of early opioid-sparing findings. Subsequent larger analyses have found the opioid-sparing effect to be small and of doubtful clinical significance, while sedation, dizziness, and, in older adults, delirium and respiratory depression in combination with opioids are meaningful harms. Several guidelines and reviews now advise against routine use. They retain a role in selected patients with a neuropathic pain component, and they should not be a default component of a postoperative order set.

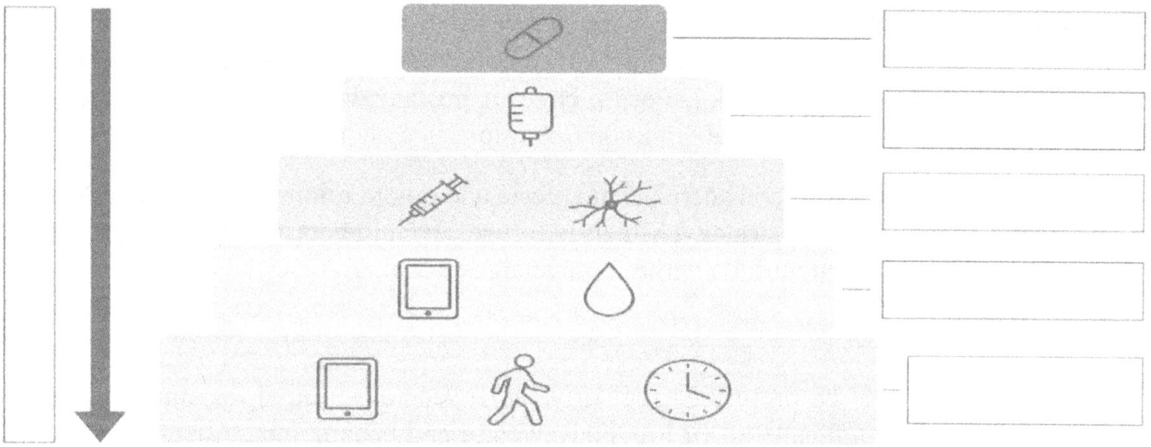

8.7.3 Opioid stewardship

Opioids remain necessary for many postoperative patients, and the aim is proportionate use rather than avoidance.

Principles for the inpatient period:

- Use the oral route where possible; reserve parenteral opioids for patients unable to take oral medication or with severe acute pain.
- Avoid long-acting and extended-release preparations in opioid-naive patients for acute postoperative pain.
- Avoid concurrent benzodiazepines, which substantially increase respiratory depression risk.

- Be cautious in obstructive sleep apnoea, obesity, older age, renal impairment, and respiratory disease, and ensure monitoring is proportionate.
- Reassess function rather than only a numerical score. The relevant questions are whether the patient can breathe deeply, cough, sit out, and mobilise, and a score-driven approach that escalates opioids toward a target number produces sedation without function.
- Prescribe an aperient with any opioid, since constipation is universal and itself causes complications.

Principles for discharge, which is where the greatest population-level harm arises:

- Prescribe the smallest quantity likely to be needed. Evidence consistently shows that a large proportion of postoperative opioid tablets dispensed are never used, and unused supplies are a major source of diversion.
- Set an expectation with the patient that opioids are for a short defined period and that pain will decrease.
- Provide a taper or stop plan explicitly.
- Continue the non-opioid components at discharge rather than discharging on opioids alone, which is a common and counterproductive pattern.
- Advise on safe storage and disposal.
- Communicate the plan to the primary care clinician, as in Chapter 3, section 3.4.2.

8.7.4 The opioid-tolerant patient

Patients on chronic opioid therapy, and patients with opioid use disorder, are systematically undertreated for acute postoperative pain, and the reasons are a mixture of dosing misconception and stigma.

Principles.

Continue the baseline requirement. A patient's usual opioid dose treats their chronic pain and prevents withdrawal; it provides no analgesia for the new surgical injury. Acute pain must be treated in addition to the baseline, not within it. Withholding or reducing the baseline dose perioperatively produces withdrawal, agitation, and worse pain.

Expect higher requirements, sometimes considerably higher, and involve an acute pain service where available.

Emphasise multimodal and regional techniques, which are more valuable in this population than in any other.

Do not attempt opioid tapering or detoxification during the perioperative period. It is the wrong setting and the wrong time, and it should be planned electively with the prescribing clinician.

Buprenorphine requires specific mention because guidance has changed. Historical practice was to discontinue buprenorphine before surgery on the assumption that it would block the effect of full agonists. Current guidance generally favours **continuing buprenorphine** through the perioperative period while adding full agonist opioids and multimodal analgesia as required, since discontinuation destabilises treatment of the underlying disorder, carries relapse and overdose risk, and is frequently unnecessary. Involve the prescriber and an addiction or acute pain service. Chapter 19 develops the management of opioid use disorder.

Methadone should be continued at the usual dose, with confirmation of the dose from the dispensing programme rather than from the patient's report alone, and with attention to QT interval and interactions.

Language matters. Chapter 1, section 1.7.2, described evidence that stigmatising documentation alters subsequent analgesic prescribing. This population is the one in which that effect is most consequential.

Chapter Summary

- **The postoperative patient who is not progressing has a complication until proven otherwise**, and **tachycardia is the earliest and most reliably ignored sign** of postoperative catastrophe.
- The traditional postoperative fever mnemonic is unreliable and **the attribution of fever to atelectasis is not supported by evidence.** Use a chronological framework as a prior, distinguish the well from the unwell patient at the bedside, examine the wound, and investigate selectively.
- **A collection will not resolve on antibiotics.** Superficial wound infection requires opening; deep space infection requires drainage. Necrotising infection is diagnosed clinically and in theatre, and scoring systems cannot exclude it.
- **Do not continue antimicrobial prophylaxis after wound closure**, including in the presence of a drain.
- **Prolonged ileus is a diagnosis of exclusion after leak has been considered.** Anastomotic leak declares between days four and eight, presents subtly, and shows itself first as tachycardia, new atrial fibrillation, failure to progress, and a non-falling inflammatory marker.
- **Postoperative delirium is largely preventable** by multicomponent nonpharmacological measures. Antipsychotics neither prevent it nor shorten it. Hypoactive delirium is commoner, worse, and missed. Establish and document the cognitive baseline preoperatively.
- **D-dimer is uninterpretable after surgery.** Proceed directly to imaging when thromboembolism is suspected, and lower the threshold because clinical assessment is less reliable. An inferior vena cava filter requires a documented retrieval plan with a named owner and a date.
- **Every device requires an indication, an owner, and an exit criterion.** Routine nasogastric decompression after abdominal surgery is harmful. Any change in drain output character should be tested biochemically rather than described.
- **Undertreated pain is a complication**, and the tension between analgesia and opioid minimisation is false. Build from regular paracetamol and appropriate nonsteroidal use, favour regional techniques, and treat opioids as the capping layer. Routine perioperative gabapentinoids are no longer recommended.
- **Continue the baseline opioid requirement in tolerant patients and treat acute pain in addition to it.** Current guidance favours continuing buprenorphine perioperatively rather than discontinuing it.

Review Questions

1. A patient is febrile to 38.4 degrees Celsius six hours after elective hip arthroplasty. She is comfortable, mobile, and eating. A colleague proposes blood cultures, urine culture, chest radiograph, and incentive spirometry. State what you would do instead and justify each departure.
2. On the fifth day after anterior resection, a patient has a heart rate of 108, has not passed flatus, is not eating, and has a C-reactive protein that has risen since day three. The surgical team attribute this to ileus. Set out your assessment, your differential, and the specific action you would take.
3. A 79-year-old is withdrawn, drowsy, and uncommunicative on the second day after hip fracture repair. Explain why this presentation is high risk, list the precipitants you would systematically exclude, and state what you would not prescribe.
4. A patient develops a proximal deep vein thrombosis on the third day after craniotomy. Construct your management approach, including who must be involved, the options along the spectrum, and what you would document.
5. A patient on 80 milligrams of methadone daily and buprenorphine is admitted for emergency laparotomy. Set out your complete analgesic plan, including what you would continue, what you would add, and the errors you would specifically avoid.

CHAPTER 9: Cardinal Symptoms at the Bedside

Learning Objectives

After studying this chapter, the reader should be able to:

1. Apply high-sensitivity troponin pathways to the assessment of chest pain, recognise the non-coronary causes that must be excluded, and make a defensible disposition decision.
2. Separate cardiac, pulmonary, metabolic, and neuromuscular causes of dyspnoea, and explain why a normal oxygen saturation does not exclude serious disease.
3. Assess acute abdominal pain in the medical inpatient, accounting for the blunted presentation that comorbidity, medication, and age produce.
4. Evaluate syncope with the objective of excluding a cardiac cause, and identify the investigations that are low yield and should be omitted.
5. Apply the timing and trigger framework to dizziness, use the HINTS examination correctly, and describe the circumstances in which it must not be applied.
6. Recognise generalised weakness and falls as sentinel presentations requiring a diagnosis rather than a label.
7. Use point-of-care ultrasound to answer defined binary questions, and describe its limitations and failure modes.

Chapter Overview

Part II concerned patients whose problem was already defined by an operation. Part III returns to the situation Chapter 1 identified as characteristic of hospital medicine: an undifferentiated patient, incomplete information, and a decision required before the picture is complete.

This chapter organises that work around seven presentations that account for a substantial proportion of medical admissions and of in-hospital deterioration. Each is treated as a reasoning problem rather than as a list of causes, following the structure established in Chapter 2. The recurring task in every section is the same: to construct a problem representation, to identify the small number of diagnoses whose omission would be catastrophic, and to decide what would need to be true for each to be present.

Three cross-cutting points deserve stating here rather than repeating in each section.

The presenting complaint is a starting point, not a category. "Chest pain" and "dizziness" are what the patient says; they are not diagnoses and they map poorly onto anatomy. Section 9.5 develops the clearest example of this failure.

Comorbidity blunts presentation. Older adults, diabetic patients, immunosuppressed patients, patients on corticosteroids or beta-blockers, and patients receiving analgesia all present atypically, and the atypicality is systematic rather than random. The consequence is that in exactly the populations at highest risk, the physical signs are least reliable.

Trajectory carries more information than any single assessment. A patient reassessed at two hours is more informative than a patient investigated more thoroughly at one hour, and Chapter 2, section 2.7.4, made the case for time as a diagnostic instrument.

9.1 Chest Pain: Risk Pathways, High-Sensitivity Troponin, and the Disposition Decision

9.1.1 Framing the problem

Chest pain assessment is usually taught as a question about acute coronary syndrome. That framing is incomplete in a way that causes harm, because several non-coronary conditions presenting with chest pain are more immediately lethal and are missed more often.

The correct framing has two parallel tracks that must be pursued simultaneously rather than sequentially.

Track one: is this an acute coronary syndrome, and what is the risk if it is not? This track is highly systematised, with validated pathways and a biomarker of remarkable performance.

Track two: is this one of the other conditions that will kill this patient today? Aortic dissection, pulmonary embolism, tension pneumothorax, oesophageal rupture, cardiac tamponade, and myocarditis all present with chest pain, and none is excluded by a normal troponin. This track is not systematised and depends entirely on the clinician remembering to pursue it.

The characteristic error is to run track one thoroughly, obtain a reassuring result, and never engage track two at all. Chapter 2, section 2.4.3, described the mechanism: an early plausible label is applied, and all subsequent data are interpreted as consistent with it.

9.1.2 High-sensitivity troponin

High-sensitivity assays detect troponin at concentrations far below the older generation, which changes the interpretation in three ways.

The reference value is a percentile, not a normal range. The conventional decision threshold is the ninety-ninth percentile of a healthy reference population, and **sex-specific thresholds** apply because the distribution differs between men and women. Using a single threshold underdiagnoses infarction in women, and this has been demonstrated repeatedly.

Detectable is not the same as elevated. Most healthy people have a measurable concentration. A result above the limit of detection but below the ninety-ninth percentile is normal.

The change over time carries more information than the single value. A rising or falling pattern indicates acute myocardial injury; a stable elevation suggests a chronic cause, and chronic elevation is common in renal impairment, heart failure, structural heart disease, and older age. The delta between two samples is therefore the key measurement, and its interpretation depends on the specific assay.

Rapid rule-out and rule-in algorithms using samples at presentation and at one, two, or three hours have been validated extensively and permit safe discharge of a large proportion of patients within a short interval. Some pathways permit a single-sample rule-out where the initial concentration is below the assay's limit of detection, the electrocardiogram is non-ischaemic, and symptoms have been present for a sufficient period. The specific thresholds and intervals are assay-dependent and must be taken from the local pathway rather than from memory or from a paper describing a different assay.

A critical limitation for hospitalists. These pathways were derived and validated in emergency department populations presenting with chest pain. Their performance in an already-admitted inpatient who develops chest pain, in whom the pretest probability, the competing causes, and the baseline troponin all differ, is not established. Applying an emergency department rule-out pathway to a hospitalised patient on the third day of an admission for sepsis is an extrapolation, and Chapter 6, section 6.5, addressed the related problem of perioperative troponin elevation.

9.1.3 Risk stratification instruments

Several validated instruments combine history, risk factors, electrocardiogram, and troponin to stratify risk. The HEART score is the most widely used and, when combined with serial troponin in a defined pathway, identifies a low-risk group with a very low rate of major adverse cardiac events at thirty days. Others in use include emergency department assessment scores derived in different populations.

Two practical points. The history component of these instruments carries substantial weight and is subjective, which introduces variability. And a low score is a statement about a population rate, not a guarantee about an individual, which is the general limitation of all such instruments discussed in Chapter 5, section 5.3.1.

9.1.4 The non-coronary causes

Aortic dissection. The diagnosis most often missed and the one with the steepest time-dependent mortality. Features raising suspicion: pain of abrupt onset and maximal at onset, rather than building; a tearing or ripping quality; migration of pain, classically to the back or between the scapulae; a pulse or blood pressure differential between limbs; a new aortic regurgitation murmur; focal neurological deficit; and syncope. Predisposing conditions include hypertension, connective tissue disorders, bicuspid aortic valve, pregnancy, and stimulant use.

Two cautions. The classical presentation is present in a minority of cases, and the absence of the classical features does not exclude the diagnosis. And **a raised D-dimer does not confirm dissection and a normal one does not reliably exclude it** in a patient with high clinical suspicion; where suspicion is high, proceed to computed tomographic angiography.

Pulmonary embolism, addressed in Chapter 14, and in the postoperative context in Chapter 8, section 8.5.2.

Tension pneumothorax, which is a clinical diagnosis requiring immediate decompression rather than imaging, and which is detectable in seconds by bedside ultrasound as discussed in section 9.7.

Oesophageal rupture, classically following forceful vomiting, with pain, subcutaneous emphysema, and rapid deterioration.

Pericarditis and tamponade. Pericarditic pain is characteristically pleuritic, positional, worse supine and relieved by sitting forward. Tamponade produces hypotension, elevated venous pressure, and pulsus paradoxus, and is again immediately visible on bedside ultrasound.

Myocarditis, which may present with chest pain, troponin elevation, and electrocardiographic changes that mimic infarction, and which is an important consideration in younger patients.

Non-lethal but common causes including gastro-oesophageal reflux, musculoskeletal chest wall pain, and anxiety. These are diagnoses of exclusion in a patient with risk factors, and attributing chest pain to reflux on the basis of response to an antacid is not a diagnostic test.

9.1.5 The disposition decision

Once acute coronary syndrome has been excluded by a validated pathway and the alternative lethal causes have been considered, the question is whether further cardiac testing is indicated before discharge.

The historical practice of routine non-invasive stress testing before discharge in all patients with chest pain has been substantially revised. In patients ruled out by a high-sensitivity troponin pathway with a low risk score, the yield of immediate stress testing is low, the rate of false positives generates downstream angiography and its complications, and the short-term event rate without testing is very low. Several guideline bodies and value-based recommendations now advise against routine immediate testing in this group, favouring outpatient assessment where indicated by symptom pattern and risk profile.

Computed tomographic coronary angiography has a defined role, particularly in patients with intermediate risk and no known coronary disease, where it has good negative predictive value for excluding significant coronary disease and can identify patients who would benefit from preventive therapy. It also increases downstream testing and revascularisation in some trials without corresponding mortality benefit, so the decision should be deliberate rather than routine.

The practical position. In a patient ruled out biochemically with a low risk score and no ongoing symptoms, discharge with outpatient follow-up is defensible and is the recommended course in most current pathways. In a patient with a concerning history, recurrent symptoms, known coronary disease, or an intermediate risk score, further assessment is appropriate, and the modality should be chosen with cardiology input. Chapter 13 develops the management of acute coronary syndrome.

9.2 Dyspnoea: Separating Cardiac, Pulmonary, and Metabolic Causes

9.2.1 What dyspnoea is

Dyspnoea is a conscious experience of uncomfortable breathing, arising from a mismatch between the respiratory drive generated centrally and the ventilation actually achieved. This definition is more useful than a list of causes, because it explains why the symptom arises in four quite different circumstances.

Increased drive from hypoxia, hypercapnia, acidosis, anaemia, fever, or anxiety.

Increased load, either resistive as in airflow obstruction, or elastic as in pulmonary oedema, fibrosis, pleural disease, or abdominal distension.

Reduced capacity to meet the load, from respiratory muscle weakness, hyperinflation with mechanical disadvantage, or fatigue.

Altered perception, in which the afferent signal is normal but its interpretation is amplified, as in anxiety, and which is a diagnosis of exclusion rather than a first hypothesis.

9.2.2 Two errors to avoid at the outset

A normal oxygen saturation does not exclude serious disease. This is the single most important statement in this section. Patients with pulmonary embolism, with metabolic acidosis, with severe anaemia, with neuromuscular respiratory failure, and with early sepsis frequently have normal saturations while being seriously unwell. Saturation measures oxygenation, and several lethal causes of dyspnoea impair ventilation, perfusion matching, oxygen delivery, or respiratory mechanics without initially impairing oxygenation.

Respiratory rate is the most neglected vital sign and the most informative. It is frequently estimated rather than counted, and estimated values cluster implausibly around round numbers. A genuinely counted respiratory rate, over a full minute, discriminates better than most other bedside measurements and is the earliest indicator of deterioration, as noted in Chapter 4, section 4.5.3.

9.2.3 Cardiac causes

Heart failure is the commonest cardiac cause. The features with the greatest discriminating value are paroxysmal nocturnal dyspnoea, orthostatic worsening, a third heart sound, elevated jugular venous pressure, and a history of prior heart failure. Peripheral oedema alone has poor discriminating value, since it has many other causes.

Natriuretic peptides are useful principally for their negative predictive value. Concentrations below the relevant threshold make heart failure unlikely; elevated values are less specific, since they rise in renal impairment, atrial fibrillation, pulmonary embolism, sepsis, and older age, and are lowered by obesity. Thresholds differ between B-type natriuretic peptide and its N-terminal fragment, and for the latter are age-stratified. Use the local assay's thresholds.

Other cardiac causes include acute coronary syndrome presenting as dyspnoea rather than pain, which is particularly common in older adults, women, and diabetic patients; valvular disease, especially aortic stenosis and mitral regurgitation; arrhythmia, particularly new atrial fibrillation with rapid ventricular response; tamponade; and pulmonary hypertension.

9.2.4 Pulmonary causes

Organising these by mechanism is more useful than by disease.

Airflow obstruction: asthma, chronic obstructive pulmonary disease, upper airway obstruction, and, importantly, the patient whose chest is silent because airflow is too low to generate wheeze. The absence of wheeze in a distressed patient is an ominous sign, not a reassuring one.

Parenchymal disease: pneumonia, interstitial disease, and acute respiratory distress syndrome.

Pulmonary vascular disease: pulmonary embolism and pulmonary hypertension. Chapter 14 develops both.

Pleural disease: effusion and pneumothorax.

Chest wall and mechanical: rib fractures, abdominal distension, massive ascites, and severe obesity.

9.2.5 Metabolic, haematological, and neuromuscular causes

Metabolic acidosis produces compensatory hyperventilation, which the patient experiences as dyspnoea. Diabetic ketoacidosis, lactic acidosis from any cause, renal failure, and toxic ingestions all present this way, and a patient with deep, rapid, unlaboured breathing and clear lungs should prompt an arterial or venous blood gas and a lactate rather than a chest radiograph alone. Chapter 12 develops acid-base analysis.

Anaemia impairs oxygen delivery with normal saturation, and severe anaemia presents with exertional dyspnoea, tachycardia, and pallor.

Sepsis commonly presents with tachypnoea before any localising feature, and the tachypnoea is frequently the only early sign.

Thyrotoxicosis and other hypermetabolic states.

Neuromuscular respiratory failure deserves particular emphasis because it is missed catastrophically. Patients with Guillain-Barré syndrome, myasthenic crisis, motor neurone disease, or high cervical cord pathology develop respiratory failure through inspiratory muscle weakness. **Oxygen saturation remains normal until immediately before decompensation**, at which point deterioration is abrupt. The correct monitoring is serial measurement of forced vital capacity and inspiratory pressures, together with observation for orthopnoea, weak cough, staccato speech, and paradoxical abdominal movement. A patient with suspected neuromuscular weakness who is monitored by pulse oximetry alone will be intubated as an emergency rather than electively. Chapter 10 addresses localisation and Chapter 14 the ventilatory management.

9.2.6 A bedside approach

Observe before touching. Position, work of breathing, use of accessory muscles, ability to speak in sentences, pattern and depth of respiration, and audible sounds. Two minutes of observation from the end of the bed frequently establishes the category.

Count the respiratory rate.

Assess the trajectory. Sudden onset over seconds to minutes suggests pneumothorax, embolism, arrhythmia, or aspiration. Onset over hours suggests pulmonary oedema, asthma, infection, or acidosis. Onset over days to weeks suggests effusion, anaemia, malignancy, or progressive parenchymal disease.

Examine for the discriminating findings: jugular venous pressure, third heart sound, crackles and their distribution, wheeze, asymmetry of air entry and percussion, calf asymmetry, and the abdomen.

Use bedside ultrasound, as in section 9.7, which resolves several of these questions in minutes.

Obtain a blood gas when acidosis, hypercapnia, or a suspected metabolic cause is plausible, and do not rely on saturation.

Reassess after intervention. The response to a diuretic, a bronchodilator, or a change in position is diagnostic information, provided the response is actually observed rather than assumed.

9.3 Acute Abdominal Pain in the Medical Inpatient

9.3.1 Why the inpatient presentation is different

Acute abdominal pain in a hospitalised medical patient differs from the same complaint in an ambulatory patient in ways that systematically increase the chance of a missed diagnosis.

The patient may not report it. Delirium, dementia, sedation, intubation, aphasia, and spinal cord pathology all prevent reporting. In these patients the presentation is a change in physiology or behaviour rather than a complaint: new tachycardia, new confusion, reduced oral intake, guarding on incidental examination, or a nurse's observation that the patient winces when moved.

The signs are blunted. Corticosteroids and immunosuppressants suppress the inflammatory response and can eliminate peritonism entirely in the presence of perforation. Opioids given for another indication mask pain. Advanced age reduces the intensity of both symptoms and signs. Diabetes with autonomic neuropathy alters visceral pain perception. Beta-blockers suppress the tachycardic response. Each of these is common in a medical inpatient population, and several coexist.

The pretest probabilities differ. Hospitalised medical patients are immobile, frequently anticoagulated, frequently on antibiotics, frequently in atrial fibrillation, and frequently hypotensive at some point. This shifts the differential toward ischaemic, iatrogenic, and complication-related causes and away from the common ambulatory diagnoses.

9.3.2 The diagnoses that must not be missed

Mesenteric ischaemia is the archetype of the diagnosis missed until it is fatal, and its features deserve specific attention. Classic teaching is pain out of proportion to the examination findings, and this is genuinely useful early, because the visceral pain of ischaemia precedes the peritoneal signs of infarction. Predisposing factors include atrial fibrillation and other embolic sources, atherosclerotic disease, hypotension or shock of any cause, vasopressor use, hypercoagulable states, and recent vascular intervention.

Two errors are common. **A normal lactate does not exclude early mesenteric ischaemia**, since lactate rises when infarction and systemic compromise are established, which is late. And plain radiography and non-contrast imaging are inadequate; the investigation is computed tomographic angiography, and it should be obtained urgently on clinical suspicion rather than after other tests have been exhausted. Chapter 7, section 7.2.4, addressed the contrast question directly.

Perforation of a viscus, which in an immunosuppressed or elderly patient may produce minimal signs. Free air may be visible on erect chest radiography but its absence does not exclude perforation, and computed tomography is more sensitive.

Obstruction with strangulation, addressed in Chapter 8, section 8.3.3.

Ruptured or expanding abdominal aortic aneurysm, which presents with pain, hypotension, and a pulsatile mass, though the classic triad is frequently incomplete. Bedside ultrasound detects the aneurysm rapidly, though not reliably the rupture.

Acute cholangitis, presenting with fever, jaundice, and right upper quadrant pain, and requiring urgent biliary drainage in addition to antimicrobial therapy. Chapter 15 develops this.

Ischaemic colitis, which is common in hospitalised patients after hypotension and presents with pain and bloody diarrhoea.

Toxic megacolon, complicating *Clostridioides difficile* infection or inflammatory bowel disease, in which examination signs may be minimal because of colonic distension and corticosteroid use.

Retroperitoneal haemorrhage, particularly in anticoagulated patients, which may present with pain, hypotension, and a falling haemoglobin without external evidence.

Extra-abdominal causes presenting abdominally: inferior myocardial infarction with epigastric pain, diabetic ketoacidosis, adrenal crisis, hypercalcaemia, lower lobe pneumonia, and pulmonary embolism.

9.3.3 Diagnoses specific to the medical inpatient

Several conditions arise principally in hospitalised patients and should be considered explicitly.

***Clostridioides difficile* colitis**, addressed in Chapter 15.

Acute colonic pseudo-obstruction, in which massive colonic dilatation occurs without mechanical obstruction, typically in an unwell, immobile, medicated inpatient. It is important because progressive caecal distension carries a risk of perforation, and management involves correction of precipitants, exclusion of mechanical obstruction, and, where distension is marked or progressive, pharmacological or endoscopic decompression.

Spontaneous bacterial peritonitis in any patient with ascites, which may present with minimal pain and requires diagnostic paracentesis. The rule is that a cirrhotic patient with ascites who becomes unwell has a diagnostic tap, and Chapter 15 develops this.

Constipation and faecal impaction, which is unglamorous, extremely common, and a genuine cause of pain, distension, delirium, and overflow diarrhoea.

Urinary retention, which is easily confirmed by bladder ultrasound in seconds and is missed regularly.

Medication-related causes, including opioid-induced constipation, nonsteroidal-related ulceration, and drug-induced pancreatitis.

9.3.4 Practical approach

Examine the patient properly, including the groins. Incarcerated femoral and inguinal hernias are missed because the examination stops at the abdominal wall.

Do not be reassured by a soft abdomen in an immunosuppressed, elderly, or opioid-treated patient. Weight the history and the physiology more heavily than the examination in these groups.

Use serial examination. Repeating the examination at two hours by the same clinician is one of the highest-yield actions available, and delegating the reassessment to a different person loses most of its value.

Obtain imaging early where a lethal cause is plausible. Chapter 2, section 2.7.4, distinguished stewardship from diagnostic restraint in the deteriorating patient; this is precisely the setting where broad and prompt investigation is correct.

Involve surgery early rather than after imaging. A surgical opinion informed by the clinical picture is more useful than one delivered after a report.

9.4 Syncope: The Rule-Out That Matters

9.4.1 Definition and the first discrimination

Syncope is transient loss of consciousness due to global cerebral hypoperfusion, characterised by rapid onset, short duration, and spontaneous complete recovery. Each element of the definition is doing work.

The first task is to establish whether the event was syncope at all, since several conditions mimic it and are managed entirely differently.

Seizure is suggested by an aura, prolonged tonic-clonic activity, lateral tongue biting, a postictal period of confusion lasting more than a few minutes, and incontinence. Brief myoclonic jerking occurs in genuine syncope and is not itself evidence of seizure, which is a common source of misdiagnosis.

Hypoglycaemia, which does not produce rapid spontaneous complete recovery unless treated.

Trauma-related loss of consciousness, where the injury preceded rather than followed the event.

Psychogenic pseudosyncope, characterised by prolonged apparent unconsciousness with normal vital signs and resistance to eye opening.

Falls without loss of consciousness, which is addressed in section 9.6 and which is frequently reported by patients as blacking out.

The collateral history from a witness is the single most valuable piece of information and is frequently not obtained. Where a witness exists, they should be contacted by telephone if not present.

9.4.2 The three mechanisms

Reflex or neurally mediated syncope, including vasovagal, situational, and carotid sinus syncope. Suggested by a prodrome of nausea, warmth, sweating, and visual dimming; an identifiable trigger such as prolonged standing, pain, emotional stress, micturition, cough, or defecation; and a benign prognosis.

Orthostatic syncope, from volume depletion, autonomic failure, or medication. Suggested by onset shortly after standing and by a documented postural fall in blood pressure. **Orthostatic vital signs are simple, informative, and routinely omitted**, and their measurement should be standard in any syncope evaluation.

Cardiac syncope, from arrhythmia or from structural disease limiting cardiac output. This is the category that matters, because it carries substantially increased mortality and because it is the one that further investigation can address.

9.4.3 The features that identify cardiac syncope

The following should be sought explicitly, and their presence changes the disposition.

- **Syncope during exertion.** Highly concerning for structural disease including aortic stenosis and hypertrophic cardiomyopathy, or for exercise-induced arrhythmia. Syncope shortly after exertion is more often reflex.
- **Syncope while supine or seated.** Reflex syncope occurs almost exclusively upright.
- **Absence of any prodrome**, with abrupt loss of consciousness.
- **Palpitations immediately preceding the event.**
- **Known structural heart disease or reduced ventricular function.**
- **Family history of sudden cardiac death**, particularly at a young age.
- **An abnormal electrocardiogram.**
- **Syncope causing significant injury**, which suggests absence of protective prodrome.

The electrocardiogram should be obtained in every patient with syncope and reviewed specifically for: evidence of prior infarction, conduction disease including bifascicular block and prolonged PR interval, prolonged or short QT interval, Brugada pattern, pre-excitation, features of hypertrophic cardiomyopathy, and features of arrhythmogenic right ventricular cardiomyopathy including T wave inversion in right precordial leads and an epsilon wave.

Consider also the structural causes that present with syncope and are immediately dangerous: pulmonary embolism, aortic dissection, tamponade, and severe aortic stenosis. Syncope as a presentation of pulmonary embolism is well described and under-recognised.

9.4.4 Investigations of low yield

Several investigations are ordered routinely in syncope and have consistently poor yield, and omitting them is a defensible and evidence-supported position.

Neuroimaging in a patient with syncope and no neurological symptoms or signs and no head injury. Syncope is a cardiovascular event, not a neurological one, and routine computed tomography of the head in unselected syncope has a very low yield of clinically relevant findings.

Carotid imaging. Carotid disease does not cause syncope; it causes focal ischaemia. Routine carotid ultrasound in syncope is not indicated.

Electroencephalography in the absence of features suggesting seizure.

Routine echocardiography in all patients, as distinct from patients with an abnormal examination, an abnormal electrocardiogram, exertional syncope, or known or suspected structural disease, in whom it is clearly indicated.

Several of these appear in value-based care recommendations precisely because they are ordered reflexively.

9.4.5 Disposition and monitoring

Risk stratification instruments exist, including scores derived in emergency department populations, and they are useful for structuring assessment. As always, they inform rather than determine.

Admission is warranted for patients with features suggesting cardiac syncope, significant structural disease, an abnormal electrocardiogram, syncope causing serious injury, ongoing symptoms, or significant comorbidity making outpatient assessment unsafe.

Duration of monitoring should match the frequency of symptoms. Inpatient telemetry captures arrhythmia only if it recurs during the admission, which for infrequent events it will not. Where an arrhythmic cause is suspected but not captured, ambulatory monitoring of appropriate duration, external event recorders, or an implantable loop recorder are the correct escalation, and the choice depends on symptom frequency. Keeping a patient in hospital for several days of telemetry to capture an event that occurs monthly is a common and unproductive practice.

Driving and occupational advice should be given and documented, since regulations differ by jurisdiction and by cause, and patients are frequently discharged without it.

9.5 Dizziness and Vertigo: HINTS and the Localisation Trap

9.5.1 The localisation trap

Traditional teaching asks the patient to describe the *type* of dizziness, and sorts them into vertigo suggesting vestibular disease, presyncope suggesting cardiovascular disease, disequilibrium suggesting neurological disease, and non-specific lightheadedness suggesting psychiatric or metabolic causes.

This approach has been examined empirically and performs poorly. Patients are inconsistent in describing their symptom type, frequently endorse multiple types, and change their description when asked again minutes later. Worse, the symptom type does not map reliably onto the underlying cause: patients with posterior circulation stroke frequently describe lightheadedness rather than spinning, and patients with orthostatic hypotension frequently describe vertigo.

The consequence is that a diagnostic approach built on symptom quality generates confident and wrong conclusions, which is the specific failure mode described in Chapter 2, section 2.5.1.

9.5.2 The timing and trigger framework

The alternative, developed principally by Newman-Toker and colleagues, asks two different questions: **how long does it last, and what brings it on?** These are reported far more reliably and map onto the pathology much better.

Three syndromes emerge.

Acute vestibular syndrome. Dizziness of acute onset that is **continuous**, persisting for days, usually with nausea, vomiting, nystagmus, and gait instability. The differential is essentially vestibular neuritis versus posterior circulation stroke, and distinguishing them is the subject of section 9.5.3.

Episodic vestibular syndrome, triggered. Brief episodes reliably provoked by a specific movement or position. The dominant cause is benign paroxysmal positional vertigo, provoked by head position change and lasting seconds to a minute. Orthostatic hypotension is the other principal triggered syndrome, provoked by standing.

Episodic vestibular syndrome, spontaneous. Episodes occurring without a trigger, lasting minutes to hours. The differential includes vestibular migraine, Ménière disease, transient ischaemic attack, cardiac arrhythmia, panic disorder, and hypoglycaemia.

Establishing which of the three syndromes applies is the entire first step, and it is done by history alone.

9.5.3 The HINTS examination

For patients with **acute vestibular syndrome only**, a three-component oculomotor examination distinguishes peripheral from central causes with performance that, in trained hands, exceeds that of early magnetic resonance imaging with diffusion weighting, which misses a meaningful proportion of posterior circulation strokes within the first day or two.

Head Impulse. The examiner rapidly rotates the patient's head a small amplitude while the patient fixates on a target. In peripheral vestibular loss, the vestibulo-ocular reflex fails and the eyes make a visible corrective saccade back to the target: an abnormal test. In central disease, the reflex is intact and no corrective saccade occurs. **A normal head impulse test in a patient with acute continuous vertigo is the worrying result**, which is the counterintuitive element and the one most often misremembered.

Nystagmus. Peripheral nystagmus is unidirectional, horizontal, and beats away from the affected side regardless of gaze direction, and it is suppressed by visual fixation. **Direction-changing nystagmus on lateral gaze, or vertical or purely torsional nystagmus, indicates a central cause.**

Test of Skew. Alternate cover testing is performed, looking for vertical corrective movement of the covered eye when uncovered. **The presence of skew deviation indicates a central cause**, most often brainstem.

The pattern indicating a peripheral cause is therefore an abnormal head impulse, unidirectional nystagmus, and absent skew. Any deviation from that pattern indicates a central cause and mandates urgent imaging and stroke pathway management.

HINTS plus adds bedside testing of hearing, since new unilateral hearing loss with acute vestibular syndrome, contrary to intuition, raises rather than lowers concern for stroke in the anterior inferior cerebellar artery territory.

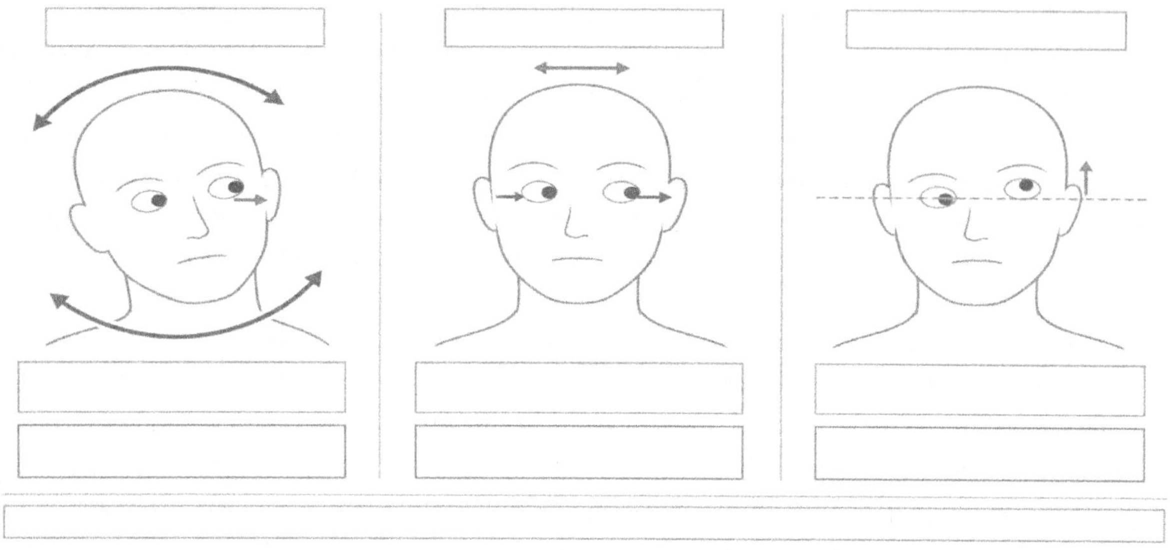

9.5.4 Where HINTS goes wrong

Three misapplications are common and all are dangerous.

Applying it to the wrong syndrome. HINTS was derived and validated in acute vestibular syndrome with nystagmus. Applying it to a patient with episodic triggered dizziness, to a patient without nystagmus, or to a patient whose symptoms have resolved produces uninterpretable results and false reassurance. This is the commonest error.

Performing it without training. The head impulse test in particular requires practice, and a poorly performed test yields a false peripheral pattern. Clinicians who have not been trained in it should not use it to exclude stroke.

Relying on the absence of other focal deficits. Isolated vertigo can be the sole manifestation of cerebellar or brainstem infarction, and the absence of limb weakness, dysarthria, or sensory change does not exclude it. Gait should be tested in every patient with acute dizziness who can stand, since severe truncal ataxia with inability to walk unaided is a central sign regardless of the oculomotor findings.

9.5.5 The triggered and spontaneous syndromes

Benign paroxysmal positional vertigo is diagnosed by the Dix-Hallpike manoeuvre for posterior canal involvement, which reproduces brief vertigo with characteristic upbeating torsional nystagmus after a short latency, fatiguing on repetition. It is treated by a repositioning manoeuvre, which is effective, takes minutes, and is substantially underused in hospital practice, where vestibular sedatives are prescribed instead. Vestibular suppressants impair central compensation and should be limited to short-term symptom control rather than used as treatment.

Orthostatic hypotension is diagnosed by measuring lying and standing blood pressure properly, which means after several minutes lying and at intervals after standing, and is a common and correctable cause in hospitalised patients, frequently medication-related.

Spontaneous episodic dizziness requires consideration of vestibular migraine, which is common and under-diagnosed, Ménière disease, arrhythmia, and transient ischaemic attack. A patient with recurrent spontaneous episodes and vascular risk factors warrants urgent assessment, since these may be posterior circulation transient ischaemic attacks preceding infarction.

9.6 Weakness and Falls as Sentinel Presentations

9.6.1 Weakness is a syndrome, not a symptom

When a patient or a referring clinician says weakness, they may mean any of several distinct things, and the first task is to establish which.

True neuromuscular weakness, meaning reduced power in a definable distribution. This is a localisation problem, addressed in Chapter 10, section 10.3, and the pattern of involvement identifies the level of the lesion.

Generalised asthenia or fatigue, meaning reduced capacity for effort without focal power loss. This is the commoner meaning and is a systemic rather than a neurological finding.

Functional decline, meaning a reduced ability to perform accustomed activities, which may reflect either of the above or neither.

Instability or falls, addressed below, which patients frequently describe as weakness.

The distinction is made by history and by examination of power against resistance. The clinical consequence is complete divergence of the differential, and the common error is to investigate a patient with systemic asthenia neurologically, or to dismiss a patient with early neuromuscular weakness as deconditioned.

9.6.2 Generalised weakness in the older adult

Generalised weakness in an older person presenting to hospital is a **presentation of acute illness until proven otherwise**, and the illnesses it most often represents are not neurological.

The differential to work through systematically:

- **Infection**, which in older adults frequently presents without fever, without localising symptoms, and with functional decline as the only manifestation. Chapter 18 addresses this.
- **Dehydration and electrolyte disturbance**, particularly hyponatraemia, hypokalaemia, hypercalcaemia, and hypomagnesaemia. Chapter 12 develops these.
- **Medication effects**, including recently added agents, accumulation in renal impairment, and polypharmacy. Chapter 3, section 3.2.1, made the case for the medication list as a diagnostic instrument.
- **Anaemia**, acute or chronic, including occult gastrointestinal blood loss.
- **Cardiac causes**, including acute coronary syndrome presenting without chest pain, new arrhythmia, and decompensating heart failure.
- **Endocrine causes**, principally hypothyroidism, hyperthyroidism in older adults which may present apathetically, adrenal insufficiency, and hyperglycaemia or hypoglycaemia.

- **Depression**, which is common, under-recognised, and presents with fatigue and functional decline.
- **Malignancy**, particularly with new weight loss.
- **Delirium**, in which hypoactive presentation is easily labelled as weakness. Chapter 8, section 8.4.4, addressed the detection problem.

9.6.3 A fall is an event with a cause

The phrase "mechanical fall" appears frequently in clinical records and is not a diagnosis. It states that the patient fell for a physical reason, which is true of all falls, and it terminates inquiry.

Every fall should be approached with three questions.

Why did the patient fall? The task is to distinguish a fall from a trip or slip in a person with normal balance, from a fall due to impaired gait, balance, vision, or strength, from a fall due to syncope, and from a fall due to a neurological event. The distinction is made by asking about the moments before the fall specifically: was there warning, was there loss of consciousness, was there a trip, and what does a witness report? A patient who cannot recall the fall itself should be presumed to have had loss of consciousness until established otherwise, and section 9.4 then applies.

What did the fall cause? This is the injury assessment, and several injuries are missed routinely.

What does the fall predict? Falls are a marker of frailty and predict further falls, fracture, functional decline, institutionalisation, and mortality. A first fall is a sentinel event and warrants a multifactorial assessment, addressed in Chapter 4, section 4.4.1, and Chapter 19.

9.6.4 The injuries missed after a fall

Intracranial haemorrhage in the anticoagulated patient. Any patient on an anticoagulant with a head strike requires imaging, and the threshold should be low even without a clear history of head strike in a patient who cannot recall the event. **Delayed intracranial haemorrhage** is a recognised phenomenon in anticoagulated patients with an initially normal scan, and a period of observation with repeat imaging on clinical change is appropriate. Local protocols vary, and clinical decision rules for head injury imaging were largely derived in populations excluding or under-representing anticoagulated patients.

Occult hip fracture. A patient with hip pain and a normal plain radiograph after a fall may still have a fracture, and continued inability to weight-bear should prompt cross-sectional imaging rather than reassurance and mobilisation.

Pelvic and sacral fractures, which are frequently invisible on plain films in osteoporotic bone.

Rib fractures, which cause splinting, atelectasis, and pneumonia, particularly in older adults, and which change analgesic and respiratory management.

Cervical spine injury, particularly central cord syndrome in a patient with cervical spondylosis after a hyperextension injury, which presents with disproportionate upper limb weakness.

Rhabdomyolysis and pressure injury after a long lie. A patient who was on the floor for hours may have significant muscle injury, acute kidney injury, hypothermia, dehydration, and pressure damage. Creatine kinase should be measured where a long lie is suspected. Chapter 16 addresses the renal management.

9.6.5 The systematic post-fall assessment

A structured approach that takes fifteen minutes and prevents most of the missed diagnoses above:

- Obtain the account of the event from the patient and from any witness, focusing on the preceding moments.
- Measure lying and standing blood pressure.
- Obtain an electrocardiogram.
- Review every medication, with particular attention to antihypertensives, sedatives, anticholinergics, hypoglycaemic agents, and any recently added drug.
- Examine for injury, including the head, the cervical spine, the ribs, the hips, the pelvis, and the wrists.
- Assess vision and hearing, and check that glasses and hearing aids are present and used.
- Assess gait and balance where safe to do so, using a timed test if available, and note the use and appropriateness of any walking aid.
- Check for cognitive impairment and delirium.
- Check feet and footwear.
- Consider bone health, including whether the patient has an untreated osteoporosis risk that this fall has now made evident, and Chapter 19 develops this.
- Review the environment where relevant, including the bed height, the call bell, the lighting, and the route to the bathroom, since Chapter 4, section 4.4.1, noted that a substantial proportion of inpatient falls occur en route to the toilet.

9.7 Bedside Ultrasound as an Extension of the Physical Examination

9.7.1 What point-of-care ultrasound is and is not

Point-of-care ultrasound is the use of ultrasound by the treating clinician, at the bedside, to answer a specific clinical question in real time. It differs from a formal departmental study in scope, in purpose, and in the standard to which it should be held.

It answers binary questions. Is there free fluid in the abdomen? Is there a pericardial effusion? Is the bladder full? Is there lung sliding? Is the inferior vena cava collapsing? These are questions with yes or no answers that can be established in seconds and that change immediate management.

It is not a comprehensive study, and should never be documented or communicated as though it were. A point-of-care cardiac view that shows no pericardial effusion has not excluded valvular disease, regional wall motion abnormality, or intracardiac thrombus.

The correct conceptual placement is as an extension of the physical examination. It answers the questions percussion and auscultation attempt to answer, and it answers them far better.

9.7.2 The applications with the greatest yield

Cardiac. Detection of pericardial effusion and tamponade physiology; gross assessment of left ventricular systolic function; assessment of right ventricular size and function, where a dilated right ventricle in a hypotensive or hypoxic patient substantially raises the probability of pulmonary embolism; and assessment of volume status in combination with other views.

Lung. This is the highest-yield application for a hospitalist and the one that most changes practice. **B-lines** in a bilateral, dependent, symmetric distribution indicate interstitial fluid and support pulmonary oedema. **Absence of lung sliding** with a lung point supports pneumothorax with performance exceeding supine chest radiography. **Pleural effusion** is identified and quantified far better than by percussion, and the presence of septations or debris is visible. **Consolidation** is identifiable. In an undifferentiated dyspnoeic patient, a lung ultrasound performed in three or four minutes frequently distinguishes pulmonary oedema from pneumonia from pneumothorax from effusion, and section 9.2 lists that as the central diagnostic task.

Inferior vena cava. Diameter and respiratory variation give an approximate indication of filling status, with the important caveat that it performs poorly as a standalone measure of fluid responsiveness and should be interpreted alongside the clinical picture and other views rather than as a number driving fluid administration.

Abdominal. Free fluid, hydronephrosis, gallbladder assessment including stones and wall thickening, aortic diameter for aneurysm, and bladder volume. The last is the simplest and among the most useful, resolving the question of urinary retention immediately and preventing unnecessary catheterisation, which returns to Chapter 4, section 4.4.4.

Vascular. Compression ultrasound of the proximal veins for deep vein thrombosis, which in trained hands has good performance for proximal thrombosis, though it does not replace a formal study in most institutional pathways.

Procedural guidance. This is the application with the strongest evidence for reducing harm. Ultrasound guidance for central venous access reduces failed attempts and complications and is a standard of care. Guidance for thoracentesis and paracentesis reduces complications and is similarly established. A hospitalist performing these procedures without ultrasound in an institution where it is available should be able to justify that choice.

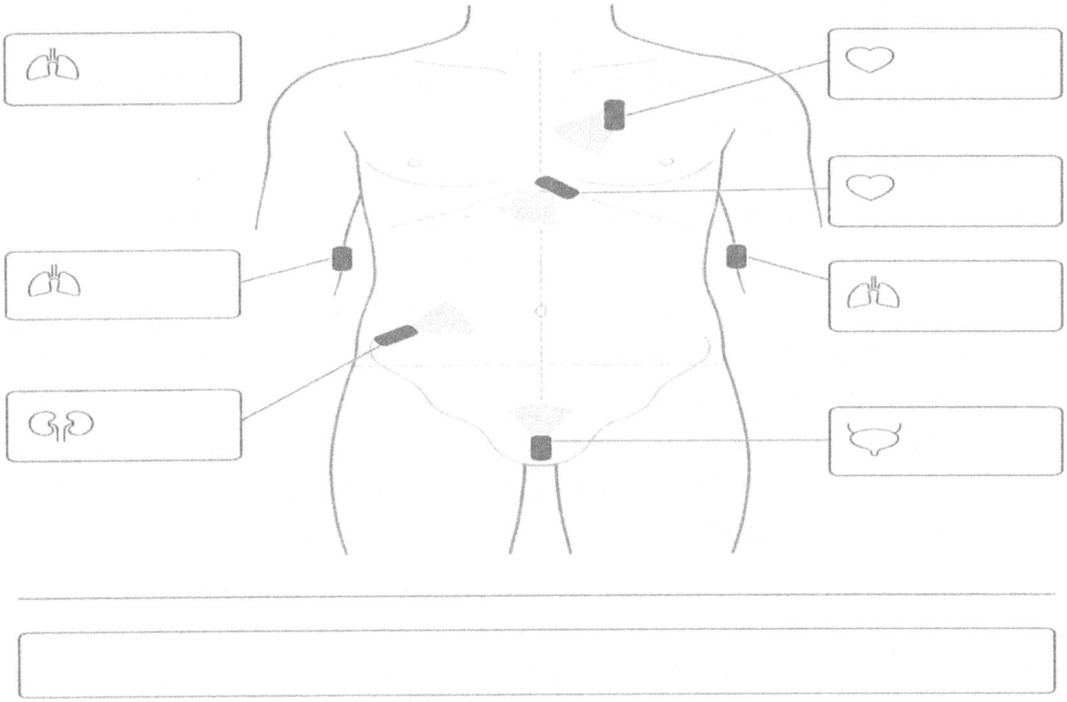

9.7.3 Limitations and failure modes

Point-of-care ultrasound generates its own errors, and the enthusiasm surrounding it has tended to under-emphasise them.

Operator dependence. Image acquisition and interpretation are skills with a genuine learning curve, and competence is not conferred by attending a course. Institutions should have credentialing pathways, and individual clinicians should have an honest sense of which questions they can answer reliably and which they cannot.

False reassurance from a negative study. A limited study answers a limited question. Not seeing a finding may mean it is absent, or that the window was inadequate, or that the operator did not look in the right place.

Anchoring. An early ultrasound finding is highly salient and can terminate the diagnostic process prematurely, which is the mechanism described in Chapter 2, section 2.4.3. A patient with visible B-lines has interstitial fluid; they may also have pneumonia, and they may also have a pulmonary embolism.

Incidental findings, which generate the cascades described in Chapter 2, section 2.7.

Documentation. Findings should be recorded with the question asked, the views obtained, the limitations, and explicitly that this was a focused study rather than a comprehensive one. Images should be stored where the system permits.

It does not replace clinical reasoning. The scan answers the question the clinician thought to ask. Constructing the right question remains the work of Chapter 2.

9.7.4 Integrating it into practice

Two habits make the difference between a device that gathers dust and one that changes care.

Scan with a question. Before placing the probe, state what is being asked and what each possible answer would change. This is the same discipline as Chapter 2, section 2.7.2, applied to imaging, and it prevents the aimless scanning that generates incidental findings.

Scan the patients you are worried about, early. The value is greatest in the undifferentiated, unstable, or deteriorating patient, where the alternative is a delay while a formal study is arranged. A hypotensive patient can have a cardiac, lung, inferior vena cava, and abdominal assessment completed in the time it takes to speak to the radiology department.

Chapter Summary

- **The presenting complaint is a starting point, not a category**, comorbidity systematically blunts presentation in the highest-risk populations, and trajectory carries more information than any single assessment.
- In **chest pain**, run two tracks simultaneously. High-sensitivity troponin pathways are excellent for coronary syndrome and exclude none of the other lethal causes. Use sex-specific thresholds, interpret the delta rather than the single value, and recognise that these pathways were derived in emergency populations. Routine immediate stress testing after a negative pathway is low yield.
- **A normal oxygen saturation does not exclude serious dyspnoea**, and respiratory rate is the most neglected and most informative vital sign. Neuromuscular respiratory failure is monitored by vital capacity, not oximetry, because saturation falls only immediately before decompensation.
- **Abdominal pain in the medical inpatient is blunted** by corticosteroids, opioids, age, and diabetes. A normal lactate does not exclude early mesenteric ischaemia. Serial examination by the same clinician is among the highest-yield actions available.
- In **syncope**, the objective is to exclude a cardiac cause. Obtain a collateral history, measure orthostatic vitals, and read the electrocardiogram systematically. Routine neuroimaging, carotid studies, and electroencephalography in unselected syncope are low yield. Match monitoring duration to symptom frequency.
- **Do not classify dizziness by symptom quality.** Use timing and triggers. HINTS applies only to acute vestibular syndrome, a normal head impulse is the concerning result, and misapplication to episodic dizziness is the commonest and most dangerous error. Test gait in every patient who can stand.
- **A mechanical fall is not a diagnosis.** Establish why the patient fell, what it caused, and what it predicts. Anticoagulated patients with head strike need imaging and consideration

of delayed haemorrhage; occult hip fracture, rib fractures, and rhabdomyolysis after a long lie are routinely missed.

- **Point-of-care ultrasound answers binary questions** and is an extension of the physical examination, not a substitute for a formal study. Its strongest evidence is for procedural guidance. Scan with a question, and document the study as focused.

Review Questions

1. A 58-year-old woman has chest pain with a high-sensitivity troponin below the ninety-ninth percentile on presentation and at two hours, and a normal electrocardiogram. State what has and has not been excluded, what features you would specifically seek before discharge, and your position on immediate stress testing.
2. A patient with suspected Guillain-Barré syndrome has an oxygen saturation of 97 per cent on air and reports feeling breathless. Explain why the saturation is reassuring in the wrong way, and state exactly what you would monitor and how often.
3. An 82-year-old on prednisolone 20 milligrams daily has vague abdominal discomfort, a soft abdomen, a heart rate of 104, and a normal lactate. Set out your reasoning and the specific action you would take.
4. A patient reports three days of continuous dizziness with nausea and nystagmus. Describe how you would establish the syndrome, what examination you would perform, and which single finding would most concern you.
5. A 79-year-old on apixaban is found on the floor and cannot recall the event. List the injuries you would specifically exclude, the investigations you would order, and the diagnosis you must not record.

CHAPTER 10: Altered Mental Status and Neurologic Localisation

Learning Objectives

After studying this chapter, the reader should be able to:

1. Describe the pathophysiology of delirium, implement a prevention bundle, and state what the pharmacological evidence does and does not support.
2. Assess the comatose patient systematically, distinguish structural from metabolic causes at the bedside, and recognise herniation syndromes.
3. Localise a neurological deficit to cortex, subcortical structures, brainstem, cerebellum, spinal cord, root, peripheral nerve, neuromuscular junction, or muscle.
4. Recognise stroke occurring in a hospitalised patient inside the therapeutic window, and describe why in-hospital stroke is treated later and worse than community stroke.
5. Manage seizure and status epilepticus with correctly dosed therapy, and recognise nonconvulsive status as a cause of unexplained altered consciousness.
6. Identify toxic and metabolic encephalopathies and the principal drug-induced neurological syndromes.
7. Assess decision-making capacity as a functional, decision-specific judgement, and act appropriately when it is absent.

Chapter Overview

Altered mental status is among the most common reasons a hospitalist is called and among the most poorly handled. The reasons are structural rather than a matter of individual knowledge.

The complaint arrives as a summary already interpreted: the patient is confused, agitated, drowsy, or not themselves. That summary conflates several distinct clinical states with different differentials and different urgencies. Delirium, coma, aphasia, psychosis, depression, and the postictal state are all reported as confusion, and the first task is always to establish which is present.

The second difficulty is that the highest-stakes diagnoses in this chapter present as the lowest-drama findings. Nonconvulsive status epilepticus presents as a drowsy patient. Posterior circulation stroke presents as dizziness. Wernicke encephalopathy presents as confusion in someone whose confusion is already being attributed to alcohol. Hypoactive delirium presents as a patient who is finally settled and causing no difficulty. In each case, the presentation that ought to trigger urgency instead triggers relief.

Three principles run through the chapter.

Establish the baseline before interpreting the present. Acute change is the defining feature of delirium and the reference point for everything else, and it cannot be established without a collateral history.

Glucose, oxygen, and thiamine come before diagnosis. Three treatable causes of altered consciousness can be excluded or corrected in minutes and are the first actions in every case.

Localise before you name. Chapter 2 argued that diagnostic error is dominated by hypotheses never generated. In neurology, localisation is the discipline that generates them, and a clinician who has localised the lesion has already narrowed the differential enormously.

10.1 Delirium: Pathophysiology, Prevention Bundles, and Pharmacology

10.1.1 Definition and why the definition matters

Delirium is an acute disturbance of attention and awareness, developing over hours to days, representing a change from baseline, fluctuating in severity, and accompanied by additional cognitive disturbance, occurring as a physiological consequence of a medical condition, substance, or withdrawal.

Four elements of that definition do practical work.

Attention is the core deficit, not memory or orientation. A patient who is oriented but cannot sustain attention through a simple task is delirious. Testing orientation alone misses a large proportion of cases.

Acuity and change from baseline distinguish delirium from dementia. This requires knowing the baseline, which requires a collateral history.

Fluctuation means a single normal assessment does not exclude the diagnosis. A patient lucid on the ward round may be delirious at four in the afternoon, and the nursing observations across the day are more informative than the physician's single encounter.

It is a physiological consequence of somcthing. Dclirium is a symptom of an underlying disturbance, in the same way that a fever is. Diagnosing delirium without seeking its cause is an incomplctc diagnosis.

10.1.2 Pathophysiology

No single mechanism explains delirium, and the current understanding is of several interacting pathways operating on a vulnerable brain.

Neuroinflammation. Peripheral inflammatory signalling from infection, tissue injury, or surgery is transmitted to the central nervous system, increases blood-brain barrier permeability, and activates microglia. The resulting central inflammatory response disrupts neuronal function. This mechanism explains why delirium accompanies conditions with no direct neurological involvement, and why an ageing brain with existing microglial priming is more susceptible.

Neurotransmitter imbalance. The most consistently implicated is cholinergic deficiency, which explains the potency of anticholinergic medications as precipitants and the association between delirium and conditions of reduced cholinergic reserve. Relative dopaminergic excess is also implicated, which provides the rationale, though not the evidence, for antipsychotic use. Gamma-aminobutyric acid, serotonin, noradrenaline, and melatonin systems are all involved.

Impaired oxidative metabolism. Reduced cerebral oxidative capacity from hypoxia, hypoperfusion, hypoglycaemia, or mitochondrial dysfunction impairs neuronal function directly.

Aberrant stress response. Sustained cortisol elevation with loss of normal feedback contributes, which links delirium to the physiology of acute illness generally.

Network disconnection. Functional imaging and electroencephalographic studies show disrupted connectivity between the networks subserving attention and awareness, which is a description of the final common pathway rather than an independent mechanism.

Circadian disruption, which is both a consequence and a contributor, and which explains the value of sleep-protective interventions.

10.1.3 The vulnerability model

The most useful clinical framework, established by Inouye and colleagues, holds that delirium arises from the interaction of **predisposing vulnerability** and **precipitating insult**, and that the relationship is multiplicative.

A highly vulnerable patient, meaning one with advanced age, established cognitive impairment, frailty, sensory impairment, and polypharmacy, develops delirium from a trivial insult such as constipation or a single dose of a sedative. A robust patient requires a major insult such as sepsis or major surgery.

The practical consequences are two. Vulnerability is assessable on admission and identifies who needs prevention. And in a highly vulnerable patient, the precipitant may be so minor that clinicians dismiss it, which leads to the erroneous conclusion that no cause was found.

Chapter 8, section 8.4.2, listed the predisposing and precipitating factors in the perioperative context, and the same lists apply to medical admissions.

10.1.4 Subtypes and detection

Hyperactive delirium, with agitation, restlessness, and hallucination, is the minority presentation and the one that gets recognised because it disrupts the ward.

Hypoactive delirium, with withdrawal, drowsiness, reduced movement, and reduced speech, is the more common presentation, carries a worse prognosis, and is missed in a large majority of cases. The patient is quiet, compliant, and causing no trouble, and is frequently described as tired or depressed.

Mixed presentations fluctuate between the two.

Detection requires systematic screening with a validated instrument applied at defined intervals by nursing staff, not physician suspicion. Brief tools suitable for ward use include the 4AT and short forms of the Confusion Assessment Method, with an adapted version for ventilated patients. The instrument matters less than the systematic application.

Every case requires a search for the cause. The systematic review should cover infection, medication including recent additions and withdrawals, metabolic and electrolyte disturbance, hypoxia, pain, urinary retention, constipation, alcohol and sedative withdrawal, and a neurological event. Sections 10.4, 10.5, and 10.6 address the last of these, and the point deserves emphasis: **new delirium can be the presentation of stroke, of nonconvulsive status, and of Wernicke encephalopathy**, and none of these will be found unless considered.

10.1.5 Prevention

Multicomponent nonpharmacological prevention has the strongest evidence in delirium, with meta-analyses showing meaningful reductions in incidence and in falls. The components are individually mundane, which is precisely why they are omitted.

- Orientation and cognitive engagement, with visible clocks and calendars.
- Sleep protection, including clustering of overnight observations and reduction of nocturnal noise and light. This requires unit-level change rather than individual effort.
- Early and repeated mobilisation.
- Sensory optimisation: glasses and hearing aids present, clean, and worn. This is close to free and routinely neglected.
- Hydration and nutrition.
- Adequate analgesia, since untreated pain is a potent precipitant.
- Avoidance of deliriogenic drugs, principally benzodiazepines and anticholinergics.
- Removal of tethers: catheters, lines, telemetry, and restraints.
- Bowel and bladder care.

In critical care settings, bundled approaches combining pain assessment, spontaneous awakening and breathing trials, analgesia and sedation choice, delirium monitoring, early mobility, and family engagement have been associated with improved outcomes, and are the intensive care expression of the same principles.

10.1.6 Pharmacology: an honest account

This section states clearly what the evidence supports, because practice diverges from it widely.

Antipsychotics do not prevent delirium. Trials of prophylactic haloperidol and of atypical agents have not shown reduced incidence.

Antipsychotics do not shorten delirium or improve outcomes. A large randomised trial in critically ill patients comparing haloperidol, ziprasidone, and placebo found no difference in days alive without delirium or coma, and systematic reviews in other settings have reached similar conclusions.

Antipsychotics may be appropriate for severe agitation or distress where the patient is at risk of harm to themselves or others, or where distress is severe. This is symptomatic treatment of agitation, not treatment of delirium, and the distinction should be explicit in the notes. Where used, the principle is a single agent, the lowest effective dose, the shortest duration, and daily review for discontinuation. Attend to QT interval, extrapyramidal effects, and the increased mortality associated with antipsychotic use in older adults with dementia.

Benzodiazepines worsen delirium and should be avoided except where they are the specific treatment: alcohol and sedative-hypnotic withdrawal, and certain toxidromes.

Physical restraint worsens delirium, prolongs it, and causes injury. It should be a last resort with a documented rationale and frequent review.

Cholinesterase inhibitors are not indicated. A trial of rivastigmine in critically ill delirious patients was stopped early because of increased mortality in the treatment group. This is worth remembering because the cholinergic hypothesis makes the intervention seem obviously reasonable, and it is not.

Dexmedetomidine has evidence for lower delirium rates compared with benzodiazepine-based sedation in ventilated patients, and its use is an intensive care decision rather than a ward one.

Melatonin and melatonin receptor agonists have been studied for prevention with mixed results. They are low risk, and their use is defensible but not established.

10.1.7 Prognosis and communication

Delirium is not benign. It is associated with increased mortality, prolonged stay, functional decline, institutionalisation, and an increased subsequent risk of dementia. A meaningful proportion of patients have persistent symptoms at discharge and beyond, and the assumption that delirium resolves by the time the patient leaves is frequently wrong.

Families should be told what is happening, told that it is common and usually reversible, told that fluctuation is expected, and involved in the nonpharmacological measures, since a familiar presence is among the more effective interventions available. Patients frequently recall the experience, including hallucinations and fear, and should be offered the opportunity to discuss it afterwards.

Document the cognitive status at discharge, and state explicitly whether the delirium has resolved. Chapter 3, section 3.7.4, addressed the general failure to record cognition in usable form, and delirium that has not resolved is a specific and important discharge finding.

10.2 Coma and Impaired Consciousness: A Systematic Bedside Approach

10.2.1 The first three minutes

Coma is a medical emergency in which the assessment and the treatment proceed simultaneously.

Airway, breathing, circulation. A patient with a reduced conscious level may not protect their airway, and positioning, suction, and airway support precede everything.

Capillary glucose. Hypoglycaemia is common, rapidly fatal, immediately reversible, and mimics almost any neurological presentation including focal deficit. It is checked in every case, without exception.

Thiamine before glucose in any patient in whom thiamine deficiency is plausible, which includes alcohol use, malnutrition, malabsorption, hyperemesis, and prolonged parenteral nutrition. Administering glucose to a thiamine-deficient patient can precipitate Wernicke encephalopathy, and the sequence matters.

Oxygenation and ventilation. Hypoxia and hypercapnia both cause reduced consciousness and both are correctable.

Consider opioid toxicity where the pupils are pinpoint and the respiratory rate is depressed, and give naloxone with the recognition that it precipitates withdrawal in dependent patients and that its duration of action is shorter than that of many opioids.

Consider the immediately reversible structural emergency, meaning raised intracranial pressure with impending herniation, discussed in section 10.2.5.

10.2.2 Describing the conscious level

Terms such as stuporous, obtunded, and lethargic are used inconsistently and transmit little. **Describe what the patient does in response to defined stimuli** rather than applying a label.

The Glasgow Coma Scale remains the common currency, and its limitations should be understood: it was derived for traumatic brain injury, the verbal component is uninterpretable in intubated or aphasic patients, and identical total scores can reflect very different clinical states. **Always record the three components separately** rather than only the total.

The FOUR score was developed to address several of these limitations, incorporating eye response, motor response, brainstem reflexes, and respiration, and is usable in intubated patients.

10.2.3 The examination that localises

Four elements, examined systematically, distinguish structural from metabolic causes and localise structural lesions.

Pupils. The pupillary pathways are relatively resistant to metabolic insult, which produces the single most useful rule in this section: **preserved pupillary light reflexes in a deeply comatose patient point strongly to a metabolic or toxic cause.**

Specific patterns: **pinpoint and reactive** suggests pontine lesion or opioid effect; **midposition and fixed** suggests midbrain involvement; **unilateral dilated and unreactive** in a patient with declining consciousness suggests third nerve compression from uncal herniation and is an emergency; **bilaterally fixed and dilated** suggests severe midbrain injury, though it also occurs with anticholinergic toxicity, severe hypothermia, and after certain drugs, so the finding is not by itself a statement of irreversibility.

Eye movements. Spontaneous roving conjugate movements imply an intact brainstem. Conjugate gaze deviation suggests a hemispheric lesion, with the eyes typically looking toward the side of a destructive hemispheric lesion and away from a seizure focus. The oculocephalic response, and where the cervical spine is cleared and the finding is needed, caloric testing, assess brainstem integrity, and should be performed by a clinician trained in their interpretation.

Motor response. Asymmetry of spontaneous movement, of withdrawal, or of tone indicates a structural lesion. Decorticate flexion suggests dysfunction above the midbrain; decerebrate extension suggests lower midbrain or upper pontine involvement; the progression from one to the other indicates deterioration.

Respiratory pattern. Of limited localising value in practice and frequently confounded by sedation and by metabolic derangement, but Cheyne-Stokes breathing, central hyperventilation, and ataxic breathing patterns each suggest particular levels.

10.2.4 Structural against metabolic

The distinction directs the immediate investigation.

Favouring a structural cause: focal or asymmetric findings; cranial nerve abnormalities; abnormal pupillary responses; abnormal brainstem reflexes; a progressive course; and a history of trauma, headache, or focal onset.

Favouring a metabolic or toxic cause: symmetric findings; preserved pupillary reflexes; the presence of asterixis, tremor, or multifocal myoclonus; a fluctuating course; and a background of organ failure, drug exposure, or endocrine disturbance.

The distinction is not absolute. Metabolic causes, particularly hypoglycaemia and hyperosmolar states, can produce focal signs, and structural lesions can present symmetrically. It is a prior rather than a conclusion.

10.2.5 Herniation syndromes

Recognising these determines whether the patient survives the next thirty minutes.

Uncal herniation. The medial temporal lobe displaces over the tentorial edge, compressing the third nerve and the midbrain. The classic sequence is a progressively dilating, unreactive pupil ipsilateral to the lesion, declining consciousness, and then contralateral hemiparesis, though ipsilateral hemiparesis occurs when the opposite cerebral peduncle is compressed against the tentorium.

Central herniation. Downward displacement of the diencephalon, producing a rostral to caudal deterioration through progressively lower brainstem levels.

Subfalcine herniation. Cingulate gyrus displacement beneath the falx, which may compress the anterior cerebral artery and produce lower limb weakness.

Tonsillar herniation. Cerebellar tonsils through the foramen magnum, compressing the medulla, producing bradycardia, hypertension, and respiratory arrest.

The Cushing response, meaning hypertension with bradycardia and irregular respiration, is a late sign of raised intracranial pressure and demands immediate action.

Immediate measures while arranging definitive management: elevate the head of the bed to approximately thirty degrees, ensure the neck is not obstructing venous drainage, optimise oxygenation and ventilation, treat fever and seizures, avoid hypotonic fluids, and consider hyperosmolar therapy with mannitol or hypertonic saline. Neurosurgical involvement is immediate, not after imaging is reported.

10.2.6 Investigation

Computed tomography of the head is the first imaging study in almost all cases of unexplained coma, principally to exclude haemorrhage, mass effect, and hydrocephalus. A normal study does not exclude a structural cause, and early ischaemic stroke, particularly in the posterior fossa, is frequently invisible.

Magnetic resonance imaging is superior for ischaemia, posterior fossa pathology, encephalitis, and diffuse axonal injury, and should follow where the diagnosis remains unclear.

Lumbar puncture where meningitis, encephalitis, or subarachnoid haemorrhage is suspected, after appropriate consideration of raised intracranial pressure. **Do not delay antimicrobial therapy for suspected bacterial meningitis while awaiting imaging or lumbar puncture.**

Electroencephalography. This is the investigation most often omitted and the omission is consequential. **Unexplained persistent impairment of consciousness requires an electroencephalogram**, because nonconvulsive status epilepticus is a recognised and treatable cause that is invisible to every other test. Section 10.5.5 develops this.

Laboratory studies covering glucose, electrolytes including sodium and calcium, renal and hepatic function, ammonia, thyroid function, blood gas with carboxyhaemoglobin where relevant, toxicology, and cultures.

Consider the diagnoses that are missed: nonconvulsive status; Wernicke encephalopathy; central nervous system infection; posterior reversible encephalopathy syndrome; autoimmune encephalitis; basilar artery occlusion; and, in a patient who appears unresponsive but is not, **locked-in syndrome**, in which a ventral pontine lesion abolishes movement while consciousness and vertical eye movement are preserved. Every apparently unresponsive patient should be asked to look up and to blink, because failing to do so leaves a fully conscious person unable to communicate.

10.3 Localisation: Cortex, Brainstem, Cord, Root, Nerve, Junction, and Muscle

10.3.1 Why localisation comes first

Neurological diagnosis proceeds in two steps, and reversing them produces most diagnostic error in this domain. **First establish where the lesion is; then establish what it is.** The differential for a lesion at each level is short and largely non-overlapping, so localisation converts an unbounded problem into a manageable one.

Three discriminators do most of the work, and a clinician who applies them consistently will localise correctly in the great majority of cases.

Upper against lower motor neurone signs. Upper motor neurone lesions produce weakness with increased tone, brisk reflexes, extensor plantar response, and a pyramidal distribution favouring extensors in the arm and flexors in the leg. Lower motor neurone lesions produce weakness with reduced tone, reduced or absent reflexes, wasting, and fasciculation. The distinction separates lesions above the anterior horn cell from those at or below it.

Presence or absence of sensory involvement. Neuromuscular junction disorders and myopathies do not cause sensory loss. If sensory findings are present, the lesion is not at the junction or in muscle.

The distribution. Whether the pattern is hemispheric, crossed, level-defined, dermatomal, length-dependent, or proximal and symmetric.

10.3.2 Cortex

Features. Contralateral deficit, and, crucially, the presence of **cortical signs**: aphasia, neglect, apraxia, agnosia, cortical sensory loss such as astereognosis and impaired two-point discrimination, and visual field defects. Seizures arise from cortex. Consciousness is preserved unless the lesion is bilateral or produces mass effect.

Vascular territories. Middle cerebral artery territory produces face and arm predominant weakness with cortical signs, with aphasia in dominant hemisphere lesions and neglect in non-dominant. Anterior cerebral artery territory produces leg predominant weakness. Posterior cerebral artery territory produces visual field loss with relative motor sparing.

The key discriminator against subcortical lesions is the presence of cortical signs. Their absence in a dense hemiparesis suggests a subcortical lesion.

10.3.3 Subcortical structures and internal capsule

A small lesion in the internal capsule produces a **pure motor hemiparesis** affecting face, arm, and leg approximately equally, without cortical signs, because the descending fibres are densely packed there. Similar small vessel lesions produce the other classical lacunar syndromes: pure sensory stroke from thalamic lesions, sensorimotor stroke, ataxic hemiparesis, and the dysarthria clumsy hand syndrome.

The clinical significance is that a dense hemiparesis without aphasia or neglect suggests a small deep lesion rather than a large cortical one, which has implications for aetiology and for prognosis.

10.3.4 Brainstem

The defining feature is crossed findings: an ipsilateral cranial nerve deficit with a contralateral deficit of the body. This occurs because cranial nerve nuclei act ipsilaterally at their level while the long tracts have not yet decussated or have already done so.

Additional features pointing to brainstem involvement: diplopia, dysarthria, dysphagia, vertigo, nystagmus, ataxia, Horner syndrome, hiccup, and impaired consciousness through involvement of the reticular activating system.

Practical rule. Any combination of cranial nerve findings with long tract findings, or any of the symptoms above occurring together, should be treated as brainstem until proven otherwise, and posterior circulation stroke should be considered urgently. Chapter 9, section 9.5, addressed the specific problem of isolated vertigo as a brainstem presentation.

10.3.5 Cerebellum

Features. Ipsilateral limb ataxia, intention tremor, dysdiadochokinesis, nystagmus, dysarthria of scanning quality, and truncal or gait ataxia. Crucially, **there is no weakness and no sensory loss**, and reflexes are normal or pendular.

A patient who cannot stand or walk unaided but has full power and normal sensation has a cerebellar or vestibular problem, and cerebellar stroke is the diagnosis not to miss because of the risk of swelling and brainstem compression.

10.3.6 Spinal cord

Features. A **sensory level** is the cardinal finding and should be sought explicitly in any patient with bilateral leg symptoms. Bilateral involvement, bladder and bowel dysfunction, and upper motor neurone signs below the lesion with lower motor neurone signs at the level.

Specific syndromes. Complete transverse lesions produce loss of all modalities below the level. **Brown-Séquard** hemisection produces ipsilateral motor and dorsal column loss with contralateral spinothalamic loss. **Central cord** syndrome, classically after hyperextension injury in a spondylotic neck, produces disproportionate upper limb weakness. **Anterior cord** syndrome spares dorsal column function. **Cauda equina** syndrome produces lower motor neurone signs, saddle anaesthesia, and sphincter disturbance, and is a surgical emergency.

The emergency to exclude is cord compression, from malignancy, abscess, haematoma, or disc. New back pain with any neurological symptom, urinary retention, or saddle sensory change requires urgent magnetic resonance imaging of the whole spine, not a plain radiograph and not a delay until the morning. In a patient with an epidural catheter, Chapter 8, section 8.6.5, applies.

10.3.7 Nerve root

Features. Pain in a **radicular** distribution, sensory disturbance in a dermatome, weakness in a myotome, and reduction or loss of the corresponding reflex. Symptoms are frequently exacerbated by manoeuvres that increase root tension or intraspinal pressure, including coughing and straight leg raising.

Because muscles receive innervation from more than one root, single root lesions cause weakness that is partial rather than complete, which distinguishes them from peripheral nerve lesions.

10.3.8 Peripheral nerve

Mononeuropathy produces deficit in the distribution of a single named nerve, which differs from the dermatomal and myotomal patterns of a root lesion. Common examples encountered in hospitalised patients include ulnar neuropathy at the elbow from positioning, peroneal neuropathy at the fibular head from prolonged bed rest or a cast, radial neuropathy from compression, and lateral cutaneous nerve of thigh compression.

Polyneuropathy is typically **length-dependent**, producing symmetric distal sensory loss in a glove and stocking distribution with distal weakness and lost ankle reflexes, and progressing proximally as it worsens.

Acute inflammatory demyelinating polyradiculoneuropathy, meaning Guillain-Barré syndrome, is the important acute presentation: ascending, relatively symmetric weakness with areflexia, frequently with preceding infection, and with the risks of respiratory failure and autonomic instability. **Monitor forced vital capacity, not oxygen saturation**, for the reasons in Chapter 9, section 9.2.5. Autonomic involvement causes arrhythmia and blood pressure lability and is a cause of death.

Critical illness polyneuropathy and myopathy develop in patients after prolonged critical illness and present as failure to wean or as profound weakness on recovery.

10.3.9 Neuromuscular junction

Features. Weakness that is **fatigable**, worsening with sustained effort and improving with rest. **No sensory involvement.** Reflexes are typically preserved. Ocular and bulbar muscles are frequently involved early, producing ptosis, diplopia, dysarthria, and dysphagia.

Myasthenia gravis worsens with certain drugs, including several antibiotics, notably aminoglycosides and fluoroquinolones, magnesium, and some cardiac agents, and this is a recurrent and preventable cause of inpatient deterioration. **Myasthenic crisis** is respiratory failure requiring ventilatory support, and again is monitored by vital capacity.

Lambert-Eaton myasthenic syndrome produces proximal weakness with reduced reflexes that facilitate after brief exercise, and is associated with malignancy.

Botulism produces descending paralysis with prominent autonomic and pupillary involvement.

10.3.10 Muscle

Features. Proximal, symmetric weakness without sensory involvement, with preserved or reduced reflexes proportional to the weakness, and frequently with elevated creatine kinase. Patients report difficulty rising from a chair, climbing stairs, and lifting objects above the head.

Causes relevant to inpatient practice include inflammatory myopathies, corticosteroid myopathy, statin-associated myopathy, thyroid disease, electrolyte disturbance including severe hypokalaemia and hypophosphataemia, rhabdomyolysis, and critical illness myopathy.

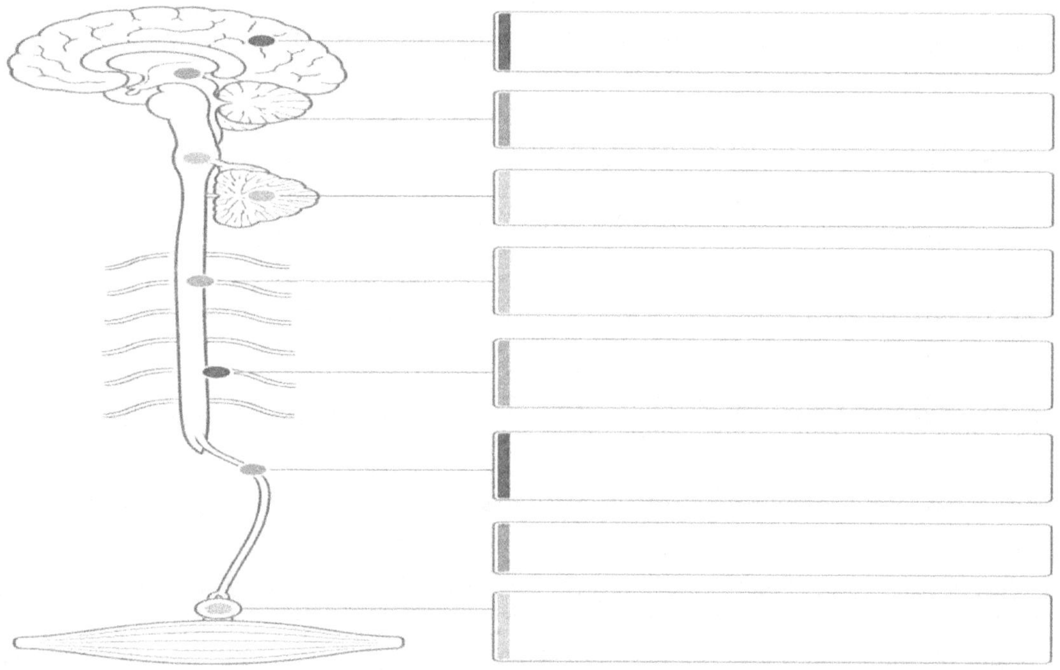

10.4 Stroke and Transient Ischaemic Attack on the Ward

10.4.1 Why in-hospital stroke is treated worse

Stroke occurring in a patient already in hospital carries worse outcomes and substantially longer delays to imaging and treatment than stroke presenting from the community. This is counterintuitive, since the patient is already surrounded by clinicians, and the reasons are worth understanding because each is correctable.

Attribution. The patient is already unwell, often sedated, postoperative, delirious, or receiving analgesia, so new neurological findings are attributed to the existing illness or its treatment. This is the anchoring mechanism from Chapter 2, section 2.4.3.

Detection delay. Ward observations do not include neurological assessment at a frequency sufficient to establish onset time, so the patient is frequently found with a deficit of unknown duration.

Process delay. The community pathway is highly optimised and begins with ambulance pre-notification. The inpatient pathway frequently has no equivalent, and the ward team must improvise access to imaging and to stroke expertise.

Contraindications. Recent surgery, anticoagulation, and active bleeding are more common in inpatients, and their presence is sometimes assumed to preclude any intervention when in fact it precludes only intravenous thrombolysis.

The correctives are an in-hospital stroke pathway with the same activation mechanism as the emergency pathway, ward staff trained to recognise and escalate, and documented neurological observations at a frequency appropriate to risk in patients at elevated risk.

10.4.2 Recognition

Public recognition tools capture face, arm, and speech, and extended versions add balance and eyes, which is important because the original tools miss posterior circulation events. Chapter 9, section 9.5, addressed dizziness as a stroke presentation.

Presentations easily missed in a hospitalised patient: isolated confusion or delirium; isolated vertigo or gait instability; a reduced conscious level; new dysphagia; visual field loss, which the patient may not report; and neglect, which by its nature the patient does not complain of.

Establish the time last known well, which is the operative variable, not the time the deficit was noticed. For an inpatient this requires asking nursing staff, family, and anyone who interacted with the patient, and it should be pursued actively rather than recorded as unknown.

10.4.3 Mimics

Before activating a pathway, and certainly before administering thrombolysis, consider the mimics, though the consideration should not delay imaging.

Hypoglycaemia, which can produce dense focal deficit and is excluded in seconds.

Seizure with postictal deficit, meaning Todd paresis, which resolves over hours.

Migraine with aura.

Recrudescence of an old deficit in the context of sepsis, metabolic derangement, or fever. This is important and common: a patient with a previous stroke develops apparent recurrence when systemically unwell, and the deficit resolves as the systemic illness is treated. It is a diagnosis of exclusion.

Functional neurological disorder.

Structural lesions including tumour, subdural haematoma, and abscess, which imaging identifies.

10.4.4 Treatment windows

Intravenous thrombolysis is indicated within a defined window from symptom onset, conventionally up to four and a half hours in most guidelines, with eligibility determined by imaging, blood pressure, coagulation status, and a list of contraindications in which recent major surgery features prominently.

Endovascular thrombectomy for large vessel occlusion has transformed outcomes and has a longer window. Standard eligibility extends to six hours from onset, and selected patients identified by perfusion or clinical-core mismatch imaging benefit up to twenty-four hours. This matters enormously for inpatients, because a postoperative patient ineligible for thrombolysis may still be an excellent thrombectomy candidate, and the assumption that recent surgery precludes intervention is a serious error.

Stroke of unknown onset, including on waking, may still be treatable, with imaging-based selection using mismatch between diffusion and fluid-attenuated inversion recovery sequences, or perfusion imaging, identifying patients likely to benefit.

The operational consequence for a hospitalist is simple: activate the stroke pathway and let the stroke service determine eligibility. Deciding at the bedside that a patient is ineligible, and therefore not activating, is the mechanism by which treatable inpatients are not treated.

10.4.5 Transient ischaemic attack

Transient ischaemic attack is a warning with a short fuse, and the risk of subsequent stroke is highest in the first days.

Risk scores have been used historically to stratify urgency, and their discrimination is modest; current guidance in most systems is for urgent specialist assessment and investigation of all patients rather than score-based triage.

Investigation should establish the vascular territory and the mechanism: brain imaging, vascular imaging of the extracranial and intracranial circulation, cardiac rhythm assessment of adequate duration to detect paroxysmal atrial fibrillation, and assessment of vascular risk factors.

Early dual antiplatelet therapy for a defined short period, followed by single agent therapy, reduces recurrent stroke after minor stroke or high-risk transient ischaemic attack, with the benefit concentrated early and the bleeding risk increasing with duration. The regimen and duration should follow current guidance.

Carotid intervention for significant symptomatic stenosis should be performed early, and the benefit falls with delay.

10.4.6 Acute stroke ward care

Several elements of early care influence outcome and are the hospitalist's responsibility where a stroke unit is not immediately available.

Dysphagia screening before anything is given by mouth, including medications and water. This is the single most important early nursing and medical action, and aspiration pneumonia is a leading cause of post-stroke death.

Blood pressure management differs according to whether thrombolysis was given and whether the stroke is ischaemic or haemorrhagic, and current guidance should be followed precisely; aggressive lowering in untreated ischaemic stroke may extend the infarct.

Glucose and temperature control, both of which worsen outcome when deranged.

Venous thromboembolism prophylaxis, with intermittent pneumatic compression established as beneficial in immobile stroke patients and pharmacological prophylaxis determined by the stroke type and by bleeding risk.

Mobilisation, which should be early but not extreme; trial evidence found that very early, high-intensity, high-dose mobilisation produced worse outcomes than usual early care, so the target is frequent short mobilisation beginning early rather than maximal intensity.

Early rehabilitation assessment, addressed in Chapter 3, section 3.6.

10.5 Seizure, Status Epilepticus, and Nonconvulsive States

10.5.1 The first question: provoked or unprovoked

A seizure in a hospitalised patient is usually **provoked**, meaning it occurs as a consequence of an acute systemic or cerebral insult, and the management is directed at the provocation rather than at long-term antiseizure therapy.

Common provocations in inpatients: alcohol withdrawal, which characteristically occurs within the first days of admission and is a leading cause; benzodiazepine and other sedative withdrawal; hypoglycaemia; hyponatraemia, particularly when it has fallen rapidly; hypocalcaemia and hypomagnesaemia; drugs that lower the seizure threshold; sepsis; hypoxia; uraemia; hepatic failure; hypertensive encephalopathy including posterior reversible encephalopathy syndrome; and any acute structural event including stroke, haemorrhage, tumour, abscess, and trauma.

Drugs to review specifically: several antibiotic classes, notably carbapenems and fourth-generation cephalosporins in renal impairment; tramadol and pethidine; bupropion; certain antipsychotics and antidepressants; theophylline; and immunosuppressants including calcineurin inhibitors.

The practical implication is that a first seizure in hospital requires a systematic metabolic, toxicological, infective, and structural evaluation rather than a reflex prescription of an antiseizure medication.

10.5.2 Assessment of a first seizure

Establish, from a witness where possible, the events before, during, and after: any warning, the nature and progression of movements, whether there was head or eye deviation, the duration, the presence of lateral tongue biting or incontinence, and the duration and character of the recovery.

Distinguish from syncope, addressed in Chapter 9, section 9.4.1, noting that brief myoclonic jerking occurs in genuine syncope and is not evidence of seizure.

Consider psychogenic nonepileptic seizures, suggested by prolonged duration, asynchronous or side-to-side movements, pelvic thrusting, eye closure with resistance to opening, waxing and waning intensity, preserved awareness during bilateral motor activity, and absence of postictal confusion. These features are suggestive rather than definitive, the diagnosis requires specialist assessment, and patients with epilepsy may also have nonepileptic events.

Investigate with glucose, electrolytes including sodium, calcium, and magnesium, renal and hepatic function, toxicology and alcohol history, infection screen where indicated, brain imaging, and electroencephalography. Prolactin measurement has limited utility and a narrow timing window and is not recommended for routine use.

Todd paresis, the transient focal deficit following a seizure, resolves over hours and is a stroke mimic as noted in section 10.4.3.

10.5.3 Status epilepticus: definition and why the timing matters

The operational definition has two time points, and both are clinically meaningful.

At approximately five minutes of continuous convulsive seizure activity, or recurrent seizures without recovery of consciousness between them, treatment should begin. This threshold exists because most self-limiting seizures stop within a couple of minutes, so activity continuing at five minutes is unlikely to stop spontaneously.

At approximately thirty minutes, the risk of neuronal injury and long-term consequences rises substantially.

The physiological basis for urgency is that gamma-aminobutyric acid receptors are internalised during prolonged seizure activity while excitatory receptors are trafficked to the membrane, so **benzodiazepines become progressively less effective the longer the seizure continues**. Early treatment is therefore not merely preferable; it is more likely to work.

10.5.4 Treatment

First line: a benzodiazepine, adequately dosed. The commonest and most consequential error in status epilepticus management is underdosing. Repeated small doses given cautiously are less effective and no safer than a correct dose given promptly. Intravenous lorazepam, intravenous diazepam, and intramuscular midazolam are all effective, and intramuscular midazolam is a valid choice where intravenous access is not immediately available, having performed at least as well as intravenous therapy in a large prehospital trial when the time to access is accounted for. A second dose is given if seizures continue after a short interval.

Concurrent measures: airway, oxygen, monitoring, capillary glucose, intravenous access, thiamine where indicated, and correction of any identified metabolic cause. Hyponatraemic and hypoglycaemic seizures will not respond durably to antiseizure medication without correction of the cause.

Second line: an intravenous antiseizure medication. A large randomised trial compared levetiracetam, fosphenytoin, and valproate in benzodiazepine-refractory status and found them broadly equivalent in efficacy and safety, with roughly half of patients responding. The choice can therefore be made on the basis of contraindications, availability, and interactions rather than on presumed superiority. Doses must be adequate; underdosing at this stage is as common as at the first.

Third line: anaesthetic agents with intubation and continuous electroencephalographic monitoring, in an intensive care setting. Refractory status requires early involvement of neurology and critical care, and the escalation should not be delayed while further boluses of second-line agents are tried.

Do not stop looking for the cause while treating. Status epilepticus is frequently the presentation of an acute structural or metabolic event, and treatment of the seizure without treatment of the cause fails.

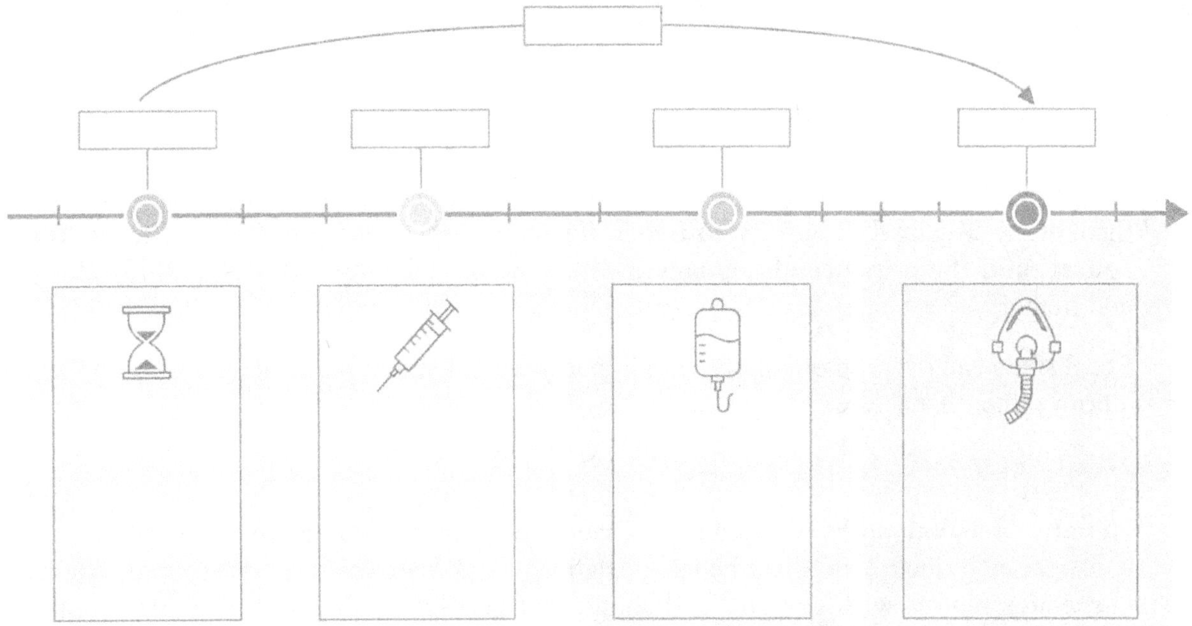

10.5.5 Nonconvulsive status epilepticus

This is the diagnosis this chapter most wants readers to remember, because it is common, treatable, and invisible without an electroencephalogram.

Consider it in:

- Any patient with **unexplained impairment of consciousness**, particularly where imaging and metabolic screening are unrevealing.
- A patient who **does not recover as expected after a convulsive seizure**. Persistent impairment beyond roughly twenty to thirty minutes after convulsions cease should raise the question, and a meaningful proportion of patients whose convulsive status has been treated remain in nonconvulsive status.
- A patient with **subtle motor phenomena**: rhythmic eyelid or facial twitching, sustained eye deviation, nystagmoid eye movements, or repetitive automatisms.
- A patient with **fluctuating confusion** without other explanation, particularly with a history of epilepsy, recent stroke, or structural brain disease.
- A patient with an unexplained **new behavioural or psychiatric presentation** in the context of brain injury.

Diagnosis requires electroencephalography, and where suspicion is high the study should be urgent rather than scheduled. Continuous monitoring is superior to a brief routine recording for detection.

Treatment follows similar principles to convulsive status, with the important qualification that the risks of aggressive treatment, particularly intubation and anaesthesia, must be weighed against the aetiology and prognosis, and this weighing requires neurological input.

10.6 Toxic-Metabolic Encephalopathies and Drug-Induced Syndromes

10.6.1 The general pattern

Toxic and metabolic encephalopathies share a characteristic clinical signature that distinguishes them from structural disease: **symmetric findings, preserved pupillary reflexes, fluctuating course, and the presence of movement phenomena** including asterixis, multifocal myoclonus, and tremor.

Focal signs can occur, particularly with hypoglycaemia and hyperosmolar states, so the pattern is a prior rather than a rule.

10.6.2 The principal metabolic causes

Hepatic encephalopathy. Graded by severity, precipitated by infection, gastrointestinal bleeding, constipation, electrolyte disturbance, sedatives, and dehydration. **Ammonia concentration correlates poorly with severity** and should not be used to diagnose, exclude, or monitor the condition, which is a common misuse. The diagnosis is clinical, and the priority is identifying the precipitant. Chapter 15 develops the management.

Uraemic encephalopathy, with asterixis, myoclonus, and, in severe cases, seizures.

Hyponatraemia, in which the rate of change matters more than the absolute value, and in which overly rapid correction causes osmotic demyelination. Chapter 12 develops the algorithm.

Hypernatraemia, hypercalcaemia, hypophosphataemia, and hypomagnesaemia.

Hypoglycaemia and hyperglycaemic states, including hyperosmolar hyperglycaemic state, addressed in Chapter 17.

Hypercapnia, which produces drowsiness, headache, and asterixis, and which is missed when oxygen saturation is normal or high. Chapter 14 addresses this.

Hypothyroidism and thyrotoxicosis, the latter presenting apathetically in older adults.

Adrenal insufficiency, addressed in Chapter 7, section 7.6.4.

10.6.3 Wernicke encephalopathy

This deserves separate treatment because it is common, devastating, easily prevented, and routinely missed.

The classical triad of confusion, ophthalmoplegia, and ataxia is present in a minority of cases. Most patients have one or two features, and confusion alone is a frequent presentation. Relying on the triad guarantees under-diagnosis.

Risk extends well beyond alcohol use: malnutrition of any cause, hyperemesis, bariatric surgery, malignancy, prolonged vomiting, dialysis, parenteral nutrition without supplementation, and severe systemic illness.

Treatment is high-dose parenteral thiamine, given promptly, for a defined course, at doses considerably higher than the oral preparations commonly prescribed. Oral thiamine is inadequate for treatment.

Give thiamine before glucose in at-risk patients, as noted in section 10.2.1.

The threshold for treatment should be very low, because thiamine is safe and inexpensive, and because untreated Wernicke encephalopathy progresses to an irreversible amnestic syndrome.

10.6.4 Drug-induced syndromes

Four hyperthermic and hypertonic syndromes are confused with one another, and distinguishing them determines treatment.

Serotonin syndrome. Onset within hours of a serotonergic drug being started, increased, or combined with another. Features: altered mental state, autonomic instability, and neuromuscular hyperactivity with **clonus and hyperreflexia that are greater in the lower limbs than the upper**. Clonus is the most useful single sign. Management is withdrawal of the offending agents, supportive care, benzodiazepines, and in severe cases cyproheptadine and cooling.

Neuroleptic malignant syndrome. Onset over days after a dopamine antagonist is started or increased, or a dopamine agonist withdrawn. Features: **lead-pipe rigidity that is generalised, hyporeflexia rather than hyperreflexia, marked hyperthermia, autonomic instability, and a**

substantially raised creatine kinase. Management is withdrawal of the offending agent, aggressive cooling and supportive care, and in severe cases dantrolene or dopamine agonists.

The discriminating features between the two are the reflexes and the tempo: hyperreflexia with clonus over hours suggests serotonin syndrome; rigidity with hyporeflexia over days suggests neuroleptic malignant syndrome.

Anticholinergic toxidrome. Confusion and agitation with dry flushed skin, dilated pupils, urinary retention, absent bowel sounds, and hyperthermia without sweating. It is common in hospitalised older adults on multiple agents with cumulative anticholinergic burden, and the treatment is removal of the agents.

Malignant hyperthermia, addressed in Chapter 8, section 8.1.2, which is triggered by specific anaesthetic agents.

10.6.5 Other drug-related presentations

Alcohol withdrawal, ranging from tremor and anxiety through hallucinosis and withdrawal seizures to delirium tremens, which carries significant mortality untreated. Treatment is benzodiazepines, ideally symptom-triggered against a validated scale, together with thiamine. Chapter 19 develops the management, and Chapter 8, section 8.4.5, made the point that benzodiazepines are the correct treatment here and the wrong one for delirium generally.

Opioid and sedative toxicity and withdrawal.

Antimicrobial neurotoxicity, particularly with cephalosporins in renal impairment, which produces encephalopathy, myoclonus, and nonconvulsive status, and which is entirely reversible on withdrawal and dose adjustment. This is worth specific vigilance because the patient population most likely to receive these agents is also the population in whom encephalopathy has many other plausible explanations.

Antiseizure medication effects, including behavioural change with levetiracetam and hyperammonaemic encephalopathy with valproate, the latter occurring with normal hepatic function and normal drug levels.

Corticosteroid-induced psychosis and mood disturbance.

Lithium toxicity, precipitated by dehydration, renal impairment, and interacting drugs.

Posterior reversible encephalopathy syndrome, presenting with headache, seizures, visual disturbance, and confusion in the context of hypertension, eclampsia, immunosuppressants, or cytotoxic agents, with characteristic imaging findings and reversibility when the precipitant is addressed.

10.7 Capacity Assessment in the Confused Patient

10.7.1 What capacity is

Decision-making capacity is the ability to make a particular decision at a particular time. Four features of that definition are frequently misunderstood and each error has consequences.

Capacity is decision-specific, not global. A patient may have capacity to decide about oral analgesia and lack it for a decision about major surgery, because the complexity and the stakes differ. A blanket statement that a patient lacks capacity is almost always wrong.

Capacity is time-specific. It fluctuates, particularly in delirium, and a patient assessed as lacking capacity in the evening may have it the following morning. Where a decision can wait, it should wait for a lucid interval.

Capacity is not determined by diagnosis. Dementia, delirium, psychiatric illness, and intellectual disability all raise the question but none answers it. The assessment is functional.

Disagreement with the recommendation is not evidence of incapacity. A patient may make a decision that clinicians consider unwise, and provided the four abilities below are intact, that decision must be respected. This is the single most important safeguard in the framework and the one most often circumvented, since capacity assessment is requested overwhelmingly when patients decline rather than when they consent.

10.7.2 The four abilities

The widely used functional standard, associated with Appelbaum and Grisso, requires that the patient can do four things.

Communicate a choice, and maintain it with sufficient consistency to be acted upon.

Understand the relevant information: the nature of the proposed intervention, the reasonably foreseeable benefits and risks, and the alternatives including doing nothing.

Appreciate the situation and its consequences, meaning apply that information to their own circumstances rather than merely reciting it. A patient who can accurately describe the risks of leaving hospital but believes those risks do not apply to them because they are not actually ill is failing at appreciation.

Reason with the information, meaning manipulate it in a way that shows a logical process connecting their values to their choice. The reasoning need not be one the clinician shares; it must be a process rather than an absence of one.

10.7.3 How to assess

Assessment is a structured conversation, and it is within the competence of the treating team. **Capacity assessment is not a psychiatric monopoly**, and referring every question to psychiatry both delays care and misallocates expertise. Psychiatric input is valuable where the presence of mental illness complicates the assessment, where the stakes are very high, or where the assessment is contested.

The technique:

- **Optimise the conditions first.** Correct reversible contributors: pain, hypoxia, hypoglycaemia, sedating medication, and delirium. Ensure hearing aids and glasses are used, use an interpreter where needed, and choose a time of day when the patient is at their best.

- **Give the information properly**, in plain language, in small pieces, with repetition, and in writing where helpful.
- **Assess each of the four abilities explicitly** with open questions. Ask the patient to explain the situation in their own words, to describe what would happen if they declined, and to explain how they reached their decision.
- **Document what you asked and what the patient said**, not merely your conclusion. A note stating that the patient lacks capacity, without the evidence, is unusable by anyone else and is indefensible if challenged.

10.7.4 When capacity is absent

The framework varies by jurisdiction and readers must know their local law, which differs substantially between systems.

Common elements across most frameworks: a documented determination that capacity is absent for the specific decision; identification of a valid advance directive or advance decision, which where applicable and valid takes precedence; identification of the appropriate surrogate decision maker, whether appointed by the patient or determined by a statutory hierarchy; and a decision made either on the standard of what the patient would have wanted, described as substituted judgement, or on the standard of the patient's best interests, with jurisdictions differing in which they apply and in how the patient's known wishes and values feed into it.

Additional principles with wide acceptance: the least restrictive option that achieves the purpose should be chosen; the patient should be involved in the decision to the greatest extent they are able, even where they cannot make it; and in a genuine emergency, treatment necessary to preserve life may proceed without consent where the patient lacks capacity and no valid refusal exists.

Practical points that recur. A patient wishing to leave against medical advice requires a capacity assessment, and if capacity is present the discharge should be managed as well as possible rather than refused, as described in Chapter 3, section 3.7.3. Family members do not automatically have decision-making authority in all jurisdictions, and their role should be established rather than assumed. And a capacity determination should be revisited as the clinical situation changes rather than treated as permanent.

Chapter 20 develops advance care planning, surrogate decision making, and the ethical framework more fully.

Chapter Summary

- **Establish the baseline, then check glucose, oxygen, and thiamine, then localise.** Confusion is a summary of several distinct states with different differentials.
- **Delirium is a symptom of an underlying disturbance**, with attention as its core deficit and fluctuation as a defining feature. Hypoactive delirium is commoner, worse, and routinely missed. **Antipsychotics neither prevent nor shorten it**, cholinesterase inhibitors have caused harm, and benzodiazepines worsen it except in withdrawal.
- In coma, **preserved pupillary light reflexes in a deeply unconscious patient point strongly to a metabolic or toxic cause.** Record the components of the coma scale separately. Ask every apparently unresponsive patient to look up, because locked-in syndrome is otherwise missed.

- **Unexplained persistent impairment of consciousness requires an electroencephalogram**, because nonconvulsive status is treatable and invisible to every other test.
- **Localise before naming.** Three discriminators do most of the work: upper against lower motor neurone signs, presence or absence of sensory involvement, and distribution. Junction and muscle disorders never cause sensory loss.
- **In-hospital stroke is treated later and worse than community stroke** through attribution, detection delay, and process delay. Activate the pathway and let the stroke service determine eligibility; recent surgery precludes thrombolysis, not thrombectomy.
- **Treat status epilepticus at five minutes**, because benzodiazepine efficacy falls as receptors are internalised, and **underdosing is the commonest error at every stage.** Second-line agents are broadly equivalent.
- **The Wernicke triad is present in a minority.** Treat on suspicion with high-dose parenteral thiamine, and give it before glucose.
- Distinguish serotonin syndrome from neuroleptic malignant syndrome by **reflexes and tempo**: clonus and hyperreflexia over hours against rigidity and hyporeflexia over days.
- **Capacity is decision-specific, time-specific, functional, and not refuted by an unwise choice.** Assess the four abilities explicitly, document what was said rather than the conclusion, and recognise that the treating team can and should perform the assessment.

Review Questions

1. A 79-year-old admitted with pneumonia is drowsy, withdrawn, and eating little on the third day. The nurse reports she is settled and comfortable. Explain why this presentation concerns you, state your assessment, and list the causes you would systematically exclude.
2. A patient is deeply unconscious with symmetric, briskly reactive pupils, intact corneal reflexes, and no focal motor asymmetry. State what this pattern suggests, what it does not exclude, and your investigation sequence.
3. A patient has weakness of the right arm and leg with a normal-appearing face, no aphasia, no neglect, and brisk reflexes on the right with an extensor plantar. Localise the lesion, justify each element of your reasoning, and state what you would exclude first.
4. A postoperative patient on day two is found with a dense left hemiparesis of unknown onset. A colleague states that recent surgery rules out any intervention. Explain why this is wrong and what you would do.
5. A patient with delirium is refusing intravenous antibiotics for a serious infection. Set out how you would assess capacity, what you would document, and how your action differs depending on the outcome.

CHAPTER 11: Fever, Inflammation, and the Hospitalised Host

Learning Objectives

After studying this chapter, the reader should be able to:

1. Describe thermoregulation and the mechanism of fever, distinguish fever from hyperthermia, and interpret the temperature record including its measurement limitations.
2. Evaluate fever in a returning traveller using incubation period, geography, and exposure, and identify the diagnoses that must be excluded urgently.
3. Manage neutropenic fever as an emergency, and adapt the differential for the principal categories of immunocompromise.
4. Apply a structured re-approach to fever that has resisted diagnosis in hospital.
5. Recognise drug fever, the hyperthermia syndromes, and the non-infectious mimics of infection.
6. Assess the patient with fever and rash, and identify the dermatological emergencies.
7. Articulate when antibiotics should be withheld or stopped, and describe the specific harms of unnecessary antimicrobial therapy.

Chapter Overview

Fever is the most common reason a hospitalist is asked to see a patient, and the request usually arrives with an implicit assumption embedded in it: that the patient has an infection and needs an antibiotic. Both parts of that assumption are frequently wrong, and this chapter is organised around dismantling them.

Chapter 8, section 8.1, addressed fever in the postoperative patient. This chapter addresses fever more generally, and it takes a particular position that should be stated at the outset. **Fever is a physiological response, not a disease.** It has a mechanism, it has adaptive functions, it is produced by infection and by many other things, and its presence tells you that inflammatory signalling is occurring rather than that a pathogen requires killing.

Four practical consequences follow, and they recur throughout the chapter.

The temperature record is data, not a diagnosis. How it was measured, at what site, and in what patient determines what it means.

Absence of fever does not exclude infection, particularly in older adults, in renal failure, in patients on corticosteroids or antipyretics, and in overwhelming sepsis, where hypothermia is a worse prognostic sign than fever.

A substantial proportion of inpatient fever is not infective. Drug fever, thromboembolism, malignancy, inflammatory disease, and the hyperthermia syndromes all present as fever in a hospitalised patient, and each is missed when the reflex is to culture and to prescribe.

Antibiotics are not a diagnostic test and they are not benign. Section 11.7 develops this and is, in a sense, the point of the chapter.

11.1 Thermoregulation and the Meaning of the Temperature Curve

11.1.1 The mechanism of fever

Core temperature is regulated around a set point maintained by the hypothalamus, principally the preoptic area, which integrates input from central and peripheral thermoreceptors and drives autonomic and behavioural responses to defend that set point.

Fever is a regulated elevation of the set point. Exogenous pyrogens, of which bacterial lipopolysaccharide is the classical example, stimulate mononuclear cells to release endogenous pyrogenic cytokines including interleukin-1, interleukin-6, tumour necrosis factor, and interferons. These act on the vascular organ of the lamina terminalis and adjacent structures to increase prostaglandin E2 synthesis, which raises the hypothalamic set point.

The patient's subsequent behaviour follows logically. With the set point raised above the current core temperature, the body perceives itself as cold and mounts heat-conserving and heat-generating responses: cutaneous vasoconstriction, which produces the pale cold peripheries seen in a rising fever; shivering, which in its extreme form is a rigor; and behavioural responses including seeking blankets. When the set point falls, either spontaneously or with an antipyretic, the reverse occurs: vasodilation, flushing, and sweating.

This explains a common bedside observation. A rigoring patient who feels cold and is piling on blankets is on the rising limb; a sweating flushed patient is on the falling limb. Rigors are not specific to bacteraemia, though they suggest a rapid rise, which is more common with bloodstream infection, biliary and urinary sepsis, and malaria.

11.1.2 Fever against hyperthermia

The distinction is not semantic and it determines treatment.

In fever, the set point is elevated and thermoregulation is intact. The body is defending a higher target. Antipyretics work because they lower the set point, principally through inhibition of prostaglandin synthesis. Physical cooling of a febrile patient is counterproductive and uncomfortable, because the body responds by shivering and vasoconstricting to defend the elevated set point.

In hyperthermia, the set point is normal and thermoregulation has failed or been overwhelmed. Heat production exceeds heat dissipation. This occurs in heat stroke, in the drug-induced hyperthermia syndromes described in Chapter 10, section 10.6.4, in thyroid storm, and in severe agitation.

The consequences for management are direct. Antipyretics do not work in hyperthermia, because there is no raised set point to lower. Active external and internal cooling is the treatment, together with removal of the cause and specific antidotes where they exist. A patient with a temperature of 41 degrees Celsius who has received paracetamol and remains hot should prompt consideration of hyperthermia rather than a second dose.

Temperatures above approximately 41.5 degrees Celsius are rarely produced by fever alone and should raise strong suspicion of a hyperthermic mechanism.

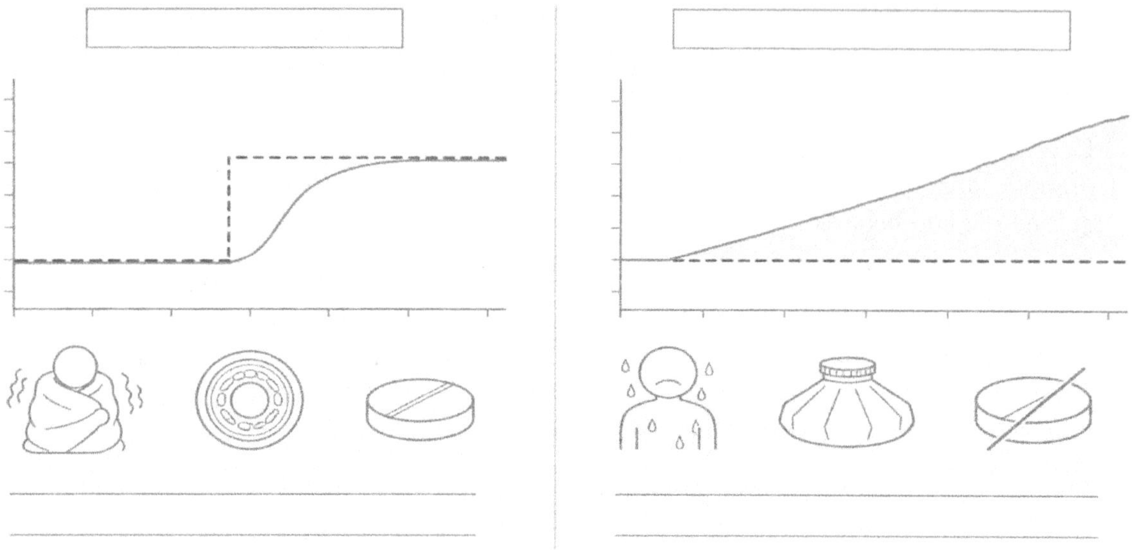

11.1.3 What the number means

Normal temperature is lower than commonly assumed. The traditional figure of 37.0 degrees Celsius derives from nineteenth-century observations and overstates the modern mean, which population studies place somewhat lower, with an apparent secular decline over the past century. More importantly, temperature varies within an individual.

Circadian variation is substantial, with a trough in the early morning and a peak in the late afternoon or early evening, spanning several tenths of a degree. A temperature of 37.6 degrees Celsius at six in the morning is more significant than the same value at six in the evening.

Site of measurement matters and peripheral sites are unreliable. Core measurements, obtained from pulmonary artery, oesophageal, bladder, or rectal sites, are accurate. Peripheral measurements, including oral, axillary, tympanic, and temporal artery devices, agree poorly with core temperature and tend to underestimate it, with the magnitude of disagreement large enough to change clinical decisions. A peripheral reading that is normal in a patient who appears septic should not be trusted, and where the answer matters, a core measurement should be obtained.

Definitions of fever conventionally use a single reading at or above approximately 38.3 degrees Celsius, or a sustained reading at or above 38.0 degrees Celsius over an hour, with lower thresholds applied in specific populations.

The older adult mounts a blunted response. Baseline temperature is lower, the febrile response to infection is attenuated, and a substantial proportion of older patients with serious infection never reach conventional fever thresholds. Geriatric-specific definitions therefore use lower absolute thresholds and, more usefully, a **rise from that individual's own baseline**. The practical rule is that in an older patient, a temperature that would be unremarkable in a younger person, or a functional decline without any fever, may represent significant infection.

Blunted responses also occur in renal failure, in patients on corticosteroids or nonsteroidal anti-inflammatory drugs, in the profoundly immunosuppressed, and in patients receiving continuous renal replacement therapy or extracorporeal support, which remove heat directly.

Hypothermia in the context of suspected infection is an adverse prognostic sign and should be treated with more concern than fever, not less.

11.1.4 Fever patterns

Classical teaching describes continuous, intermittent, remittent, and relapsing patterns, with specific associations such as the tertian and quartan periodicity of certain malarial species and the relapsing pattern historically associated with lymphoma.

An honest appraisal is that fever patterns are of limited diagnostic value in modern practice, because antipyretics, antimicrobials, corticosteroids, and cooling interventions all distort the curve before it can declare itself. The patterns remain worth recognising when they appear spontaneously and undisturbed, which is uncommon.

Two features of the curve retain genuine utility.

Relative bradycardia, in which the pulse rise is disproportionately small for the degree of fever, has recognised associations including enteric fever, legionellosis, some viral infections, drug fever, and factitious fever. It is a soft sign and is confounded by beta-blockade and conduction disease, but it is worth noticing.

The trajectory, meaning whether fever is escalating, plateauing, or resolving, and whether it correlates with an intervention. A fever that resolves within a defined interval of stopping a drug is informative, as section 11.5 develops.

11.1.5 Should fever be treated?

The reflex to normalise the temperature deserves examination, because the evidence for benefit is weak and the mechanism suggests possible harm.

Fever appears to be adaptive. It is metabolically expensive and highly conserved across species, it impairs the replication of several pathogens, and it enhances multiple immune functions.

Trial evidence has not demonstrated outcome benefit from antipyresis in infection. Randomised evaluation of routine paracetamol in critically ill patients with suspected infection did not show improvement in the principal outcomes, and systematic reviews of fever control in sepsis have not established benefit.

The reasonable position is to treat fever for **symptomatic relief** where the patient is uncomfortable, and to recognise that doing so is a comfort intervention rather than a therapeutic one. There is no obligation to treat a fever in a comfortable patient.

Specific circumstances where control is more clearly indicated: acute brain injury, including stroke and traumatic injury, where fever is consistently associated with worse outcomes; pregnancy; and patients with limited cardiac or respiratory reserve in whom the metabolic cost of fever is poorly tolerated. Hyperthermia, as distinct from fever, always requires active management.

A practical caution. Antipyretics mask the temperature record and can conceal both deterioration and response to treatment. Scheduled regular antipyretic administration in a patient under investigation for undiagnosed fever removes one of the few available signals, and section 11.4 argues for withholding it during structured reassessment.

11.2 Fever in the Returning Traveller

11.2.1 The structure of the assessment

Fever in a patient who has recently travelled is a distinct clinical problem in which a systematic history does most of the diagnostic work, and in which the differential is driven by three variables.

Incubation period, meaning the interval between exposure and symptom onset, which is the single most discriminating piece of information and which is calculated from the date of departure from the endemic area at the latest.

Geography, meaning specifically where the patient was, including rural against urban, altitude, and season, rather than the country alone.

Exposures, meaning what the patient did: freshwater contact, insect bites, animal contact, food and water sources, sexual contact, healthcare contact, caves, and mass gatherings.

To these are added **prophylaxis and vaccination history**, with the essential caveat that neither excludes the corresponding disease. Malaria chemoprophylaxis reduces but does not eliminate risk, and adherence is frequently imperfect.

11.2.2 Incubation period as the organising principle

Short incubation, under about ten days. Dengue, chikungunya, and Zika; rickettsial infections including the spotted fever and typhus groups; leptospirosis; enteric bacterial infections; respiratory viral infections including influenza; arboviral infections generally; and the earliest presentations of viral haemorrhagic fevers.

Intermediate incubation, approximately ten to twenty-one days. Malaria, which spans a very wide range; enteric fever; leptospirosis; brucellosis; Q fever; African trypanosomiasis; and viral haemorrhagic fevers.

Long incubation, beyond about twenty-one days. Malaria, particularly the relapsing species which may present months or years later; tuberculosis; viral hepatitis; acute human immunodeficiency virus infection, which presents as a seroconversion illness some weeks after exposure; amoebic liver abscess, which may present many months later; visceral leishmaniasis; schistosomiasis, including the acute Katayama syndrome; and filarial infections.

The practical use of this framework is subtractive. A fever beginning more than three weeks after return effectively excludes dengue and the other short-incubation arboviruses, which narrows the field considerably. A fever beginning within a few days of arrival in a tropical region is unlikely to be malaria acquired on that trip.

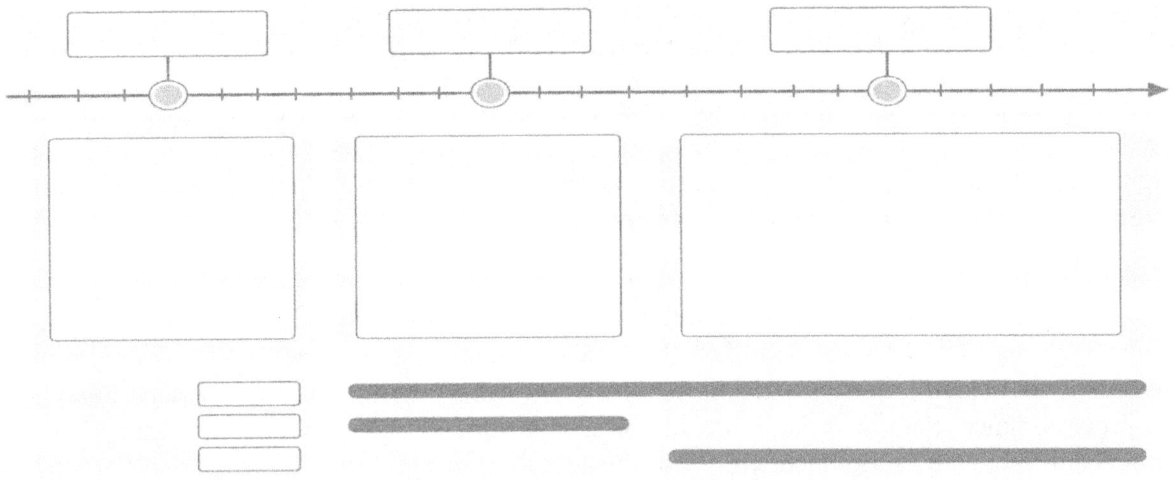

11.2.3 Malaria: the diagnosis that must not be missed

Any fever in a person who has been in a malaria-endemic area is malaria until excluded, regardless of prophylaxis, regardless of how long ago, and regardless of how convincing an alternative explanation appears.

The reason for this categorical framing is that falciparum malaria can progress from mild symptoms to death within days, that early treatment is highly effective, and that the presentation is entirely non-specific, comprising fever, headache, myalgia, and malaise with no reliable distinguishing features. Cyclical fever is neither sensitive nor early.

Diagnosis is by microscopy of thick and thin blood films, with the thick film for detection and the thin film for species identification and parasite quantification, or by a rapid diagnostic antigen test. A single negative result does not exclude the diagnosis; conventionally three sets of films at intervals over a day or two are required before malaria is excluded in a patient with a compatible exposure.

Severity assessment determines management and is defined by specific clinical and laboratory criteria including impaired consciousness, seizures, respiratory distress, acidosis, hypoglycaemia, renal impairment, jaundice, significant anaemia, shock, bleeding, and a high parasite count. Severe malaria requires parenteral therapy, with artesunate established as superior to quinine, and management in a high dependency setting.

Common errors: attributing fever to a plausible alternative without testing; accepting a single negative film; failing to recognise severity criteria in a patient who looks reasonably well; and delaying treatment while awaiting species confirmation.

11.2.4 Other specific considerations

Dengue presents with fever, severe myalgia and arthralgia, retro-orbital headache, and rash, with thrombocytopenia and leucopenia. The important clinical point is that deterioration classically occurs around the time of **defervescence**, when plasma leakage may produce haemodynamic compromise. Warning signs including abdominal pain, persistent vomiting, mucosal bleeding, lethargy, and a rising haematocrit with falling platelets indicate a patient requiring close observation. **Avoid nonsteroidal anti-inflammatory drugs and aspirin** because of bleeding risk.

Enteric fever presents with progressive fever, relative bradycardia, abdominal symptoms which may be constipation rather than diarrhoea, and, in a minority, a subtle rash. Blood culture is the diagnostic test; stool culture is less sensitive. Antimicrobial resistance patterns vary substantially by region of acquisition and determine therapy.

Viral haemorrhagic fever requires a risk assessment in any febrile patient returning from an affected region within the relevant incubation window, based on geography, exposures, and clinical features. Where risk is identified, the patient should be isolated according to local protocol and public health authorities notified immediately. **Testing for malaria must not be delayed** by this process, since malaria is far more likely and is rapidly treatable, and laboratory handling should be arranged in accordance with local biosafety guidance.

Eosinophilia in a returning traveller directs attention to helminth infection, including schistosomiasis, strongyloidiasis, filariasis, and tissue nematodes. **Strongyloides deserves specific mention**, because latent infection can persist for decades and can produce fatal hyperinfection when the patient is given corticosteroids or other immunosuppression. Any patient with relevant exposure history who is about to receive immunosuppression should be screened.

Sexual history should be taken in every returning traveller with fever, since acute human immunodeficiency virus infection and other sexually transmitted infections are common and are missed when not asked about.

Notification. Several of the conditions in this section are notifiable, and public health should be informed promptly rather than after confirmation.

11.2.5 Initial investigation

A reasonable initial panel: thick and thin films or a rapid diagnostic test for malaria, repeated as above; blood cultures; full blood count with differential, attending to thrombocytopenia, eosinophilia, and lymphopenia; liver and renal function; lactate; urinalysis and culture; chest radiography; and stored serum for later serological comparison.

Directed additions follow from the exposure history and might include stool microscopy and culture, serology for arboviral and rickettsial infections, testing for human immunodeficiency virus, and specific molecular testing where available.

Discuss with infectious diseases early, particularly where the exposure is unusual, where the patient is unwell, or where a notifiable or high-consequence infection is possible.

11.3 Neutropenic Fever and the Immunocompromised Host

11.3.1 Neutropenic fever is a medical emergency

The framing matters because the patient frequently does not look unwell. A neutropenic patient with an evolving bacterial infection may have a normal blood pressure and a comfortable appearance in the hour before profound shock, because the inflammatory response that would ordinarily produce visible illness cannot be mounted.

Definition. An absolute neutrophil count below 0.5 times ten to the ninth per litre, or below 1.0 and expected to fall below 0.5, together with a single temperature at or above approximately 38.3 degrees Celsius or a sustained temperature at or above 38.0 degrees Celsius over an hour. Local thresholds vary slightly.

The central management principle is that empirical broad-spectrum antibacterial therapy should be administered promptly, conventionally within an hour of presentation, after cultures are taken but without waiting for results and without waiting for a source to be identified. This is one of the few situations in this book where the instruction is to give antibiotics immediately, and section 11.7 should be read as compatible with it rather than contradicting it.

11.3.2 What is different about the neutropenic patient

Signs of inflammation are absent or minimal. There is no pus, because pus is neutrophils. A pneumonia may show minimal or no infiltrate on radiography until the count recovers. A urinary tract infection may show no pyuria. A soft tissue infection may show erythema without induration or fluctuance. **Absence of a localising sign does not mean absence of a source.**

The likely sources are predictable. Mucosal barrier injury from chemotherapy allows translocation of gut and oral flora, which is the commonest mechanism. Vascular access devices are a major source. The perianal region, the skin, the lungs, the sinuses, and the oropharynx should all be examined specifically.

Avoid rectal examination, rectal thermometers, and suppositories in profoundly neutropenic patients because of the risk of bacteraemia from mucosal trauma, and inspect the perianal area visually instead.

Fungal risk rises with the duration of neutropenia, which is the reason that prolonged fever changes management as described below.

11.3.3 Initial management

Take cultures without delaying therapy: peripheral blood cultures and cultures from each lumen of any indwelling vascular device, plus site-directed sampling.

Give an antipseudomonal beta-lactam as monotherapy in most protocols. This is the standard initial regimen, and choice depends on local resistance patterns and institutional guidance.

Do not add a glycopeptide routinely. Empirical vancomycin or an equivalent is reserved for specific indications: suspected catheter-related infection, skin or soft tissue infection, haemodynamic instability, known colonisation with a resistant Gram-positive organism, severe mucositis, or pneumonia in defined circumstances. Routine addition does not improve outcomes and increases toxicity and resistance.

Assess risk formally. Validated instruments identify a low-risk group with anticipated short neutropenia, no significant comorbidity, and clinical stability, who in appropriate settings can be managed with oral therapy and, in selected cases, as outpatients with careful arrangements. This is an established and evidence-supported pathway but requires reliable follow-up and clear escalation instructions.

Involve haematology or oncology immediately, since the underlying disease, the chemotherapy protocol, and the anticipated count trajectory all shape management.

11.3.4 The patient with persistent fever

Fever persisting beyond approximately four to seven days despite appropriate broad-spectrum therapy, in a patient who remains neutropenic, requires reassessment rather than escalation by reflex.

Reassess systematically: repeat examination with attention to sites not previously examined, repeat cultures, review the antimicrobial spectrum against the likely organisms, consider resistant bacteria, and consider non-infective causes including the underlying malignancy itself, drug fever, and thromboembolism.

Consider invasive fungal infection. Computed tomography of the chest is the key investigation for invasive mould disease and may show characteristic findings before they are visible on plain radiography. Serum biomarkers including galactomannan and beta-D-glucan have defined roles with important limitations in sensitivity and specificity and are affected by concurrent antifungal therapy and by certain drugs and products.

Empirical antifungal therapy is conventional in persistently febrile neutropenic patients with expected prolonged neutropenia, though a pre-emptive strategy guided by biomarkers and imaging is used in some centres. Follow institutional protocol.

Do not simply stack additional antibacterial agents onto a regimen that is not working without a hypothesis about what is being covered that was not covered before.

11.3.5 Other categories of immunocompromise

The differential shifts according to which arm of immunity is impaired, and thinking in these terms is more useful than a general category of immunosuppression.

Solid organ transplant recipients follow a broadly predictable timeline. In the first month, infections are principally nosocomial, surgical, and donor-derived. From approximately one to six months, the period of maximal immunosuppression, opportunistic infections predominate, including *Pneumocystis*, cytomegalovirus, other herpesviruses, *Aspergillus*, *Nocardia*, *Listeria*, and reactivation of latent infections including tuberculosis. Beyond six months, community-acquired infections predominate, with late opportunistic infection in those requiring continued intensive immunosuppression. Prophylaxis history modifies this substantially.

Human immunodeficiency virus infection stratifies by CD4 count. Below approximately 200 cells per microlitre, *Pneumocystis* pneumonia becomes a major consideration. Below approximately 100, cerebral toxoplasmosis and cryptococcal disease. Below approximately 50, disseminated mycobacterial disease and cytomegalovirus end-organ disease. Tuberculosis occurs at any count and is more likely to be extrapulmonary and atypical at low counts.

Biologic and targeted agents carry agent-specific risks that should be looked up rather than assumed. Tumour necrosis factor inhibitors are associated with reactivation of tuberculosis and with granulomatous fungal infections. B cell depleting agents are associated with hepatitis B reactivation and with progressive multifocal leukoencephalopathy, and blunt the antibody response including to vaccination. Complement inhibitors carry a marked risk of meningococcal disease, requiring vaccination and often prophylaxis. Several kinase inhibitors carry specific opportunistic risks.

Corticosteroids impair cell-mediated immunity in a dose and duration dependent manner, and are associated with *Pneumocystis*, fungal infection, and, as noted in section 11.2.4, strongyloides hyperinfection.

Asplenia and hyposplenism, whether surgical, congenital, or functional as in sickle cell disease and coeliac disease, confer susceptibility to encapsulated organisms and the risk of overwhelming post-splenectomy infection, which can progress from well to fatal within hours. These patients require vaccination, often antimicrobial prophylaxis, an emergency supply of antibiotics, and a very low threshold for immediate parenteral therapy when febrile. They are also at risk from babesiosis and from *Capnocytophaga* following dog bites.

Neutropenia from causes other than chemotherapy, including drug-induced agranulocytosis, should be managed with the same urgency as chemotherapy-induced neutropenia.

11.4 Undiagnosed Fever in Hospital: A Structured Re-Approach

11.4.1 The problem and the classification

Classical fever of unknown origin was defined by Petersdorf and Beeson as fever exceeding a defined threshold on several occasions over more than three weeks, remaining undiagnosed after a period of inpatient investigation. Modern definitions substitute a defined set of qualifying investigations for the fixed period of hospitalisation, and recognise distinct categories: **classical**, **nosocomial**, meaning fever arising in a hospitalised patient in whom infection was not present or incubating on admission, **neutropenic**, addressed in section 11.3, and **immunodeficiency-associated**.

The practical situation this section addresses is narrower and more common than formal fever of unknown origin: a hospitalised patient who has been febrile for several days, has been cultured and imaged, is receiving antibiotics, and has no diagnosis. The correct response is not further reflexive testing. It is a structured restart.

11.4.2 The structured re-approach

Step one: verify that the fever is real. Review how the temperature was measured and at what site, given the limitations in section 11.1.3. Confirm the readings from the chart rather than from report. Consider, rarely and carefully, factitious fever, suggested by absence of the expected physiological accompaniments such as tachycardia and diaphoresis, by temperatures recorded only when unobserved, and by a dissociation between temperature and the patient's appearance.

Step two: take the history again, completely, from the beginning. This is the highest-yield action and it is almost never done, because everyone assumes it was done on admission. Cover systematically: occupational exposures; animal and pet contact including birds and reptiles; travel over the preceding year and not merely the preceding month; freshwater and soil exposure; sexual history; injecting drug use; dental history and recent procedures; prosthetic material of any kind including joints, valves, grafts, and mesh; transfusion history; family history including periodic fever syndromes and Mediterranean or other relevant ancestry; prior tuberculosis exposure and treatment; and a complete list of every substance ingested including over-the-counter preparations, supplements, and herbal products.

Step three: examine the patient again, completely, undressed. Skin including the whole surface, the scalp, and between the toes; nails for splinter haemorrhages; mucous membranes; the oral cavity and teeth; lymph nodes in every region; temporal arteries; fundi; the thyroid; the heart for a new murmur; the abdomen for organomegaly; the spine for focal tenderness; joints; the genitals and perineum; and the prostate or pelvis as appropriate.

Step four: review every drug, including those recently stopped, those given intermittently, and those the patient regards as not medications. Section 11.5 addresses drug fever.

Step five: review every device and line, with the discipline from Chapter 8, section 8.6.1: indication, owner, exit criterion. An indwelling device is a source until excluded.

Step six: review the primary data personally. Look at the images rather than reading the reports. Look at the actual culture results including intermediate growth and organisms dismissed as contaminants. Look at the full blood film. This step frequently uncovers something that was reported but not integrated.

Step seven: consider stopping drugs rather than adding them. A deliberate interruption of antimicrobial therapy in a patient who is clinically stable serves two purposes: it may resolve a drug fever, and it permits meaningful cultures to be taken. This requires clinical judgement and should not be done in an unstable patient, but it is frequently the action that breaks the deadlock, and the reflex to continue empirical therapy indefinitely is a major obstacle to diagnosis.

11.4.3 The four diagnostic categories

Undiagnosed fever resolves into four groups, and the relative proportions have shifted over time as imaging has improved, with infection falling and non-infectious inflammatory disease rising as a proportion in developed settings.

Infection. Consider particularly the occult and the slow: infective endocarditis including culture-negative and prosthetic valve disease; intra-abdominal, pelvic, hepatic, splenic, and renal abscess; osteomyelitis and discitis, which is easily missed and requires magnetic resonance imaging; prosthetic material infection; tuberculosis including extrapulmonary and miliary forms; endovascular graft infection; dental and sinus sources; and, depending on geography, brucellosis, Q fever, and enteric fever.

Malignancy. Lymphoma is the classical cause and may present with fever, sweats, and weight loss before any mass is apparent. Renal cell carcinoma, hepatocellular carcinoma, atrial myxoma, and metastatic disease also cause fever. Haemophagocytic lymphohistiocytosis deserves specific mention and is addressed in section 11.5.4.

Inflammatory and autoimmune disease. Adult-onset Still disease, characterised by quotidian fever, an evanescent salmon-coloured rash, arthritis, and a strikingly high ferritin; giant cell arteritis and polymyalgia rheumatica, which should be considered in any patient over fifty with fever and a raised inflammatory response, and in whom temporal artery imaging or biopsy may be indicated; the systemic vasculitides; systemic lupus erythematosus; sarcoidosis; and inflammatory bowel disease.

Miscellaneous. Drug fever; venous thromboembolism, which is a genuinely common and repeatedly overlooked cause of inpatient fever; thyrotoxicosis; adrenal insufficiency; haematoma resorption; subacute thyroiditis; hereditary periodic fever syndromes, which usually present earlier in life but not always; and factitious fever.

11.4.4 Investigation in the undiagnosed patient

Imaging. Cross-sectional imaging of chest, abdomen, and pelvis is the conventional next step. **Echocardiography**, with transoesophageal study where endocarditis is suspected and the transthoracic study is inadequate or negative. **Magnetic resonance imaging of the spine** where any focal back pain exists. **Positron emission tomography** has a substantial and well-documented yield in undiagnosed fever, identifying occult infection, vasculitis, and malignancy, and is increasingly used earlier in the sequence where available.

Laboratory. Serial blood cultures taken off antibiotics where feasible; inflammatory markers with attention to the pattern rather than the value; ferritin, which when very high raises specific possibilities; lactate dehydrogenase; protein electrophoresis; autoantibody screening directed by clinical features rather than as a blanket panel, given the false positive problem discussed in Chapter 2, section 2.7.3; tuberculosis testing including interferon gamma release assay with awareness of its limitations in active disease; and directed serology.

Tissue. Biopsy of any accessible abnormality, including lymph node, temporal artery, bone marrow, or liver, guided by the clinical picture. Bone marrow examination has a defined yield in specific circumstances rather than as a routine step.

A note on empirical therapy. Empirical corticosteroids should generally be avoided before a diagnosis is established, because they obscure the clinical picture, can worsen undiagnosed infection, and may partially treat lymphoma sufficiently to prevent its diagnosis while not curing it. The exception is a patient with a strong clinical suspicion of giant cell arteritis and visual symptoms, where sight-threatening disease justifies immediate treatment with biopsy arranged promptly thereafter.

Finally, a reassurance worth giving. A meaningful proportion of undiagnosed fevers resolve spontaneously without a diagnosis ever being made, and this group has a good prognosis. Where the patient is stable and the systematic work has been done, observation with defined review is a legitimate plan rather than a failure.

11.5 Drug Fever, Hyperthermia Syndromes, and Their Mimics

11.5.1 Drug fever

Drug fever is fever attributable to a medication, resolving on its withdrawal, without an alternative explanation. It is common, it is a diagnosis of exclusion, and it is under-considered because the reflex response to fever is to add drugs rather than to remove them.

Mechanisms include hypersensitivity, which is the commonest; altered thermoregulation, as with anticholinergics and sympathomimetics; idiosyncratic reactions; direct pharmacological effects, as with the cytokine release accompanying treatment of certain infections; and administration-related effects, as with amphotericin infusion reactions and contaminated infusates.

Timing. The classical interval from starting the drug to the onset of fever is on the order of a week to ten days for a first exposure, but the range is wide. On re-exposure, fever may occur within hours. Fever may also begin after the drug has been taken uneventfully for months.

Commonly implicated agents. Beta-lactam antibiotics, sulfonamides, antiseizure medications including phenytoin and carbamazepine, allopurinol, several antiarrhythmics, minocycline, heparins, amphotericin, and many others. The general rule is that any drug can do it, and the ones most often responsible are simply the ones most often prescribed.

Clinical features. The most useful is that the patient frequently **appears well relative to the height of the fever**, and is not toxic, though this is not universal. Relative bradycardia may be present. Eosinophilia occurs in a minority and its absence does not exclude the diagnosis. Rash occurs in a minority. Mild transaminase elevation is common.

Diagnosis and management. Stop the suspected agent. Fever typically resolves within two to four days, and longer for drugs with a long half-life or active metabolites. Where several candidate drugs exist, stop those that are non-essential and those with the strongest association, rather than stopping everything at once, unless the patient is unwell. Deliberate rechallenge is not required to confirm the diagnosis and is not recommended, and the drug should be recorded as an adverse reaction in the record and communicated at discharge.

11.5.2 Serious drug reactions that present with fever

Distinguishing simple drug fever from a severe systemic drug reaction matters greatly, and the features are covered further in section 11.6.

Drug reaction with eosinophilia and systemic symptoms presents typically two to eight weeks after the culprit drug, with fever, facial oedema, a widespread rash, lymphadenopathy, eosinophilia and atypical lymphocytes, and internal organ involvement, most often hepatitis but also nephritis, pneumonitis, and myocarditis. It may relapse after apparent resolution, and it requires prolonged treatment and follow-up.

Stevens-Johnson syndrome and toxic epidermal necrolysis, addressed in section 11.6.3.

Acute generalised exanthematous pustulosis, addressed in section 11.6.3.

Drug-induced hypersensitivity to specific agents, including the well-described reactions to certain antiretroviral and antiseizure medications with defined genetic associations.

11.5.3 The hyperthermia syndromes

These were developed in Chapter 10, section 10.6.4, and are summarised here from the perspective of the febrile patient, since the distinction from fever determines treatment.

Neuroleptic malignant syndrome, developing over days after a dopamine antagonist is introduced or increased or a dopamine agonist withdrawn, with generalised lead-pipe rigidity, hyporeflexia, autonomic instability, and a markedly raised creatine kinase.

Serotonin syndrome, developing over hours, with clonus and hyperreflexia predominating in the lower limbs, agitation, and autonomic instability.

Malignant hyperthermia, triggered by specific anaesthetic agents, presenting intraoperatively or in the immediate recovery period with hypercapnia, rigidity, and rapidly rising temperature.

Anticholinergic toxicity, with hyperthermia in the absence of sweating, dry flushed skin, dilated pupils, urinary retention, and delirium.

Sympathomimetic toxicity, from stimulants, with hyperthermia, agitation, hypertension, and tachycardia.

Thyroid storm, addressed in Chapter 17, which presents with hyperthermia, tachyarrhythmia, agitation or delirium, and gastrointestinal symptoms, and which is precipitated by infection, surgery, or iodine load in a patient with untreated thyrotoxicosis.

Heat stroke, from environmental exposure or exertion, with hyperthermia and central nervous system dysfunction.

In all of these, antipyretics are ineffective and active cooling with treatment of the underlying process is required, for the reasons in section 11.1.2.

11.5.4 Non-infectious mimics of infection

These deserve a list because each is regularly treated as sepsis for several days before recognition.

Venous thromboembolism. Pulmonary embolism produces fever in a meaningful proportion of cases and is among the most frequently missed causes of unexplained inpatient fever.

Transfusion reactions. Febrile non-haemolytic reactions are common and benign; acute haemolytic reactions and transfusion-related acute lung injury are not, and the distinction requires stopping the transfusion and assessing rather than treating through it.

Tissue infarction of any kind, including myocardial infarction, bowel infarction, and large haematoma resorption.

Crystal arthropathy. Acute gout and pseudogout produce fever, a raised inflammatory response, and a hot swollen joint, and are indistinguishable from septic arthritis without joint aspiration. **Aspirate the joint**, because the two coexist and because treating one as the other is harmful in both directions.

Acute pancreatitis, which produces a systemic inflammatory response without infection in its early phase, addressed in Chapter 15.

Adrenal insufficiency, addressed in Chapter 7, section 7.6.4.

Malignancy, particularly lymphoma and renal cell carcinoma, as in section 11.4.3.

Haemophagocytic lymphohistiocytosis merits specific attention because it is rapidly fatal, is treatable, and is missed. Suspect it in a patient with persistent fever, cytopenias affecting two or more lineages, splenomegaly, a very high ferritin, raised triglycerides, low fibrinogen, and raised transaminases. It is triggered by infection, malignancy, and autoimmune disease, and the pattern of a septic-appearing patient not responding to antimicrobial therapy with a strikingly high ferritin should prompt haematology involvement urgently.

Postoperative inflammatory fever, addressed in Chapter 8, section 8.1.2.

11.6 Rash and Fever: Dermatologic Emergencies

11.6.1 A structured approach

Fever with rash is a presentation in which a small number of observations rapidly narrow a very large differential. Five questions structure the assessment.

What is the primary morphology? Macular and papular; vesicular or bullous; pustular; petechial or purpuric; or erythrodermic.

Are mucous membranes involved? Involvement of the eyes, mouth, or genitals raises the concern substantially and points toward the severe drug reactions and certain infections.

Does the skin hurt? Pain out of proportion to the visible appearance suggests necrotising infection, as in Chapter 8, section 8.2.4, or toxic epidermal necrolysis.

Is the epidermis detaching? A positive Nikolsky sign, meaning shearing of epidermis with lateral pressure on apparently uninvolved skin, indicates full-thickness epidermal separation.

How toxic is the patient? The combination of rash with hypotension, altered mental state, or organ dysfunction defines the emergencies.

Take a complete drug history with dates, since the interval between drug initiation and rash onset is a principal diagnostic discriminator.

11.6.2 Petechial and purpuric rash with fever

This combination should be treated as an emergency until proven otherwise.

Meningococcal disease. A non-blanching rash in a febrile patient, particularly one that is evolving rapidly, requires immediate parenteral antimicrobial therapy before any further investigation, before lumbar puncture, and before transfer. Progression to purpura fulminans with disseminated intravascular coagulation can occur within hours. Do not wait to confirm.

Other bacterial sepsis with disseminated intravascular coagulation, from any organism.

Rickettsial infection. Rocky Mountain spotted fever and related infections classically produce a rash beginning peripherally, including on palms and soles, and spreading centrally. The rash appears after the fever and may be absent early. **Empirical doxycycline should be given on suspicion**, since delay markedly increases mortality and confirmatory testing is retrospective.

Infective endocarditis, with splinter haemorrhages, Janeway lesions, and Osler nodes.

Viral haemorrhagic fever, in the appropriate exposure context as in section 11.2.4.

Non-infective causes including immune thrombocytopenia, thrombotic microangiopathies, and vasculitis.

11.6.3 Severe cutaneous adverse reactions

Stevens-Johnson syndrome and toxic epidermal necrolysis exist on a spectrum defined by the extent of body surface area with epidermal detachment. Onset is typically within a few weeks of starting the culprit drug. Features include prodromal fever and malaise, painful skin, a rash that may begin as targetoid or macular lesions, involvement of two or more mucosal surfaces, and progression to epidermal detachment with a positive Nikolsky sign.

Management requires immediate withdrawal of all non-essential drugs and any plausible culprit, supportive care with attention to fluid, thermoregulation, and infection, ophthalmological assessment because ocular sequelae are common and preventable, and transfer to a burns or specialist unit. Severity scoring instruments exist for prognostication. Immunomodulatory treatment remains an area of variable practice and should involve dermatology.

Drug reaction with eosinophilia and systemic symptoms, as in section 11.5.2. The key distinguishing features from a simple drug rash are the later onset, facial oedema, eosinophilia, and internal organ involvement, and it must be looked for with liver function tests, renal function, and a differential count in any patient with a widespread drug rash and fever.

Acute generalised exanthematous pustulosis, characterised by rapid onset within days of the drug, widespread small sterile pustules on an erythematous background beginning in flexures, fever, and neutrophilia, resolving with desquamation after withdrawal. It is distinguished from pustular psoriasis and from infection by history and, where necessary, biopsy.

11.6.4 Toxin-mediated and infective emergencies

Toxic shock syndrome, staphylococcal or streptococcal, presents with fever, hypotension, a diffuse macular erythroderma resembling sunburn, mucosal hyperaemia, and multiorgan involvement, with desquamation occurring later in convalescence. Sources may be occult, including retained tampons, nasal packing, and minor wounds, and a search for the source is part of the management alongside antimicrobial therapy including an antitoxin agent, and consideration of immunoglobulin in severe streptococcal disease.

Necrotising soft tissue infection, addressed in Chapter 8, section 8.2.4.

Disseminated gonococcal infection, with fever, sparse pustular or haemorrhagic lesions on distal extremities, tenosynovitis, and arthritis.

Varicella zoster, including primary varicella in an adult, which is more severe than in children, and disseminated zoster in the immunocompromised, which requires isolation and parenteral therapy.

Eczema herpeticum, meaning widespread herpes simplex infection of eczematous skin, which is painful, rapidly progressive, and requires prompt antiviral therapy.

Measles, which is resurging in several regions with falling vaccination coverage, and which should be considered in an unvaccinated patient with fever, coryza, conjunctivitis, cough, and a descending rash. It requires isolation and notification, and complications include pneumonia and encephalitis.

Erythroderma of any cause, meaning erythema involving the great majority of the body surface, which produces fluid loss, thermoregulatory failure, high-output cardiac failure, and infection risk, and which is a dermatological emergency irrespective of its cause.

Chapter 18 addresses the antimicrobial management of the infective conditions above, and the dermatological manifestations of systemic disease are developed further in the dermatology chapters of Part IV.

11.7 When Not to Give Antibiotics

11.7.1 The premise

Antibiotics are prescribed in hospitals to a substantial proportion of inpatients, and analyses consistently find that a large fraction of that prescribing is unnecessary, of inappropriate spectrum, or of excessive duration.

The reason this persists is not ignorance. It is that the perceived costs of the two errors are asymmetric. Withholding an antibiotic from a patient who turns out to have an infection is a visible, attributable, personally consequential error. Giving an antibiotic to a patient who does not need it produces harm that is delayed, diffuse, and attributable to no one. Prescribing therefore drifts in one direction, and correcting that drift requires making the second category of harm concrete.

The harms of unnecessary antimicrobial therapy are specific and worth naming: *Clostridioides difficile* infection; selection of resistant organisms in this patient and in the institution; direct adverse effects including acute kidney injury, hepatotoxicity, cytopenias, neurotoxicity, tendinopathy, QT prolongation, and anaphylaxis; disruption of the microbiome with consequences that are increasingly recognised; the requirement for intravenous access with its own infection and thrombosis risks; obscuring the diagnosis, as section 11.4.2 described; prolonged admission; and the labelling of patients with spurious allergies that constrain their care for life.

11.7.2 Situations in which antibiotics should generally be withheld

Asymptomatic bacteriuria. This is the single highest-volume opportunity. Bacteriuria without urinary symptoms should not be treated in almost all populations, including older adults, catheterised patients, and patients with diabetes. Recognised exceptions are pregnancy and before urological procedures involving mucosal trauma. Treating asymptomatic bacteriuria does not prevent symptomatic infection and does cause harm. Chapter 18 develops this.

Delirium attributed to a positive urine culture. This deserves separate mention because it is the commonest specific manifestation of the above. A confused older patient with bacteriuria and no urinary symptoms usually has delirium from another cause, and the culture has anchored the diagnosis. Chapter 10, section 10.1.4, listed the systematic search that should occur instead.

A positive respiratory culture without clinical pneumonia. Sputum and tracheal aspirate cultures grow colonising organisms routinely, particularly in patients with chronic lung disease and in the ventilated. Treat the patient, not the culture.

A positive wound swab without clinical signs of infection. All open wounds are colonised. Chronic leg ulcers in particular are swabbed and treated repeatedly with no benefit and considerable harm.

A single positive blood culture with a likely contaminant. A coagulase-negative staphylococcus in one of two culture sets, in a patient without a vascular device, without prosthetic material, and without clinical sepsis, is usually a contaminant. The correct action is assessment and, where necessary, repeat cultures rather than a course of a glycopeptide.

Clostridioides difficile **testing of formed stool**, or testing in a patient whose diarrhoea has an alternative explanation such as laxatives or enteral feeding, which detects colonisation and produces treatment of a non-disease. Chapter 2, section 2.7.3, addressed this as the archetypal stewardship problem.

Viral upper respiratory infection and acute bronchitis in patients without chronic lung disease.

Aspiration events. Aspiration of gastric contents produces a chemical pneumonitis that is not initially infective, and a proportion resolve without antimicrobial therapy. Observation for the first day or so, with treatment if fever, infiltrate, and clinical deterioration develop or persist, is a defensible approach in a stable patient. Chapter 18 develops the distinction.

Acute pancreatitis without proven infected necrosis, where prophylactic antimicrobial therapy is not indicated.

Non-infectious fever of the kinds catalogued in section 11.5.4.

11.7.3 Stopping and narrowing

Withholding is only part of the discipline. Equally important is stopping.

The antimicrobial timeout. At approximately forty-eight to seventy-two hours, when culture results are available and the clinical trajectory is apparent, every antimicrobial prescription should be actively reviewed against four questions: is there still evidence of infection; can the spectrum be narrowed; can the route be changed from intravenous to oral; and when will it stop. This review is a defined process rather than an assumption, and building it into the daily round is among the highest-yield stewardship interventions available to a hospitalist.

De-escalation. Empirical broad-spectrum therapy is appropriate at the outset in a seriously unwell patient; continuing it once an organism and its sensitivities are known is not.

Shorter courses. The evidence of the past two decades has been consistently in one direction: shorter courses are non-inferior to longer ones across a wide range of infections, including community-acquired pneumonia, hospital-acquired pneumonia, uncomplicated Gram-negative bacteraemia, pyelonephritis, intra-abdominal infection after adequate source control, and cellulitis. Specific durations should be taken from current guidance and are developed in Chapter 18. The general principle is that the historically conventional durations were arbitrary and that the burden of justification now falls on the longer course.

Intravenous to oral switch. Many agents have excellent oral bioavailability, and switching in a stable patient who is absorbing enterally removes line-associated risk and frequently permits earlier discharge.

Penicillin allergy delabelling. A large majority of patients labelled as penicillin allergic are not, and the label is associated with receipt of inferior alternative agents, more *Clostridioides difficile*, more resistant organisms, and worse outcomes. Taking a proper allergy history, distinguishing intolerance from true allergy, and referring appropriate patients for assessment is a genuine clinical intervention rather than an administrative one.

11.7.4 The counterweight

This section must end where it began in section 11.3.1, because the argument is easily misapplied.

In sepsis and septic shock, in neutropenic fever, in suspected meningococcal disease, in suspected bacterial meningitis, and in necrotising infection, antimicrobial therapy should be given immediately, empirically, broadly, and without waiting for diagnostic confirmation. Delay in these situations is associated with increased mortality, and the reasoning of this section does not apply to them.

The discipline being advocated is not restraint in the unwell patient. It is the avoidance of reflexive prescribing in the patient who is not septic, the active review of therapy already started, and the recognition that continuing an antibiotic requires as much justification as starting one.

Chapter Summary

- **Fever is a regulated elevation of the hypothalamic set point**; hyperthermia is a failure of thermoregulation. Antipyretics work in the first and not the second, and a patient who stays hot despite adequate antipyresis should prompt reconsideration.
- **Peripheral temperature measurement is unreliable**, older adults mount a blunted response, and hypothermia in suspected infection is a worse sign than fever. Fever patterns are of limited value in modern practice; relative bradycardia and trajectory retain some utility.
- **Treat fever for comfort, not as a therapeutic goal**, with specific exceptions including acute brain injury. Scheduled antipyretics remove a diagnostic signal in the undiagnosed patient.
- In the returning traveller, **incubation period, geography, and exposure** drive the differential, and the incubation period is most useful subtractively. **Any fever after exposure to a malaria-endemic area is malaria until excluded**, three negative films are required, and prophylaxis does not exclude it.
- **Neutropenic fever is an emergency requiring antibiotics within an hour.** Signs of inflammation are absent because they require neutrophils. Do not add a glycopeptide routinely, avoid rectal examination, and reassess rather than stack agents when fever persists.
- **Undiagnosed inpatient fever requires a structured restart**, not more tests: verify the fever, retake the entire history, re-examine the undressed patient, review every drug and device, look at the primary data yourself, and consider stopping drugs rather than adding them.
- **Drug fever presents in a patient who looks well for the height of the fever** and resolves within days of withdrawal. Venous thromboembolism, crystal arthropathy, transfusion reactions, and haemophagocytic lymphohistiocytosis are the mimics most often treated as sepsis.

- **Fever with a non-blanching rash is an emergency**, and empirical therapy precedes investigation. Mucosal involvement, skin pain, and a positive Nikolsky sign identify the severe cutaneous adverse reactions.
- **Antibiotics are not a diagnostic test and are not benign.** Asymptomatic bacteriuria, colonising respiratory and wound cultures, and probable blood culture contaminants should not be treated. Conduct an antimicrobial timeout at forty-eight to seventy-two hours, de-escalate, shorten, switch to oral, and delabel spurious allergies. None of this applies to sepsis, neutropenic fever, or suspected meningitis, where immediate therapy is the rule.

Review Questions

1. A patient has a temperature of 41.2 degrees Celsius, rigid limbs, and a creatine kinase of 8,000 units per litre, three days after an antipsychotic was increased. Two doses of paracetamol have had no effect. Explain why, state your diagnosis, and outline your immediate management.
2. A patient presents with fever nine days after returning from a two-week trip to sub-Saharan Africa, having taken malaria prophylaxis. The first blood film is negative and a colleague proposes discharge with outpatient follow-up. State your position and justify it.
3. A neutropenic patient with acute myeloid leukaemia has a temperature of 38.5 degrees Celsius, a normal blood pressure, and no localising signs. Set out your management in the first hour and state which antibiotic you would not add and why.
4. A patient has been febrile for eight days on broad-spectrum antibiotics with negative cultures and unremarkable computed tomography. List, in order, the seven steps of your structured re-approach, and state which of them you consider most likely to yield the diagnosis.
5. An 84-year-old with delirium has a urine culture growing *Escherichia coli* and no urinary symptoms. The ward team has started ciprofloxacin. Explain what is wrong with this, what harms it may cause, and what you would do instead.

CHAPTER 12: Fluids, Electrolytes, and Acid-Base

Learning Objectives

After studying this chapter, the reader should be able to:

1. Explain why the physical examination performs poorly for volume assessment, and distinguish preload responsiveness from the need for fluid.
2. Select an appropriate crystalloid, describe the consequences of chloride loading, and apply the principles of fluid stewardship.
3. Evaluate hyponatraemia using a tonicity-based algorithm, treat symptomatic and asymptomatic presentations appropriately, and apply correction limits to avoid osmotic demyelination.
4. Manage disorders of potassium, magnesium, and calcium, including their interdependence.
5. Perform a stepwise acid-base analysis using compensation formulae, and recognise when compensation is inappropriate.
6. Calculate and interpret the anion gap and the delta ratio, and identify mixed disturbances.
7. Identify patients at risk of refeeding syndrome and make defensible decisions about nutritional support.

Chapter Overview

Fluid and electrolyte management is the most frequently performed therapeutic activity in hospital medicine and the one most often done badly. The reasons are worth naming before the content.

Fluid is prescribed as though it were not a drug. Intravenous fluid is ordered by people who would not prescribe an unfamiliar antibiotic without thought, in volumes and compositions that are rarely calculated, frequently continued after the indication has passed, and seldom reviewed. It has a dose, a duration, a set of contraindications, and a well-documented capacity to kill.

The bedside tools do not work as well as clinicians believe. Section 12.1 addresses this directly. Volume assessment by physical examination has poor test characteristics, and the confidence with which it is performed is unrelated to its accuracy.

Electrolyte disorders are usually symptoms, not diagnoses. Hyponatraemia is a finding produced by something, and treating the number without identifying the mechanism produces both diagnostic and therapeutic error. This is the reasoning discipline of Chapter 2 applied to biochemistry.

Correction can be more dangerous than the disorder. This is the theme that recurs most. Overly rapid correction of hyponatraemia causes osmotic demyelination. Overly rapid correction of hypernatraemia causes cerebral oedema. Aggressive refeeding kills malnourished patients. In each case the derangement developed slowly and the physiological adaptation to it is now the thing that must be respected.

The chapter presents formulae where they are genuinely useful. Readers should treat them as estimates that direct the next measurement rather than as instruments of precision, and should verify all reference ranges against their own laboratory, since these vary meaningfully between analysers and institutions.

12.1 Volume Assessment: Why the Physical Examination Fails

12.1.1 The uncomfortable evidence

Clinicians assess volume status many times a day and record confident conclusions. The evidence for the individual components of that assessment is poor.

Skin turgor, dry mucous membranes, sunken eyes, and capillary refill have been examined repeatedly and perform weakly, particularly in older adults, in whom skin elasticity declines independently of hydration and in whom mouth breathing and anticholinergic medication produce dry mucous membranes regardless of volume state.

Jugular venous pressure is the most informative single sign when it is measured well and is clearly abnormal, and it is also subject to poor interobserver agreement. Its value is asymmetric: a convincingly elevated venous pressure is meaningful, whereas a venous pressure that cannot be seen is frequently uninformative rather than reassuring.

Postural vital signs detect substantial volume loss reasonably well, with a marked postural rise in pulse being the more useful component, and they detect moderate loss poorly. They are also confounded by autonomic neuropathy, by beta-blockade, and by medication.

Central venous pressure, despite decades of use, does not predict which patients will respond to fluid. Systematic reviews have consistently found essentially no relationship between static filling pressures and fluid responsiveness, and this finding has been robust across populations. A central venous pressure tells you something about the relationship between volume and cardiac compliance at that moment; it does not tell you what will happen if you give more.

Fluid balance charts are incompletely recorded, omit insensible losses, and accumulate error across days. They are useful for trend and useless for precision.

Daily weight is the most underused measurement in this domain. It is simple, quantitative, and directly reflects total body water change, and it is omitted because it requires effort from nursing staff rather than because it lacks value.

12.1.2 Preload responsiveness is not the same as needing fluid

Two concepts are routinely conflated, and separating them prevents a great deal of harm.

Preload responsiveness means that giving fluid will increase stroke volume, which occurs when the ventricle is operating on the steep portion of the Frank-Starling relationship. Roughly half of haemodynamically unstable patients are preload responsive at any given moment, which means that in the other half, fluid will raise filling pressures and cause harm without increasing output.

The need for fluid is a clinical judgement that additionally requires that increasing stroke volume would be beneficial, and that the harms of the volume load are acceptable. A patient with sepsis and a low cardiac output may be preload responsive and benefit. A patient with the same responsiveness and pulmonary oedema may be harmed by the identical intervention.

Fluid tolerance is the third concept and the one most recently emphasised: whether the patient can accommodate additional volume without pulmonary or systemic congestion. Lung ultrasound showing B-lines, as in Chapter 9, section 9.7.2, and assessment of venous congestion, indicate a patient in whom further fluid will cause harm even if it would transiently increase output.

12.1.3 Dynamic assessment

Where the question genuinely matters, dynamic measures outperform static ones.

Passive leg raising with measurement of the change in stroke volume or a surrogate is the most broadly applicable test. It transiently autotransfuses venous blood, is reversible, requires no fluid administration, and is valid in spontaneously breathing patients and in atrial fibrillation. It requires a means of measuring the response, which may be echocardiographic, and simply observing the blood pressure is considerably less reliable.

Pulse pressure variation and stroke volume variation perform well but only under restrictive conditions: sinus rhythm, controlled mechanical ventilation with adequate tidal volume, absence of spontaneous respiratory effort, and a closed chest. Most ward patients fail these conditions, and applying the measures outside them produces false results.

Inferior vena cava assessment is convenient and, used alone, performs modestly, as noted in Chapter 9, section 9.7.2. It contributes to a picture rather than answering the question.

A fluid challenge with a defined small volume given rapidly and a defined measured response remains a legitimate approach, provided the response is actually measured and the challenge is not simply repeated by default.

12.1.4 A practical position

For the hospitalist on a general ward, the following is defensible.

Use several imperfect measures together rather than relying on one. History of intake and losses, weight trend, jugular venous pressure where clearly abnormal, postural measurements, urine output, mucous membranes and axillae, and where available lung and cardiac ultrasound.

Weigh the patient daily and treat the trend as a primary measurement.

Treat each fluid administration as a test with a stated hypothesis and a measured endpoint. State what is expected to improve and check whether it did. Chapter 2, section 2.7.2, applied this discipline to diagnostic tests, and it applies equally to therapeutic ones.

Reassess before repeating. The commonest error in ward fluid management is the second and third litre given because the first was given, without any assessment in between.

12.2 Crystalloid Choice, Chloride Load, and Fluid Stewardship

12.2.1 The compositions

Understanding the differences requires knowing what is in the bags.

Sodium chloride 0.9 per cent contains sodium and chloride at approximately 154 millimoles per litre each. It is isotonic with respect to plasma osmolality but its chloride concentration is substantially above the physiological plasma concentration of roughly 100 millimoles per litre. It contains no buffer.

Balanced or buffered crystalloids, including compound sodium lactate preparations and acetate-buffered solutions, contain sodium at concentrations closer to plasma, chloride at concentrations closer to physiological, small amounts of potassium, and an organic anion buffer, either lactate, acetate, or gluconate, which is metabolised to bicarbonate. Some contain calcium or magnesium.

Glucose 5 per cent is, physiologically, free water once the glucose is metabolised. It distributes throughout total body water and contributes almost nothing to intravascular volume. It should never be used for resuscitation.

Hypertonic saline preparations are used for specific indications addressed in section 12.3.

12.2.2 The chloride problem

Administering large volumes of a solution containing supraphysiological chloride produces **hyperchloraemic metabolic acidosis**, through mechanisms best understood using the physicochemical framework: adding chloride relative to sodium reduces the strong ion difference, which obligates a fall in bicarbonate.

The concern extends beyond the biochemistry. Chloride loading has been shown experimentally to produce renal vasoconstriction and reduced renal blood flow through tubuloglomerular feedback, and observational data associated hyperchloraemia with acute kidney injury and mortality.

The trial evidence is more equivocal than the mechanism suggests, and readers should know this. Several large randomised comparisons have been conducted. One large single-centre trial in critically ill patients found a lower rate of a composite renal outcome with balanced solutions, and a companion trial in non-critically ill emergency department patients found a similar direction of effect. Two subsequent large multicentre trials found no significant difference in mortality. Meta-analyses have generally suggested either a small benefit or no difference.

The reasonable synthesis: balanced crystalloids are a sensible default for most resuscitation and replacement, the magnitude of benefit is small at most, and the choice matters more as the volume administered increases. For a patient receiving a litre, it is unlikely to matter. For a patient receiving many litres, it plausibly does.

12.2.3 When saline is the right choice

Several situations favour sodium chloride 0.9 per cent specifically.

Hypochloraemic metabolic alkalosis, most often from vomiting or from diuretic therapy, where chloride repletion is the treatment and a balanced solution containing a bicarbonate precursor would be counterproductive.

Hyponatraemia and traumatic brain injury or raised intracranial pressure, where the slight hypotonicity of some balanced solutions relative to plasma is undesirable. Compound sodium lactate solutions have a lower effective osmolality than plasma and can lower serum sodium and contribute to cerebral oedema when given in large volumes.

Where a calcium-containing solution is contraindicated in the same line, notably with citrated blood products, because of the risk of clot formation.

Conversely, a common concern about balanced solutions deserves correction: **the small potassium content of balanced crystalloids is not a reason to avoid them in hyperkalaemia.** Large volumes of saline worsen acidosis, which shifts potassium extracellularly, and comparative data have not shown balanced solutions to raise potassium more than saline.

12.2.4 Colloids

Hydroxyethyl starch preparations should not be used. Multiple large randomised trials demonstrated increased renal replacement therapy and, in some, increased mortality. This is a settled question.

Albumin has been extensively studied. In broad critical care populations it is neither better nor worse than crystalloid for mortality, at considerably greater cost. It appears harmful in traumatic brain injury. It has established specific indications in liver disease, including spontaneous bacterial peritonitis, large-volume paracentesis, and hepatorenal syndrome, addressed in Chapter 15.

12.2.5 Fluid stewardship

The most useful conceptual advance in this area has been to treat fluid as a drug with a defined prescription, and to recognise distinct phases of fluid therapy with opposite objectives.

Resuscitation. Rapid administration to restore perfusion in shock, given as defined boluses with measured response.

Optimisation. Titrated administration to support organ perfusion once the immediate emergency has passed, guided by dynamic assessment.

Stabilisation. Maintenance and replacement of ongoing losses only, with the recognition that further resuscitation fluid is now harmful.

Evacuation, or deresuscitation. Active removal of accumulated fluid, since a positive cumulative balance is consistently associated with worse outcomes across multiple populations. This phase is the one most often omitted entirely: fluid is given during the acute phase and never removed.

Every fluid prescription should specify the indication, the composition, the volume, the rate, the intended endpoint, and the point at which it will be reviewed. This is the direct analogue of the antimicrobial timeout in Chapter 11, section 11.7.3.

12.2.6 Maintenance fluids and iatrogenic hyponatraemia

Maintenance prescribing is where the most preventable harm occurs, because it is delegated, standardised, and unreviewed.

Approximate daily requirements in an adult without unusual losses are on the order of 25 to 30 millilitres of water per kilogram, approximately 1 millimole per kilogram each of sodium, potassium, and chloride, and 50 to 100 grams of glucose to limit ketosis, though this does not meet nutritional needs. These figures require adjustment for age, frailty, cardiac and renal function, and existing deficits or excesses, and older and frail patients generally require less.

Hypotonic maintenance fluid causes hospital-acquired hyponatraemia, particularly in patients with any stimulus to antidiuretic hormone release, which includes pain, nausea, postoperative state, and many medications. Since almost every hospitalised patient has such a stimulus, the practical implication is that routine hypotonic maintenance is unsafe, and isotonic or near-isotonic solutions are preferred for most patients, with the volume rather than the tonicity adjusted downward where fluid restriction is required.

Review maintenance fluid daily and stop it when the patient is drinking. Continued maintenance fluid in a patient who is eating and drinking is a common source of overload, and prescriptions written on admission are frequently still running on day four.

12.3 Hyponatraemia: A Tonicity-Based Algorithm and Correction Limits

12.3.1 What hyponatraemia is

Hyponatraemia is a disorder of **water**, not of sodium. This single reframing prevents most of the errors in its management.

Serum sodium concentration is determined by the ratio of exchangeable sodium and potassium to total body water. A low concentration therefore means relatively too much water, which in almost all cases means that water excretion is impaired, since a person with normal renal water handling can excrete a very large volume of dilute urine and will not become hyponatraemic from drinking alone unless the intake is extreme or the solute intake very low.

The clinical consequence of hypotonic hyponatraemia is movement of water into cells, and the organ that matters is the brain, constrained within the skull. The brain adapts to chronic hyponatraemia by extruding organic osmolytes, which is why chronic hyponatraemia is better tolerated than acute, and why rapid correction of chronic hyponatraemia is dangerous: the adapted brain cannot reaccumulate osmolytes quickly enough and shrinks.

12.3.2 Step one: is this hypotonic hyponatraemia?

Measure serum osmolality. This step is skipped routinely and it must not be, because two categories of hyponatraemia require entirely different management.

Pseudohyponatraemia occurs with severe hypertriglyceridaemia or paraproteinaemia, where the solid phase of plasma is expanded and indirect measurement methods report a falsely low sodium concentration. Measured osmolality is normal. There is no disorder of water and no treatment is required beyond addressing the lipid or protein abnormality.

Hypertonic hyponatraemia occurs when an additional effective osmole draws water out of cells, diluting sodium. The classical cause is hyperglycaemia; others include mannitol and absorbed irrigation solutions. Measured osmolality is high. Treatment is directed at the responsible osmole, and a correction factor is applied to interpret the sodium: sodium falls by approximately 2.4 millimoles per litre for each 5.5 millimoles per litre that glucose is elevated above normal, though published factors vary and the relationship is not linear across the range.

If the measured osmolality is low, this is true hypotonic hyponatraemia and the algorithm proceeds.

12.3.3 Step two: urine osmolality

This step establishes whether the kidney is diluting appropriately.

Urine osmolality below approximately 100 milliosmoles per kilogram indicates maximally dilute urine and therefore appropriate suppression of antidiuretic hormone. Water excretion is intact, and the hyponatraemia results from either water intake exceeding a normal excretory capacity, as in primary polydipsia, or from a reduced excretory capacity due to inadequate solute intake, as in beer potomania and the so-called tea and toast diet, where the limited solute load caps the volume of water that can be excreted. Reset osmostat also produces relatively dilute urine at a lower set point.

Urine osmolality above approximately 100 milliosmoles per kilogram indicates that water excretion is impaired, which is the situation in the great majority of cases, and the algorithm continues.

12.3.4 Step three: urine sodium and volume assessment

Urine sodium below approximately 30 millimoles per litre suggests avid sodium retention and therefore a low effective circulating volume. This occurs in true hypovolaemia, and in the oedematous states of heart failure and cirrhosis, where the circulating volume is sensed as low despite total body sodium excess.

Urine sodium above approximately 30 millimoles per litre suggests that sodium retention is not occurring, which points to the syndrome of inappropriate antidiuresis, to diuretic therapy, to renal salt wasting, to adrenal insufficiency, or to hypothyroidism.

Diuretics confound this measurement substantially and thiazides in particular are a leading cause of hyponatraemia. Where a diuretic is in use, urine sodium is uninterpretable and the diuretic should be considered the likely cause until excluded.

Volume assessment is the fourth input, with the caveats of section 12.1 fully in force. It is the weakest step in the algorithm and should not be allowed to override the biochemistry.

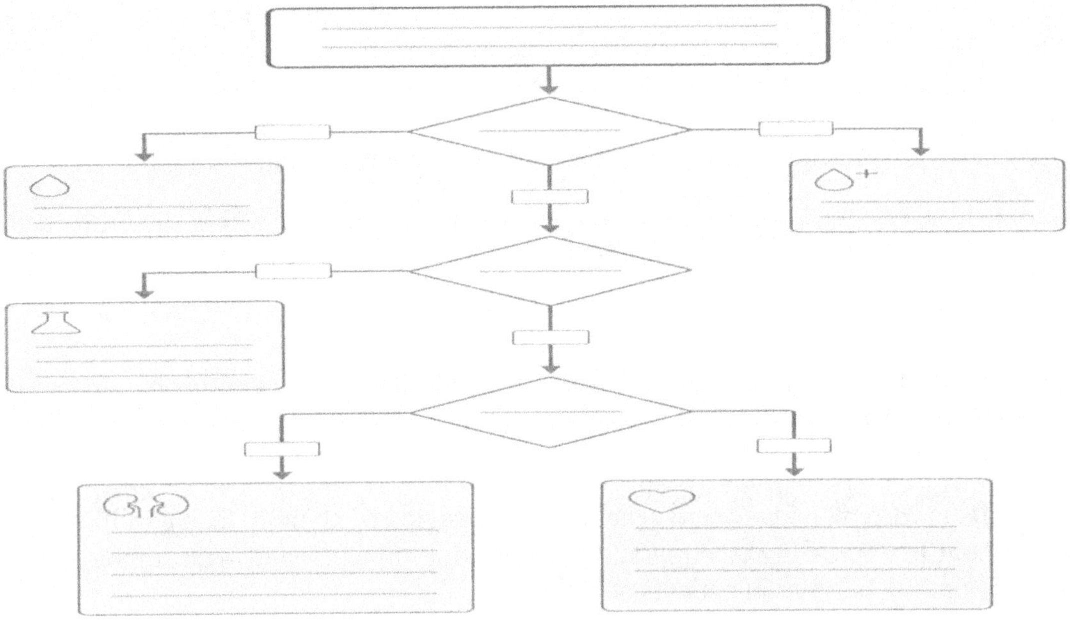

12.3.5 The syndrome of inappropriate antidiuresis

This is the commonest cause of euvolaemic hyponatraemia in hospitalised patients, and it is a diagnosis with criteria rather than a label applied by exclusion of the obvious.

The essential features are hypotonic hyponatraemia, urine that is inappropriately concentrated for the degree of hypotonicity, clinical euvolaemia, urine sodium that is not low in the context of normal salt and water intake, and the **exclusion of adrenal insufficiency and hypothyroidism**, both of which produce an identical biochemical picture and both of which are missed routinely because the diagnosis is assumed rather than established.

Causes are grouped usefully as malignancy, particularly small cell lung carcinoma; pulmonary disease including pneumonia and tuberculosis; central nervous system disease including stroke, haemorrhage, infection, and trauma; drugs, of which the most important are selective serotonin reuptake inhibitors, antipsychotics, antiseizure medications including carbamazepine, cyclophosphamide, and desmopressin; pain, nausea, and the postoperative state; and human immunodeficiency virus infection.

Cerebral salt wasting is a contested entity that resembles the syndrome of inappropriate antidiuresis biochemically but occurs with true volume depletion, principally after subarachnoid haemorrhage. The distinction matters because the treatments are opposite, and where it is suspected, specialist input is warranted.

12.3.6 Treatment: the acute symptomatic patient

Severe symptoms, meaning seizures, coma, or a markedly reduced conscious level attributable to hyponatraemia, constitute an emergency in which cerebral oedema is causing harm now, and the correction limits described below are secondary to raising the sodium quickly enough to relieve it.

The established approach is **hypertonic saline given as a small rapid bolus**, conventionally in the region of 100 to 150 millilitres of 3 per cent saline over ten to twenty minutes, repeated up to a small number of times as required, with the target being a **prompt rise of approximately 4 to 6 millimoles per litre**, which is sufficient to reverse cerebral oedema. Doses, concentrations, and protocols vary between guidelines and institutions and must be taken from local guidance.

Once symptoms have resolved, further correction should proceed slowly within the limits below, and the amount already given counts toward the daily total.

12.3.7 Correction limits and osmotic demyelination

Osmotic demyelination syndrome results from overly rapid correction of chronic hyponatraemia, produces a delayed and frequently devastating neurological syndrome appearing days after the correction, and is largely preventable.

Correction limits in current guidance are generally in the region of no more than 8 millimoles per litre in any 24-hour period, with some guidelines permitting up to 10 and with tighter limits of around 4 to 6 millimoles per litre in patients at high risk.

High-risk features include a serum sodium below approximately 105 millimoles per litre, hypokalaemia, alcohol use disorder, malnutrition, advanced liver disease, and hypoxia.

Two practical points determine whether the limit is respected.

First, **measure frequently**. Two-hourly sodium measurement during active correction is appropriate. Formulae, including the widely used equation estimating the change in serum sodium from a litre of a given infusate, systematically underestimate the actual rise, principally because they do not account for the water diuresis that follows once the stimulus to antidiuretic hormone is removed. Use them to select an initial rate and then measure.

Second, **anticipate autocorrection**. The commonest cause of overcorrection is not the fluid given but the sudden onset of a large water diuresis when the underlying stimulus resolves, as occurs when hypovolaemia is corrected, when a causative drug is stopped, or when adrenal insufficiency is treated. A urine output that becomes suddenly large and dilute is a warning that the sodium is about to rise rapidly.

If overcorrection occurs, it can be reversed, and doing so promptly appears to reduce the risk of demyelination. The approach involves administration of free water as glucose 5 per cent, with desmopressin to abolish the water diuresis. Some centres now use a proactive strategy in high-risk patients, giving desmopressin from the outset to prevent unpredictable diuresis and controlling the rise entirely with hypertonic saline. Either approach requires specialist input and close monitoring.

12.3.8 Treatment: the chronic asymptomatic patient

Management is directed at the cause.

Hypovolaemic hyponatraemia is treated with isotonic saline and correction of the losses, with the expectation of autocorrection as described above.

Hypervolaemic hyponatraemia, in heart failure and cirrhosis, is treated with treatment of the underlying disorder, sodium and water restriction, and diuresis. It is a marker of disease severity and prognosis in both conditions.

The syndrome of inappropriate antidiuresis is treated first by removing the cause where possible, including stopping the responsible drug. Fluid restriction is first-line, and its likely success can be predicted from the ratio of urine to serum electrolytes: a very concentrated urine predicts failure of restriction alone. Increasing solute intake, with oral urea or with salt tablets combined with a loop diuretic, increases free water clearance. Vasopressin receptor antagonists are effective and are constrained by cost, by hepatotoxicity concerns with prolonged use of one agent, and by the risk of rapid overcorrection, and their use should generally involve specialist input.

12.3.9 Hypernatraemia in brief

Hypernatraemia is almost always a water deficit, and in a conscious person with access to water it should not occur, which means its presence usually indicates impaired thirst, impaired access, or impaired consciousness. It is common in older hospitalised patients and is associated with high mortality, largely reflecting the underlying condition.

Calculate the free water deficit, replace it with the sodium content of any replacement fluid taken into account, and **correct slowly**, conventionally at no more than approximately 10 to 12 millimoles per litre in 24 hours in chronic hypernatraemia, because the adapted brain accumulates idiogenic osmoles and rapid correction causes cerebral oedema. Ongoing losses must be replaced in addition to the deficit, and the commonest reason for failure to correct is failure to account for continuing losses.

Diabetes insipidus, central or nephrogenic, should be considered where the urine is inappropriately dilute in the face of hypernatraemia.

12.4 Potassium, Magnesium, and Calcium Disorders

12.4.1 Hyperkalaemia

Establish that it is real. Pseudohyperkalaemia is common and arises from haemolysis during sampling, prolonged tourniquet time and fist clenching, delayed sample processing, and marked thrombocytosis or leucocytosis, in which potassium is released during clotting. A markedly elevated potassium in a well patient with no cause should prompt a repeat sample, taken carefully, before treatment, and where available a blood gas potassium provides a rapid check.

Assess the risk. The danger is cardiac arrhythmia, and the risk depends on the absolute concentration, the rate of rise, and the presence of other conditions affecting membrane excitability including acidosis, hypocalcaemia, hyponatraemia, and hypothermia. A chronically elevated potassium in a dialysis patient carries less immediate risk than the same value arising acutely.

The electrocardiogram is helpful when abnormal and unreliable when normal. The classically described sequence of peaked T waves, PR prolongation, QRS widening, and a sine wave pattern does not occur reliably in order, and cardiac arrest can occur without preceding electrocardiographic change. A normal tracing therefore does not permit a relaxed approach in a patient with a markedly elevated potassium.

Management has three components, and they must be understood as separate.

Stabilise the myocardium with intravenous calcium, as gluconate or chloride, where there are electrocardiographic changes or the potassium is markedly elevated. This does not lower potassium; it raises the threshold for arrhythmia, and its effect is short-lived and may require repetition.

Shift potassium into cells with intravenous insulin given with glucose, which is the mainstay, with the essential caveat that **hypoglycaemia is a frequent and under-recognised complication** requiring scheduled glucose monitoring for several hours afterwards, and with attention to the glucose dose in patients who are already hyperglycaemic or who have renal impairment. Nebulised beta-2 agonists provide an additional shifting effect and are additive to insulin. Sodium bicarbonate has a limited role and is of most value in the presence of significant metabolic acidosis rather than as a routine measure.

Remove potassium from the body, which is the only definitive step. Options are a loop diuretic in a patient with adequate renal function and volume, gastrointestinal potassium binders, and dialysis where the elevation is severe, refractory, or accompanied by other indications. Newer binding agents act more rapidly and are better tolerated than older resins, whose use has been constrained by concerns about gastrointestinal adverse effects.

Address the cause. Review every drug that raises potassium, including renin-angiotensin system blockers, mineralocorticoid receptor antagonists, potassium-sparing diuretics, nonsteroidal anti-inflammatory drugs, trimethoprim, heparin, and calcineurin inhibitors, and consider tissue breakdown, acidosis, adrenal insufficiency, and potassium load from any source.

12.4.2 Hypokalaemia

Establish the mechanism, which falls into three categories that are usually distinguishable from history and urine studies.

Redistribution into cells, from insulin, beta-2 agonists, alkalosis, refeeding as in section 12.7, and periodic paralysis. Total body potassium is normal and aggressive replacement risks rebound hyperkalaemia.

Gastrointestinal loss, from diarrhoea, which also produces a non-anion-gap acidosis, or from vomiting and nasogastric drainage, where the loss is largely renal, driven by the accompanying alkalosis and volume depletion, rather than direct loss in the vomitus.

Renal loss, from diuretics, hyperaldosteronism, hypomagnesaemia, renal tubular acidosis, and several drugs including amphotericin and some antimicrobials.

Replace magnesium first or concurrently. This is the single most useful practical point in this section. Hypomagnesaemia causes renal potassium wasting and renders hypokalaemia refractory to replacement. A patient whose potassium will not rise despite adequate supplementation almost always has an unmeasured or untreated magnesium deficit.

Route and rate. Oral replacement is preferred where the patient can absorb and the deficit is not severe. Intravenous replacement requires attention to concentration and rate, with peripheral administration limited by phlebitis and higher rates requiring central access and cardiac monitoring. Local protocols specify these limits and must be followed.

Recognise the size of the deficit. The relationship between serum concentration and total body potassium is non-linear, and a serum potassium of 3.0 millimoles per litre typically represents a total body deficit of several hundred millimoles. Replacement is therefore usually more prolonged than a single dose.

12.4.3 Magnesium

Magnesium is the most neglected electrolyte in hospital practice and the one whose deficiency most often explains a failure to correct something else.

Hypomagnesaemia causes refractory hypokalaemia, refractory hypocalcaemia through impaired parathyroid hormone secretion and action, arrhythmia including torsades de pointes, tremor, weakness, tetany, and seizures.

Causes relevant to inpatients include gastrointestinal losses, alcohol use disorder, malnutrition and refeeding, diuretics, proton pump inhibitors with prolonged use, and a group of drugs producing renal magnesium wasting including aminoglycosides, amphotericin, platinum agents, calcineurin inhibitors, and epidermal growth factor receptor antagonists.

Measurement is imperfect, since serum magnesium reflects a small fraction of total body magnesium and can be normal in the presence of deficiency. A low-normal value in a patient with a compatible clinical picture should be treated.

Hypermagnesaemia occurs principally in renal impairment with magnesium administration, including magnesium-containing laxatives and antacids, and in the treatment of pre-eclampsia. It produces reduced reflexes, weakness, hypotension, and, at high concentrations, respiratory depression and cardiac arrest. Treatment is cessation of the source, intravenous calcium for cardiac protection, and dialysis where severe.

12.4.4 Calcium

Measure it correctly. Total calcium must be interpreted in relation to albumin, since roughly half of circulating calcium is protein bound. Correction formulae adjusting total calcium for albumin are widely used and are imprecise, particularly in critical illness, and **ionised calcium is preferable where the answer matters** and where a blood gas analyser is available. Acid-base status alters the bound fraction independently of total calcium, with alkalosis increasing binding and reducing the ionised fraction, which is the mechanism of tetany during hyperventilation.

Hypercalcaemia. The overwhelming majority of cases are due to primary hyperparathyroidism, which is commoner in outpatients, or malignancy, which is commoner in inpatients. Malignant hypercalcaemia occurs through humoral mechanisms mediated by parathyroid hormone-related peptide, through osteolytic metastases, and through calcitriol production in some lymphomas. Other causes include granulomatous disease, thyrotoxicosis, immobilisation, thiazides, lithium, vitamin D and calcium excess, and milk-alkali physiology.

Distinguishing the cause rests principally on the parathyroid hormone concentration, which is elevated or inappropriately normal in primary hyperparathyroidism and suppressed in malignancy and most other causes.

Management of symptomatic or severe hypercalcaemia: intravenous isotonic saline to restore volume and promote urinary calcium excretion, which is the first and most important step; a bisphosphonate or denosumab to inhibit bone resorption, recognising that the onset of effect takes a couple of days; calcitonin for a rapid but transient additional effect in the interim; and corticosteroids where the mechanism is calcitriol-mediated, as in granulomatous disease and some lymphomas. **Loop diuretics should not be used routinely** and are reserved for managing volume overload during saline administration, since their historical use for calciuresis is not supported and they worsen volume depletion. Dialysis is available for severe refractory cases.

Hypocalcaemia. Causes relevant to inpatients include post-surgical hypoparathyroidism after thyroid or parathyroid surgery; vitamin D deficiency; hypomagnesaemia as above; acute pancreatitis; rhabdomyolysis and tumour lysis, through phosphate binding; citrate from massive transfusion or regional anticoagulation; hungry bone syndrome; and certain drugs including bisphosphonates and denosumab.

Clinical features include perioral and acral paraesthesia, cramps, tetany with the classical carpopedal spasm, laryngospasm, seizures, and QT prolongation with risk of arrhythmia. The Chvostek and Trousseau signs are traditional and imperfect, with the former in particular occurring in a proportion of normal individuals.

Treatment is intravenous calcium for symptomatic or severe hypocalcaemia with cardiac monitoring, oral replacement with vitamin D or its activated forms for chronic management, and correction of magnesium, without which calcium will not correct.

Phosphate deserves brief mention here and is developed in section 12.7. Severe hypophosphataemia causes muscle weakness including respiratory muscle weakness, haemolysis, rhabdomyolysis, arrhythmia, and encephalopathy, and it is the hallmark of refeeding syndrome.

12.5 The Stepwise Acid-Base Analysis with Compensation Formulae

12.5.1 Why a fixed sequence matters

Acid-base interpretation performed by pattern recognition works for simple disturbances and fails for mixed ones, which are common in hospitalised patients and are precisely the cases where the answer changes management. A fixed sequence, applied every time, detects the second and third disorder that pattern recognition misses.

A note on samples. For pH and bicarbonate, a venous sample is adequate for most purposes and agrees closely with arterial values. Venous carbon dioxide runs higher than arterial and is useful for screening rather than precision. Venous samples do not assess oxygenation. Arterial sampling is required where oxygenation or precise carbon dioxide measurement matters, as in respiratory failure, which is developed in Chapter 14.

12.5.2 The six steps

Step one: is the pH abnormal, and in which direction? Acidaemia below the reference range, alkalaemia above it. A normal pH does not exclude a disturbance and frequently indicates two opposing ones.

Step two: identify the primary disorder. Compare the direction of the pH change with the bicarbonate and the carbon dioxide. In a metabolic disorder the bicarbonate moves in the same direction as the pH. In a respiratory disorder the carbon dioxide moves in the opposite direction to the pH.

Step three: is the compensation appropriate? This is the step most often omitted and it is where mixed disorders are found. Compensation follows predictable quantitative relationships, and the formulae are given below.

Two rules govern interpretation. Compensation never fully returns the pH to normal, so a normal pH in the presence of clear metabolic and respiratory abnormalities indicates two primary disorders rather than complete compensation. And compensation never overshoots, so a compensatory response greater than predicted indicates a second primary disorder in that direction.

Step four: calculate the anion gap, in every case, regardless of the pH, because a raised gap may be present with a normal or even alkalaemic pH in a mixed disorder. Section 12.6 develops this.

Step five: if the anion gap is raised, calculate the delta ratio, addressed in section 12.6.4.

Step six: for a metabolic alkalosis, measure the urine chloride, which distinguishes saline-responsive from saline-resistant causes.

12.5.3 The compensation formulae

The following are the conventional formulae. They are expressed in millimetres of mercury for carbon dioxide, since the classical formulae are stated in those units; where blood gases are reported in kilopascals, convert by dividing the millimetre of mercury value by approximately 7.5. Reference ranges and expected values vary slightly between sources.

Metabolic acidosis. Expected arterial carbon dioxide equals 1.5 multiplied by the bicarbonate, plus 8, with a tolerance of about 2 in either direction. An alternative approximation is that the carbon dioxide in millimetres of mercury approximates the last two digits of the pH.

Metabolic alkalosis. Carbon dioxide rises by approximately 0.7 millimetres of mercury for each 1 millimole per litre rise in bicarbonate above normal. Respiratory compensation for metabolic alkalosis is limited by hypoxic drive and is frequently incomplete.

Acute respiratory acidosis. Bicarbonate rises by approximately 1 millimole per litre for each 10 millimetres of mercury rise in carbon dioxide above normal.

Chronic respiratory acidosis. Bicarbonate rises by approximately 3.5 to 4 millimoles per litre for each 10 millimetres of mercury rise in carbon dioxide, reflecting renal bicarbonate retention that takes several days to develop.

Acute respiratory alkalosis. Bicarbonate falls by approximately 2 millimoles per litre for each 10 millimetres of mercury fall in carbon dioxide.

Chronic respiratory alkalosis. Bicarbonate falls by approximately 4 to 5 millimoles per litre for each 10 millimetres of mercury fall in carbon dioxide.

The clinical use of the acute and chronic respiratory formulae is to establish the time course, which is frequently unknown from the history. A patient with a carbon dioxide of 70 millimetres of mercury and a bicarbonate of 26 has an acute problem; the same carbon dioxide with a bicarbonate of 38 indicates chronic retention with acute worsening. This distinction directs management, as Chapter 14 develops.

12.5.4 Metabolic alkalosis and urine chloride

Metabolic alkalosis requires both a generating process and a maintaining process, since the normal kidney excretes excess bicarbonate readily. The maintaining process is usually chloride depletion, volume depletion, potassium depletion, or mineralocorticoid excess.

Saline-responsive alkalosis, indicated by a urine chloride below approximately 20 millimoles per litre, arises from vomiting, nasogastric suction, diuretic therapy after the diuretic has worn off, and post-hypercapnic states. Treatment is repletion with sodium chloride and potassium.

Saline-resistant alkalosis, with a urine chloride above approximately 20 millimoles per litre, arises from mineralocorticoid excess including primary hyperaldosteronism and Cushing syndrome, severe potassium depletion, current diuretic effect, and rare tubular disorders. Treatment is directed at the cause and includes potassium repletion and mineralocorticoid antagonism where appropriate.

Severe alkalaemia impairs oxygen unloading, lowers ionised calcium, and can cause arrhythmia and reduced respiratory drive, and warrants active management rather than observation.

12.6 Anion Gap, Delta-Delta, and Mixed Disturbances

12.6.1 The anion gap

The anion gap is the difference between the measured principal cation and the measured principal anions, calculated as serum sodium minus the sum of chloride and bicarbonate. It represents the unmeasured anions, principally albumin, phosphate, sulphate, and organic acids.

The reference range depends on the analyser. Older methods produced a conventional normal range of approximately 8 to 12 millimoles per litre; modern ion-selective electrode methods measure chloride differently and produce lower normal ranges, commonly in the region of 3 to 11. **Use your own laboratory's range**, because applying an outdated reference range causes both false-positive and false-negative interpretation.

Include potassium or not, consistently. Some formulations add potassium to the cation side, which raises the reference range accordingly. Either is acceptable provided the matching reference range is used.

Correct for albumin. This step is essential and frequently omitted. Albumin is the dominant unmeasured anion, so hypoalbuminaemia, which is near-universal in hospitalised patients, lowers the measured gap and can conceal a significant organic acidosis. The conventional correction adds approximately 2.5 millimoles per litre to the calculated gap for every 10 grams per litre that albumin falls below approximately 40 grams per litre. A patient with an albumin of 20 grams per litre and an apparently normal anion gap of 12 has a corrected gap of about 17, which is clearly raised.

12.6.2 High anion gap metabolic acidosis

The traditional mnemonic taught for decades includes entities that are now rare or that have been reclassified. A more contemporary framework covers the causes actually encountered.

- **Glycols**, meaning ethylene glycol and propylene glycol, the latter being an important and under-recognised cause in patients receiving prolonged infusions of certain intravenous drug preparations in which it is the diluent.
- **Oxoproline**, also called pyroglutamic acid, which accumulates in patients on chronic therapeutic paracetamol who are malnourished, female, or have renal impairment, and which is a genuinely under-diagnosed cause of unexplained high anion gap acidosis in hospitalised patients.
- **L-lactate**, addressed below.
- **D-lactate**, in short bowel syndrome, producing acidosis with encephalopathy and a normal conventional lactate assay, since standard assays measure only the L-isomer.
- **Methanol.**
- **Aspirin and other salicylates**, which characteristically produce a mixed picture of high anion gap acidosis with a primary respiratory alkalosis.
- **Renal failure**, through retention of sulphates, phosphates, and organic anions.
- **Ketoacidosis**, diabetic, alcoholic, or starvation, addressed in Chapter 17.

The osmolar gap should be calculated where toxic alcohol ingestion is plausible. It is the difference between the measured and the calculated osmolality, and a raised gap suggests the presence of an unmeasured osmole. Its limitations matter: the normal range is wide, the gap may be normal late in the course once the parent alcohol has been metabolised to its acid metabolites, and a normal gap therefore does not exclude toxic alcohol poisoning in a patient presenting late.

Lactate deserves specific comment. Elevated lactate is not synonymous with tissue hypoperfusion. Type A lactic acidosis reflects inadequate oxygen delivery, as in shock and ischaemia. Type B occurs without global hypoperfusion and includes the effect of beta-2 agonists, adrenaline, metformin in the context of renal impairment, thiamine deficiency, liver failure with impaired clearance, malignancy, seizures, and severe exertion. **The trend matters more than the single value**, and lactate clearance over the first hours is more prognostically useful than the presenting concentration.

12.6.3 Normal anion gap metabolic acidosis

Also called hyperchloraemic acidosis, this arises from loss of bicarbonate or from failure to excrete acid, with chloride retained to preserve electroneutrality.

Causes: gastrointestinal bicarbonate loss, principally diarrhoea, and also high-output stomas, fistulae, and ureteric diversions; renal tubular acidoses; carbonic anhydrase inhibitors; early renal failure; and, importantly for this chapter, **administration of large volumes of chloride-rich fluid**, as described in section 12.2.2.

The urine anion gap helps distinguish renal from gastrointestinal causes where the history does not, being negative when renal ammonium excretion is appropriate, as in diarrhoea, and positive when it is impaired, as in renal tubular acidosis.

12.6.4 The delta ratio

When a high anion gap acidosis is present, the delta ratio detects whether a second metabolic disorder coexists.

The principle. In a pure high anion gap acidosis, each unit of added organic acid consumes one unit of bicarbonate and adds one unit to the anion gap, so the rise in the gap should approximately match the fall in bicarbonate.

The calculation is the change in the anion gap from its normal value divided by the change in bicarbonate from its normal value, using the corrected anion gap.

Interpretation:

- **Ratio below approximately 0.4**: the bicarbonate has fallen much more than the gap has risen, indicating a coexisting normal anion gap acidosis, or predominantly a normal anion gap acidosis.
- **Ratio approximately 0.4 to 0.8**: a mixed high and normal anion gap acidosis.
- **Ratio approximately 1 to 2**: a pure high anion gap acidosis.
- **Ratio above approximately 2**: the gap has risen more than the bicarbonate has fallen, indicating either a coexisting metabolic alkalosis or a pre-existing elevated bicarbonate, most often from chronic respiratory acidosis.

Practical caveats. The ratio is an approximation and behaves differently across acidoses, being closer to 1 in ketoacidosis and often higher in lactic acidosis, because the anions are handled differently by the kidney. It should be used to raise a question rather than to make a diagnosis, and the question it raises is frequently the useful one: a patient with diabetic ketoacidosis and a ratio above 2 has probably been vomiting.

12.6.5 Worked reasoning

A patient presents with vomiting, abdominal pain, and hypotension. The blood gas shows a pH of 7.30, carbon dioxide of 26 millimetres of mercury, and bicarbonate of 13 millimoles per litre. Sodium is 138, chloride 96, albumin 22 grams per litre, and lactate is 5.

Step one. Acidaemia.

Step two. The bicarbonate is low and moves with the pH, so the primary disorder is metabolic acidosis.

Step three. Expected carbon dioxide by the metabolic acidosis formula is approximately 1.5 times 13 plus 8, which is about 27.5, with a tolerance of 2. The measured value of 26 falls within this, so respiratory compensation is appropriate and there is no additional respiratory disorder.

Step four. The anion gap is 138 minus the sum of 96 and 13, which is 29. Correcting for an albumin of 22, add approximately 4.5, giving a corrected gap of about 33.5. This is markedly raised.

Step five. The delta ratio, using a normal gap of 12 and a normal bicarbonate of 24, is the change in gap of about 21.5 divided by the change in bicarbonate of 11, which is approximately 1.95. This is at the upper end, suggesting a possible coexisting metabolic alkalosis, which fits the history of vomiting.

Conclusion. A high anion gap metabolic acidosis, most consistent with lactic acidosis in the context of hypoperfusion, with appropriate respiratory compensation and a probable coexisting metabolic alkalosis from vomiting. The alkalosis is masking the severity of the acidosis, which means the underlying process is worse than the bicarbonate alone suggests.

That final sentence is the reason the sequence is worth performing.

12.7 Refeeding Syndrome and Nutritional Support Decisions

12.7.1 The physiology

Refeeding syndrome is the constellation of metabolic disturbances that follows the reintroduction of nutrition in a person who has been starved, and understanding the mechanism makes the management self-evident.

During starvation, insulin secretion falls, glucagon rises, and metabolism shifts to fat and protein catabolism. Intracellular stores of phosphate, potassium, and magnesium are depleted progressively, and thiamine stores are consumed. Crucially, **serum concentrations of these electrolytes remain within the reference range** because they are maintained at the expense of the intracellular pool. A normal phosphate before feeding therefore provides no reassurance.

On refeeding, carbohydrate administration triggers insulin release. Insulin drives glucose, phosphate, potassium, and magnesium into cells, and the shift is superimposed on a depleted total body pool, so serum concentrations fall abruptly. Simultaneously, the shift to carbohydrate metabolism increases thiamine demand in an already depleted patient. Insulin also promotes sodium and water retention, which produces oedema and can precipitate cardiac failure in a patient with reduced cardiac mass from prolonged malnutrition.

Hypophosphataemia is the hallmark, and its consequences are the principal source of harm: respiratory muscle weakness and failure to wean, cardiac dysfunction and arrhythmia, haemolysis, rhabdomyolysis, impaired oxygen delivery through reduced red cell 2,3-diphosphoglycerate, seizures, and encephalopathy.

12.7.2 Identifying the at-risk patient

Widely used criteria, of which the version issued by national guidance bodies is the most familiar, identify high risk by the presence of a single major factor or a combination of lesser ones.

Single high-risk features include a very low body mass index, unintentional weight loss exceeding roughly 15 per cent over three to six months, negligible nutritional intake for more than about ten days, and low concentrations of potassium, phosphate, or magnesium before feeding begins.

Combinations of moderate features include a moderately low body mass index, weight loss exceeding roughly 10 per cent, negligible intake for more than about five days, and a history of alcohol use disorder or of drugs including insulin, chemotherapy, antacids, and diuretics.

Populations to think of specifically: patients with alcohol use disorder; patients with eating disorders; patients with malignancy, particularly of the upper gastrointestinal tract; patients after prolonged critical illness; patients with dysphagia; older patients with prolonged poor intake; postoperative patients who have been nil by mouth for extended periods; and patients presenting after periods of social deprivation or homelessness.

12.7.3 Management

Give thiamine and other B vitamins before or with the first feed, and continue for a defined period. This is inexpensive, safe, and prevents Wernicke encephalopathy, addressed in Chapter 10, section 10.6.3.

Start feeding at a low energy level and increase gradually. Conventional guidance begins at a low intake per kilogram per day in high-risk patients, with an even lower starting point in extreme cases, and increases over several days to the target. Local protocols specify the figures.

Measure and replace electrolytes before and during feeding, with daily or more frequent measurement of phosphate, potassium, magnesium, calcium, sodium, and glucose during the first days.

An important point of emphasis has changed. Historical practice sometimes withheld feeding until electrolytes were normalised. Contemporary consensus is that **electrolyte abnormalities should be corrected concurrently with feeding rather than by delaying it**, since prolonged withholding of nutrition in an already malnourished patient causes its own harm. The correct action is to start low, replace aggressively, and monitor closely, not to wait.

Monitor fluid balance and cardiac status, since fluid retention is part of the syndrome and cardiac reserve is reduced.

A note on evolving evidence. In some populations, notably adolescents and young adults with anorexia nervosa managed in specialist settings with intensive monitoring, more rapid refeeding has been shown to be safe and to shorten admission. This does not generalise to the unmonitored general medical ward, and hospitalists should follow local protocol and involve dietetic and, where relevant, specialist eating disorder services.

12.7.4 Nutritional support decisions

Screen every admitted patient with a validated screening instrument, since malnutrition is present in a substantial proportion of medical inpatients, is associated with worse outcomes, and is routinely undetected.

Enteral nutrition is preferred over parenteral wherever the gut is functional and accessible, because it maintains gut mucosal integrity, is associated with fewer infectious complications, and is substantially cheaper and simpler.

Indications for parenteral nutrition are essentially a non-functioning or inaccessible gastrointestinal tract, including obstruction, high-output fistula, severe malabsorption, and prolonged ileus. Timing of initiation in critically ill patients has been the subject of substantial trial evidence and should follow current critical care guidance.

Nasogastric against post-pyloric feeding. Gastric feeding is simpler and adequate for most patients. Post-pyloric access is used where gastric feeding is not tolerated or where aspiration risk is high, though the evidence that it reduces pneumonia is less strong than commonly assumed.

Percutaneous endoscopic gastrostomy is appropriate where prolonged enteral feeding is anticipated in a patient expected to benefit. It is not appropriate reflexively for dysphagia, and one situation deserves explicit statement: **in advanced dementia, tube feeding has not been shown to prolong survival, prevent aspiration pneumonia, improve pressure injury healing, or improve quality of life**, and careful hand feeding is the recommended alternative. This is a well-established position in geriatric and palliative guidance and is frequently unknown to families and to clinicians. Chapter 20 develops the conversation.

Artificial nutrition and hydration are medical treatments and are subject to the same considerations of benefit, burden, and patient goals as any other. Where they are not achieving their purpose, or where the goals of care have changed, they can be withheld or withdrawn, and Chapter 20 addresses this.

Chapter Summary

- **Fluid is a drug** with an indication, dose, duration, and review point, and it moves through phases with opposing objectives, of which deresuscitation is the one most often omitted.
- **The physical examination performs poorly for volume assessment**, and static filling pressures do not predict fluid responsiveness. Distinguish preload responsiveness, need for fluid, and fluid tolerance. Weigh the patient daily.
- **Balanced crystalloids are a sensible default**, with saline preferred in hypochloraemic alkalosis and where hypotonicity is undesirable. Hydroxyethyl starch should not be used. **Routine hypotonic maintenance fluid causes hospital-acquired hyponatraemia.**
- **Hyponatraemia is a disorder of water.** Measure osmolality first to exclude pseudohyponatraemia and hypertonic hyponatraemia, then urine osmolality, then urine sodium. Exclude adrenal insufficiency and hypothyroidism before diagnosing inappropriate antidiuresis.
- **Severe symptoms warrant prompt hypertonic saline** to raise sodium by 4 to 6 millimoles per litre. Otherwise respect correction limits, measure two-hourly, and anticipate autocorrection when the underlying stimulus resolves, which is the commonest cause of overcorrection.
- **Replace magnesium first** in refractory hypokalaemia and hypocalcaemia. In hyperkalaemia, stabilise, shift, and remove are three separate actions, and only the third lowers total body potassium. Monitor glucose for hours after insulin.

- **Apply the six-step acid-base sequence every time.** Compensation never normalises the pH fully and never overshoots. Calculate the anion gap in every case and **correct it for albumin**, since hypoalbuminaemia conceals significant organic acidosis.
- **The delta ratio detects the second metabolic disorder**, and a ratio above 2 in a patient with a high anion gap acidosis usually means a coexisting alkalosis masking the severity.
- **In refeeding syndrome, serum electrolytes are normal before feeding despite depleted intracellular stores.** Give thiamine first, start low, increase slowly, and correct electrolytes concurrently with feeding rather than by delaying it.
- **Tube feeding in advanced dementia does not prolong survival, prevent aspiration, or improve quality of life.**

Review Questions

1. A patient with sepsis has received three litres of crystalloid and remains hypotensive. A colleague proposes a fourth litre on the basis of a central venous pressure of 6. Explain what the measurement does and does not tell you, and describe how you would decide.
2. A patient has a serum sodium of 118 millimoles per litre, is alert, and has been taking sertraline and a thiazide. Set out your diagnostic sequence, stating what each measurement would change, and your management plan including correction targets.
3. A patient with a serum potassium of 3.1 millimoles per litre has received 120 millimoles of potassium over two days with no change. State the most likely explanation and what you would do.
4. Interpret the following and state the complete diagnosis: pH 7.47, carbon dioxide 30 millimetres of mercury, bicarbonate 21 millimoles per litre, sodium 140, chloride 96, albumin 25 grams per litre.
5. A 48-year-old with alcohol use disorder has eaten almost nothing for two weeks. Phosphate, potassium, and magnesium are all at the lower limit of normal. The dietitian proposes starting full-rate enteral feeding tomorrow once the electrolytes are replaced. State your position and your plan.

CHAPTER 13: Cardiovascular Emergencies and Haemodynamics

Learning Objectives

After studying this chapter, the reader should be able to:

1. Distinguish type 1 from type 2 myocardial infarction and from non-ischaemic myocardial injury, and explain why the distinction changes management.
2. Classify acute decompensated heart failure by perfusion and congestion, and construct a decongestion strategy including the management of diuretic resistance.
3. Make rate, rhythm, and anticoagulation decisions in atrial fibrillation, including new atrial fibrillation arising during acute illness.
4. Manage bradyarrhythmias and tachyarrhythmias on the ward, and describe the practical management of implanted cardiac devices.
5. Distinguish hypertensive emergency from asymptomatic severe hypertension, and apply condition-specific blood pressure targets.
6. Differentiate the four categories of shock at the bedside and support the circulation appropriately.
7. Deliver and lead in-hospital resuscitation, and manage the post-arrest patient including the principles of neuroprognostication.

Chapter Overview

Part IV addresses the emergencies that arise on the ward, and it opens with the cardiovascular system because cardiovascular deterioration is the commonest final pathway of in-hospital decline regardless of the admitting diagnosis.

Three themes structure this chapter.

Mechanism determines treatment. The recurring failure in ward cardiology is applying a protocol derived for one mechanism to a patient with another. Anticoagulating a type 2 infarction, rate-controlling the atrial fibrillation of septic shock while the sepsis goes untreated, and diuresing the hypotensive patient with right ventricular failure are all instances of the same error. Sections 13.1, 13.2, and 13.6 are structured around getting the mechanism right first.

The number is not the emergency. A blood pressure of 210 over 120 in an asymptomatic patient, a heart rate of 140 in a patient with sepsis, and a troponin of 200 nanograms per litre in a patient with pneumonia are all findings that generate reflex intervention and that frequently require none. Section 13.5 develops this most directly.

Recognition precedes rescue. Chapter 4, section 4.5, established that the difference between institutions lies in detection and response rather than in treatment. Everything in this chapter is treatable; most of the deaths follow from late recognition.

13.1 Acute Coronary Syndrome on the Medical Ward: Type 1 Against Type 2 Infarction

13.1.1 The definitional framework

The universal definition of myocardial infarction distinguishes several entities that are frequently conflated in ward practice, and the distinctions are clinically consequential rather than academic.

Myocardial injury is present when cardiac troponin is elevated above the ninety-ninth percentile upper reference limit. It is acute when there is a rise or fall in the concentration, and chronic when the elevation is stable.

Myocardial infarction requires acute myocardial injury **plus clinical evidence of acute myocardial ischaemia**. The supporting evidence may be symptoms of ischaemia, new ischaemic electrocardiographic changes, development of pathological Q waves, imaging evidence of new loss of viable myocardium or a new regional wall motion abnormality in a pattern consistent with an ischaemic aetiology, or identification of coronary thrombus.

The essential point is that an elevated troponin is not a diagnosis of infarction. Troponin is a marker of myocyte injury from any cause, and its interpretation requires the clinical context. Chapter 6, section 6.5, made this argument in the perioperative setting; it applies with equal force on the medical ward.

Type 1 myocardial infarction results from acute atherothrombotic coronary artery disease, usually precipitated by plaque rupture or erosion with superimposed thrombus. This is the process that antiplatelet therapy, anticoagulation, and revascularisation are designed to treat.

Type 2 myocardial infarction results from a mismatch between myocardial oxygen supply and demand in the absence of acute atherothrombosis. Mechanisms include tachyarrhythmia, bradyarrhythmia, hypotension and shock, severe hypertension, hypoxaemia, severe anaemia, sepsis, coronary spasm, coronary embolism, and spontaneous coronary artery dissection.

Types 3 to 5 cover infarction with death before biomarkers could be obtained, and infarction related to percutaneous coronary intervention and to coronary artery bypass surgery respectively.

Non-ischaemic myocardial injury covers the many conditions that damage myocytes without ischaemia: myocarditis, takotsubo syndrome, heart failure, pulmonary embolism with right ventricular strain, sepsis, renal failure with impaired clearance, infiltrative disease, arrhythmia, cardiac contusion, and cardiotoxic drugs.

13.1.2 Why this matters on the ward

Type 2 infarction and non-ischaemic injury together account for a large proportion of troponin elevations in hospitalised medical patients, and considerably outnumber type 1 events in that population.

The prognosis is not benign. Patients with type 2 infarction have high mortality, frequently exceeding that of type 1 patients, though the deaths are predominantly non-cardiac and reflect the severity of the precipitating illness rather than the coronary event itself.

The management is different, and applying the type 1 pathway causes harm. Dual antiplatelet therapy and anticoagulation in a patient with type 2 injury from sepsis or gastrointestinal bleeding adds bleeding risk with no established benefit. Urgent invasive investigation in an acutely septic patient adds contrast, transfer, and procedural risk. The evidence base for antithrombotic and invasive management in type 2 infarction is limited, and the default should therefore be to treat the precipitant.

The management of type 2 infarction is treatment of the supply and demand imbalance. Control the arrhythmia. Restore the blood pressure. Correct the anaemia where significant. Treat the hypoxia and the sepsis. Relieve the pain. These interventions address the mechanism directly.

Secondary prevention still applies. A patient with type 2 infarction has demonstrated that their coronary circulation cannot meet increased demand, which frequently means underlying coronary disease. Outpatient cardiovascular assessment and risk factor management are appropriate, and this is a finding that must survive the discharge summary, as Chapter 3, section 3.4.2, required.

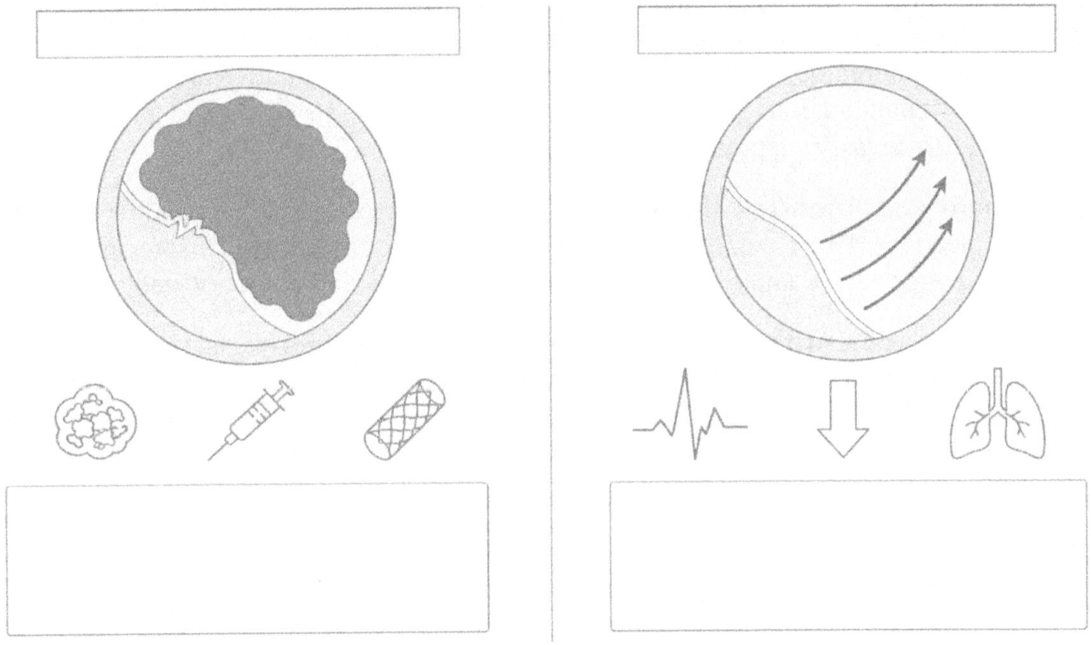

13.1.3 Distinguishing them in practice

No single test separates the two, and the judgement is clinical.

Features favouring type 1: typical ischaemic symptoms; dynamic ischaemic electrocardiographic change, particularly ST elevation or new ST depression and T wave inversion in a coronary territory; a large and rapidly rising troponin; a regional wall motion abnormality in a coronary distribution; known coronary disease; and absence of an adequate alternative explanation.

Features favouring type 2: an identifiable and sufficient precipitant, such as sustained tachyarrhythmia, hypotension, severe anaemia, or hypoxaemia; a modest troponin rise; absence of ischaemic symptoms, though this is unreliable in the acutely unwell; and improvement in the troponin trend as the precipitant is corrected.

Where the distinction is unclear, and particularly where the patient is stable and the precipitant is treatable, a reasonable approach is to treat the precipitant, monitor the troponin trend and electrocardiogram, involve cardiology, and defer the decision about invasive investigation until the acute illness has settled.

13.1.4 Managing type 1 acute coronary syndrome on the ward

ST elevation myocardial infarction occurring in a hospitalised patient requires activation of the primary percutaneous coronary intervention pathway immediately, exactly as for a community presentation, with the same time targets. The delays that affect in-hospital stroke, described in Chapter 10, section 10.4.1, apply here too.

Non-ST elevation acute coronary syndrome requires antithrombotic therapy, anti-ischaemic therapy, and risk stratification determining the timing of invasive assessment. Validated risk scores are used to categorise patients, with very high-risk features including haemodynamic instability, cardiogenic shock, refractory or recurrent chest pain despite treatment, life-threatening arrhythmia, and mechanical complications mandating immediate invasive strategy, and high-risk features indicating an early invasive approach.

Antithrombotic and adjunctive therapy should follow current guidelines and be selected with attention to bleeding risk, renal function, and any planned procedure. Chapter 6, section 6.2, addressed the perioperative implications of antiplatelet therapy and coronary stents.

Myocardial infarction with non-obstructive coronary arteries is an important category encountered when angiography does not show significant epicardial disease despite a genuine infarct pattern. It is a working diagnosis requiring further evaluation rather than an endpoint, with cardiac magnetic resonance imaging and other investigations directed at identifying plaque disruption, spasm, embolism, dissection, myocarditis, or takotsubo syndrome.

Takotsubo syndrome deserves specific mention in a hospital medicine text because it is frequently precipitated by acute physical illness and by the emotional stress of hospitalisation, presents identically to acute coronary syndrome including with electrocardiographic changes and troponin elevation, and is diagnosed by the characteristic regional wall motion abnormality extending beyond a single coronary territory with unobstructed arteries. It is not benign, carrying real rates of acute heart failure, arrhythmia, and mortality.

13.2 Acute Decompensated Heart Failure: Phenotypes and Decongestion

13.2.1 Classify before treating

The single most useful step in acute heart failure is to place the patient into one of four categories defined by two bedside questions, an approach derived from the haemodynamic profiles described by Stevenson and colleagues.

Is the patient congested? Orthopnoea, elevated jugular venous pressure, peripheral oedema, ascites, hepatic congestion, and pulmonary crackles indicate a wet profile. Bedside lung ultrasound showing bilateral B-lines is more sensitive than auscultation, as noted in Chapter 9, section 9.7.2.

Is the patient perfusing? Narrow pulse pressure, cool peripheries, altered mental state, oliguria, hyponatraemia, and rising lactate or worsening renal function indicate a cold profile.

The four combinations that result have different treatments.

Warm and wet is by far the commonest presentation and is treated with decongestion, principally diuresis, with vasodilators where blood pressure permits.

Cold and wet is the highest-risk profile, requiring cautious decongestion with consideration of inotropic support, and carrying the worst prognosis.

Cold and dry indicates hypoperfusion without congestion, requiring careful assessment for hypovolaemia and consideration of inotropes rather than further diuresis.

Warm and dry is the compensated state and is the target of treatment.

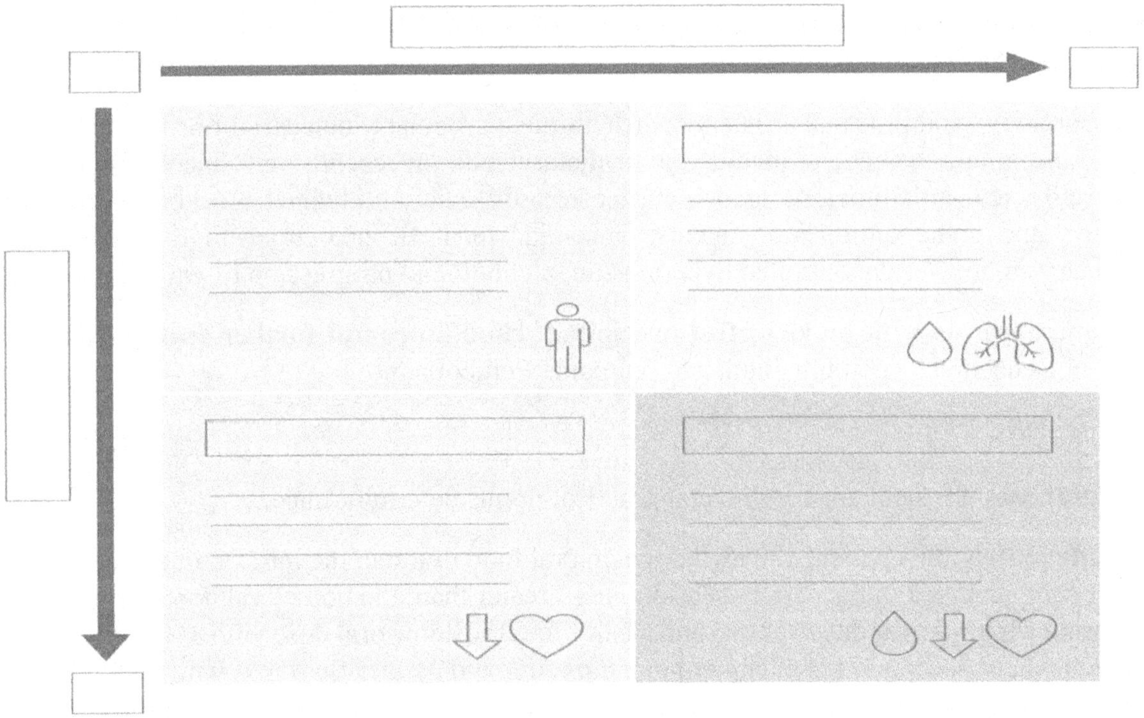

13.2.2 Presentation phenotypes

Beyond the four profiles, several distinct presentations warrant different initial management.

Gradual decompensation of chronic heart failure develops over days to weeks with progressive fluid accumulation and weight gain. Total body volume is genuinely increased, and diuresis is the principal treatment.

Acute pulmonary oedema with hypertension, sometimes called sympathetic crashing acute pulmonary oedema, develops over minutes to hours in a patient who is often not volume overloaded. The mechanism is redistribution of fluid into the lungs driven by a sudden rise in afterload and sympathetic activation, rather than accumulation. **The treatment is therefore**

vasodilation and non-invasive ventilation rather than large-dose diuresis, and high-dose nitrate therapy with positive pressure support produces rapid improvement. Aggressive diuresis in a patient who is euvolaemic in total body terms produces hypovolaemia and renal injury.

Cardiogenic shock, addressed in section 13.6.4.

Isolated or predominant right ventricular failure, from pulmonary hypertension, right ventricular infarction, or pulmonary embolism. This phenotype is dangerous to mismanage, because the right ventricle is preload dependent and aggressive diuresis or vasodilation can precipitate collapse. Chapter 6, section 6.4.4, addressed the physiology.

High-output failure, from severe anaemia, thyrotoxicosis, arteriovenous fistula, sepsis, or thiamine deficiency, in which the treatment is the underlying cause.

13.2.3 Identify the precipitant

Decompensation nearly always has a cause, and finding it is as important as treating the congestion. The list to work through:

Acute coronary syndrome and ischaemia; arrhythmia, particularly new atrial fibrillation; infection of any kind; non-adherence to medication or dietary sodium; recently introduced drugs, notably nonsteroidal anti-inflammatory agents, corticosteroids, calcium channel blockers with negative inotropy, and some antidiabetic agents; anaemia; renal deterioration; thyroid dysfunction; pulmonary embolism; uncontrolled hypertension; alcohol; and progression of valvular disease.

A decompensation with no identified precipitant should prompt further search, particularly for silent ischaemia, occult infection, and pulmonary embolism.

13.2.4 Decongestion

Loop diuretics are the mainstay. Several practical points determine success.

Dose adequately. In a patient already taking an oral loop diuretic, the intravenous dose should be at least equivalent to, and generally substantially greater than, the home oral dose. Trial evidence comparing a high-dose strategy at two and a half times the home oral dose with a low-dose strategy at an equivalent dose found greater symptomatic relief and greater fluid loss with the higher dose, at the cost of a transient rise in creatinine, without difference in the primary endpoints.

Bolus and infusion appear broadly equivalent in the same trial, so either is acceptable, and the choice can be made on practical grounds.

Assess the response early rather than the following day. Two approaches are used. Urine output over the first hours is simple and informative. **A spot urine sodium measured a couple of hours after the dose** predicts the diuretic response well, with a low value indicating an inadequate natriuretic response requiring dose escalation. This is a simple, cheap, and underused measurement that permits same-day escalation rather than a wasted day.

Escalate promptly if the response is inadequate, by doubling the dose rather than by adding a second agent first.

Add sequential nephron blockade where high-dose loop therapy alone is insufficient. Options with trial support include a carbonic anhydrase inhibitor, which improved decongestion when added to loop therapy in a randomised trial, and a thiazide-type diuretic, which increased weight loss in another. Mineralocorticoid receptor antagonists have a role, and sodium-glucose cotransporter-2 inhibitors have evidence for benefit when initiated during the admission.

Monitor daily weight, fluid balance, electrolytes including potassium and magnesium, and renal function.

13.2.5 Diuretic resistance and worsening renal function

Mechanisms of diuretic resistance include inadequate dosing, poor oral absorption due to gut wall oedema, hypoalbuminaemia reducing delivery to the tubule, reduced renal perfusion, distal tubular hypertrophy with chronic loop diuretic use, competing organic anions in renal impairment, high dietary sodium, and concurrent nonsteroidal anti-inflammatory drugs.

Worsening renal function during decongestion requires careful interpretation. A modest rise in creatinine during effective decongestion is common and, in a patient who is improving symptomatically and becoming less congested, does not necessarily indicate harm and should not automatically stop the diuresis. The physiological insight underlying this is that **venous congestion, rather than low cardiac output, is the dominant driver of renal dysfunction in most decompensated heart failure**, so relieving congestion frequently improves renal function overall despite a transient rise.

The judgement therefore rests on the trajectory of congestion rather than on the creatinine alone. A patient who is becoming less congested with a rising creatinine is usually being treated correctly. A patient whose creatinine is rising while congestion is unchanged or worsening is not, and requires reassessment for hypoperfusion, obstruction, or an alternative cause.

Ultrafiltration has been compared with stepped pharmacological therapy and was not superior, with more adverse events, so it is reserved for genuine diuretic refractoriness with specialist involvement.

13.2.6 Disease-modifying therapy during admission

Continue guideline-directed therapy wherever possible. Discontinuation of beta-blockade during decompensation is associated with worse outcomes and should be reserved for patients with low output states or symptomatic bradycardia; dose reduction is preferable to cessation.

Renin-angiotensin system inhibitors and mineralocorticoid antagonists may need temporary adjustment in the context of hypotension or renal deterioration, and should be restarted before discharge wherever possible.

Initiation of disease-modifying therapy during the admission, rather than deferral to outpatient follow-up, is now supported for several agent classes, and the admission represents a reliable opportunity that outpatient care frequently misses.

Discharge readiness requires that the patient is close to euvolaemia rather than merely improved, has been transitioned to an oral regimen with an observed response, has stable renal function and electrolytes, has an explicit weight target and instructions on what to do if the weight rises, and has early follow-up arranged. Chapter 3, sections 3.4 and 3.5, addressed the transition, and heart failure is the condition in which those principles are tested most often.

13.3 Atrial Fibrillation: Rate, Rhythm, and Anticoagulation Decisions

13.3.1 New atrial fibrillation in the acutely unwell patient

Atrial fibrillation arising during an acute medical illness is a different clinical problem from atrial fibrillation presenting to an outpatient clinic, and treating it as the same produces error.

It is usually secondary. Sepsis, pneumonia, pulmonary embolism, thyrotoxicosis, alcohol, electrolyte disturbance particularly of potassium and magnesium, hypoxia, pain, surgery, and myocardial ischaemia all precipitate atrial fibrillation, and in a substantial proportion the rhythm reverts when the precipitant is treated.

The commonest error is treating the rhythm and ignoring the cause. A patient with a heart rate of 150 in septic shock does not primarily have an arrhythmia problem; they have sepsis with a compensatory and partly maladaptive response. Aggressive rate control in that patient removes a compensatory tachycardia and can precipitate haemodynamic collapse.

The correct sequence is to treat the precipitant, correct potassium and magnesium, address hypoxia and pain, and address the rate only where it is contributing to haemodynamic compromise or myocardial ischaemia.

New atrial fibrillation during acute illness is not benign in the longer term. These patients have a substantially increased risk of recurrent atrial fibrillation and of stroke over subsequent years, which means the episode must be communicated at discharge with a plan for follow-up rhythm assessment rather than dismissed as a transient event.

13.3.2 Rate control

Targets. A lenient strategy targeting a resting rate below approximately 110 beats per minute was found non-inferior to a strict strategy in a randomised trial, and lenient control is therefore acceptable as an initial target in stable patients, with tighter control pursued if symptoms persist or ventricular function deteriorates.

Agents. Beta-blockers are first-line in most patients. Non-dihydropyridine calcium channel blockers are effective and are **contraindicated in heart failure with reduced ejection fraction** because of negative inotropy. Digoxin is useful as an adjunct, particularly in patients with heart failure or hypotension, and is limited by slow onset, narrow therapeutic index, accumulation in renal impairment, and poor rate control during exertion. Amiodarone provides rate control and some rhythm effect and is useful in critically ill patients with hypotension, at the cost of a substantial adverse effect profile and the possibility of unintended cardioversion.

Practical cautions. Avoid combining intravenous beta-blockers and calcium channel blockers because of profound bradycardia and hypotension. Correct magnesium, which both aids rate control and is frequently depleted. In pre-excited atrial fibrillation, meaning atrial fibrillation with an accessory pathway producing an irregular broad complex tachycardia, **atrioventricular nodal blocking agents are contraindicated** because they can accelerate conduction down the pathway and precipitate ventricular fibrillation; the treatment is electrical cardioversion.

13.3.3 Rhythm control

Immediate electrical cardioversion is indicated in haemodynamic instability attributable to the arrhythmia, with the recognition that in a patient with septic shock and atrial fibrillation, the instability is frequently attributable to the sepsis and cardioversion will not fix it and will not hold.

Elective rhythm control has been re-examined. A large trial of early rhythm control initiated within a year of diagnosis found lower rates of cardiovascular outcomes compared with usual care, which has shifted practice toward earlier consideration of rhythm control, particularly in symptomatic patients and those with heart failure.

The thromboembolic considerations around cardioversion are important and frequently misapplied. The traditional teaching permits cardioversion without prior anticoagulation when the arrhythmia has been present for less than a defined period, conventionally 48 hours. Observational data have shown that thromboembolic events occur even within this window, particularly in patients with higher stroke risk profiles, and current guidance is more cautious. Where duration is uncertain or exceeds the window, either a period of therapeutic anticoagulation beforehand or transoesophageal echocardiography to exclude atrial thrombus is required.

Anticoagulation is required for a defined period after cardioversion regardless of the pre-cardioversion strategy, conventionally at least four weeks, because atrial mechanical function recovers more slowly than electrical function and thrombus can form after the rhythm has been restored. This is one of the most consistently forgotten points in ward practice.

13.3.4 Anticoagulation

Risk stratification uses a validated clinical score incorporating heart failure, hypertension, age, diabetes, prior stroke or thromboembolism, vascular disease, and sex, with more recent guidance from some bodies removing the sex category as a determinant of the treatment threshold. Local guidance should be followed.

Bleeding risk scores should be used to identify and correct modifiable risk factors and to flag patients requiring closer review, not to withhold anticoagulation. Patients at high bleeding risk are frequently also at high thromboembolic risk, and the absolute benefit of anticoagulation in that group is often greater rather than smaller.

Direct oral anticoagulants are preferred to vitamin K antagonists for most patients, with the specific exceptions of mechanical heart valves and moderate to severe mitral stenosis, where a vitamin K antagonist remains indicated.

Inappropriate dose reduction is a common and harmful error. Direct oral anticoagulants have specific licensed dose-reduction criteria based on combinations of age, weight, and renal function. Reducing the dose outside those criteria, usually from an intuition about bleeding risk, is associated with increased thromboembolic events without a corresponding reduction in bleeding. Check the criteria rather than estimating.

Left atrial appendage occlusion is an option for patients with a genuine long-term contraindication to anticoagulation and should be a specialist decision.

Chapter 7, section 7.4, addressed perioperative interruption.

13.4 Bradyarrhythmias, Tachyarrhythmias, and Device Interrogation

13.4.1 Bradyarrhythmia: establish whether it is intrinsic or extrinsic

The first question in symptomatic bradycardia is whether the conduction system is damaged or suppressed, because the reversible causes are common and are frequently missed.

Extrinsic and reversible causes: drugs, principally beta-blockers, non-dihydropyridine calcium channel blockers, digoxin, antiarrhythmics, and centrally acting agents including clonidine and some ophthalmic preparations that are systemically absorbed; hyperkalaemia; hypothyroidism; hypothermia; hypoxia; raised intracranial pressure; obstructive sleep apnoea; and vagal stimulation from pain, vomiting, or instrumentation.

Intrinsic causes: sinus node dysfunction, conduction system fibrosis, myocardial ischaemia particularly inferior infarction, infiltrative disease including amyloid and sarcoid, infection including Lyme carditis and endocarditis with abscess, and post-surgical or post-procedural injury.

13.4.2 Atrioventricular block

First-degree block, meaning prolonged conduction without dropped beats, is usually benign in isolation.

Second-degree Mobitz type I, with progressive PR prolongation before a dropped beat, is usually at the level of the atrioventricular node, frequently responds to atropine, and rarely progresses to complete block.

Second-degree Mobitz type II, with constant PR intervals and sudden dropped beats, is usually infranodal, does **not** reliably respond to atropine, and carries a meaningful risk of progression to complete heart block. It requires monitoring and usually pacing.

High-grade and complete block require pacing support, temporary or permanent depending on reversibility.

Practical points. Atropine acts on the atrioventricular node and is therefore of limited use in infranodal block, where it may occasionally worsen the situation by increasing atrial rate without improving conduction. Transcutaneous pacing is a bridge that is painful and frequently fails to capture; capture must be confirmed mechanically by pulse or ultrasound rather than assumed from the monitor. Chronotropic infusions provide temporary support. Transvenous pacing is definitive as a bridge.

Specific antidotes are worth knowing: intravenous calcium for calcium channel blocker toxicity, glucagon and high-dose insulin with glucose for beta-blocker and calcium channel blocker toxicity, and digoxin-specific antibody fragments for digoxin toxicity. Toxicology advice should be sought early in significant overdose.

13.4.3 Tachyarrhythmia: the two questions

Classify by **width** and **regularity**, which generates a manageable differential.

Narrow and regular: sinus tachycardia, atrial tachycardia, atrial flutter with fixed conduction, and paroxysmal supraventricular tachycardia by reentry involving the atrioventricular node or an accessory pathway. Vagal manoeuvres, performed properly, and adenosine are both diagnostic and therapeutic. Adenosine has a very short half-life, requires rapid administration with a flush, causes a brief but unpleasant sensation that patients should be warned about, and is relatively contraindicated in severe asthma and in the presence of pre-excitation with irregular broad complex tachycardia.

Narrow and irregular: atrial fibrillation, atrial flutter with variable conduction, and multifocal atrial tachycardia, the last of which is characteristically associated with severe pulmonary disease and is treated by treating the lung disease.

Broad and regular: assume ventricular tachycardia. This is the most important rule in this section. The prior probability of ventricular tachycardia in a broad complex regular tachycardia is high, and it is very much higher in a patient with structural heart disease or previous myocardial infarction. Morphological criteria exist to distinguish ventricular tachycardia from supraventricular tachycardia with aberrancy and are useful in expert hands, and the safe default in a ward setting is to treat as ventricular tachycardia. **Verapamil must not be given to an undifferentiated broad complex tachycardia**, as it can cause catastrophic haemodynamic collapse in ventricular tachycardia.

Broad and irregular: atrial fibrillation with bundle branch block, pre-excited atrial fibrillation, and polymorphic ventricular tachycardia.

13.4.4 Management of ventricular arrhythmia

Unstable ventricular tachycardia is treated by immediate synchronised cardioversion; pulseless ventricular tachycardia by defibrillation as in section 13.7.

Stable monomorphic ventricular tachycardia may be treated pharmacologically. Comparative trial evidence has favoured procainamide over amiodarone for acute termination with fewer adverse cardiac events, though availability and familiarity vary; amiodarone and lidocaine remain in wide use. Correct electrolytes and identify ischaemia.

Polymorphic ventricular tachycardia requires the QT interval to be assessed. In the setting of a prolonged QT, meaning torsades de pointes, treatment is intravenous magnesium, correction of potassium, withdrawal of all QT-prolonging agents, and increasing the heart rate by isoprenaline or overdrive pacing to shorten the QT. In the setting of a normal QT, polymorphic ventricular tachycardia usually indicates acute ischaemia and requires urgent assessment for that.

Electrical storm, meaning multiple episodes within a short period, requires sedation, beta-blockade, antiarrhythmic therapy, correction of precipitants, and urgent electrophysiology involvement.

13.4.5 Implanted cardiac devices

Hospitalists encounter these frequently and are often uncertain, so the practical essentials are set out here.

Establish what the device is. A permanent pacemaker, an implantable cardioverter defibrillator, and a cardiac resynchronisation device with or without defibrillator function behave differently.

The patient's device card, the chest radiograph appearance, and device interrogation all establish this. A defibrillator generator is larger and the leads have visible shock coils on radiography.

Magnet response differs between device types, and this is the point most often confused. Placing a magnet over a **pacemaker** generally causes asynchronous pacing at a fixed rate, which is used to prevent inappropriate inhibition by electromagnetic interference. Placing a magnet over an **implantable cardioverter defibrillator** generally suspends tachyarrhythmia detection and therapy, and **does not** alter the pacing mode. Responses are manufacturer-specific and programmable, so a magnet is a temporising measure and not a substitute for interrogation.

Interrogation provides the arrhythmia history, the number and appropriateness of any therapies delivered, battery and lead status, and the programmed parameters. It should be obtained in any patient with a device who presents with syncope, palpitations, shocks, heart failure decompensation, or suspected device malfunction.

A patient who has received a shock requires assessment of whether it was appropriate, meaning delivered for a genuine ventricular arrhythmia, or inappropriate, most often for rapidly conducted atrial fibrillation, sinus tachycardia, or lead noise. Multiple shocks constitute an emergency requiring urgent electrophysiology involvement, sedation, and consideration of magnet application while awaiting it.

Perioperative management was addressed in Chapter 6, and **deactivation at the end of life** is addressed in Chapter 20. The latter deserves a note here: a patient dying with an active defibrillator may receive repeated shocks during the dying process, which is distressing and avoidable, and deactivation should be discussed as part of any decision to limit escalation.

13.5 Hypertensive Urgency and Emergency: The Treatment Threshold

13.5.1 The distinction that matters

Hypertensive emergency is severe blood pressure elevation accompanied by **acute target organ damage**. The organ damage defines the emergency; the number does not.

Recognised presentations include hypertensive encephalopathy, intracerebral haemorrhage, acute ischaemic stroke in specific contexts, acute coronary syndrome, acute pulmonary oedema, aortic dissection, acute kidney injury, eclampsia and pre-eclampsia, microangiopathic haemolytic anaemia, and severe retinopathy with haemorrhages and papilloedema.

Asymptomatic severe hypertension, sometimes called hypertensive urgency, is severe elevation without evidence of acute organ damage. This is the far commoner scenario on the ward and in the emergency department.

13.5.2 Why asymptomatic severe hypertension should not be treated acutely

This deserves emphasis because the reflex to lower a frightening number is strong and the harm from doing so is real.

The autoregulation argument. Cerebral and renal blood flow are autoregulated across a range of perfusion pressures, and in chronic hypertension that range shifts upward. A patient habituated to a mean arterial pressure of 130 may become ischaemic at a pressure that would be entirely normal in someone else. Rapid pharmacological lowering, particularly with agents whose effect is unpredictable, can precipitate cerebral, myocardial, and renal ischaemia.

The evidence argument. Studies of asymptomatic severe hypertension have not shown benefit from acute blood pressure reduction, and have identified harm from aggressive treatment. Short-term cardiovascular event rates in asymptomatic patients are low.

The practical approach. Confirm the measurement with an appropriately sized cuff, in both arms, after a period of rest. Look for and treat the reversible contributors that are common in hospitalised patients: pain, anxiety, urinary retention, missed usual medication, withdrawal states, stimulant use, and drugs including nonsteroidal anti-inflammatory agents and corticosteroids. Assess for target organ damage with history, examination including fundoscopy where indicated, electrocardiogram, renal function, and urinalysis. Then, if no acute damage is present, **restart or adjust oral therapy and arrange follow-up**, aiming for gradual control over days to weeks. Rapid-acting oral or sublingual agents given to produce a fall in the ward are not appropriate.

13.5.3 Targets in hypertensive emergency

Where acute organ damage is present, treatment is urgent, controlled, and monitored, usually with a titratable intravenous agent and frequently with arterial monitoring.

The general target in most hypertensive emergencies is a reduction in mean arterial pressure of no more than approximately 25 per cent in the first hour, then to approximately 160 systolic and 100 to 110 diastolic over the next several hours, then gradual normalisation over the following day or two. The principle is controlled reduction rather than normalisation.

Condition-specific exceptions are important and differ substantially:

Aortic dissection requires rapid reduction of both blood pressure and the rate of rise of pressure, with a systolic target typically below 120 and a heart rate target typically below 60, achieved quickly. **A rate-controlling agent must be given before or with a vasodilator**, because a vasodilator alone produces reflex tachycardia and increased shear stress, which propagates the dissection.

Acute ischaemic stroke requires permissive hypertension in most cases, with treatment reserved for extreme elevation or for patients undergoing reperfusion therapy, where lower thresholds apply. Chapter 10, section 10.4.6, addressed this.

Intracerebral haemorrhage is managed with a moderate systolic target, with evidence supporting controlled reduction and cautioning against very large or very rapid drops.

Acute pulmonary oedema is treated with vasodilator therapy, principally nitrates, alongside non-invasive ventilation, as in section 13.2.2.

Eclampsia and severe pre-eclampsia require magnesium sulphate for seizure prophylaxis alongside specific antihypertensive agents, with obstetric involvement, and the definitive treatment is delivery.

Phaeochromocytoma crisis requires alpha blockade before any beta blockade, since unopposed alpha stimulation from beta blockade alone can produce severe hypertension.

Agents commonly used include labetalol, nicardipine or clevidipine, esmolol, glyceryl trinitrate for pulmonary oedema and coronary ischaemia, and phentolamine for catecholamine excess. Sodium nitroprusside is highly effective and titratable and is limited by cyanide and thiocyanate toxicity with prolonged use. **Hydralazine has an unpredictable and prolonged effect and should be avoided in dissection and used cautiously generally**, and short-acting sublingual nifedipine capsules should not be used at all because of uncontrolled falls in pressure.

13.6 Shock States: Differentiating and Supporting

13.6.1 Definition and the four categories

Shock is circulatory failure resulting in inadequate cellular oxygen utilisation. It is a physiological state, not a blood pressure, and **a normal blood pressure does not exclude shock**, particularly in young patients and in chronic hypertensives whose compensated pressure is high.

The four categories are defined by the mechanism of circulatory failure, and each has a characteristic physiological profile.

Category	Preload	Cardiac output	Systemic vascular resistance	Typical periphery
Hypovolaemic	Low	Low	High	Cold
Cardiogenic	High	Low	High	Cold
Obstructive	Variable, often high	Low	High	Cold
Distributive	Low or normal	High or normal	Low	Warm early

These profiles are a framework rather than a rule, and mixed shock is common in hospitalised patients. A patient with septic shock and a septic cardiomyopathy has distributive and cardiogenic components simultaneously, and a patient with cardiogenic shock who becomes infected acquires a distributive component.

13.6.2 Differentiating at the bedside

History and context do most of the work. A patient with melaena is hypovolaemic; a patient with a new murmur and pulmonary oedema is cardiogenic; a patient with fever and a source is distributive.

Examination. Peripheral temperature and capillary refill separate warm from cold shock reasonably well early in the course, though late distributive shock becomes cold. Jugular venous pressure is elevated in cardiogenic and obstructive shock and low in hypovolaemic shock, and this single sign is among the more discriminating available.

Point-of-care ultrasound is the highest-yield bedside investigation in undifferentiated shock, as Chapter 9, section 9.7.2, described. A focused examination establishes left ventricular function, right ventricular size, pericardial effusion, inferior vena cava appearance, lung sliding and B-lines, and the presence of free abdominal fluid or aortic aneurysm, and this combination usually identifies the category within minutes.

Laboratory. Lactate reflects the severity and, more usefully, its clearance over hours reflects the response, as Chapter 12, section 12.6.2, discussed. Central venous oxygen saturation, where available, is low in low output states and normal or high in distributive shock and in states of impaired oxygen utilisation.

13.6.3 Obstructive shock requires a mechanical answer

This category is separated because recognising it is time-critical and the treatment is not pharmacological.

Cardiac tamponade presents with hypotension, elevated venous pressure, and muffled heart sounds, with pulsus paradoxus, and is confirmed by echocardiography. The treatment is drainage. Fluid may temporise; vasopressors do not fix it.

Tension pneumothorax is a clinical diagnosis requiring immediate decompression, and is visible on bedside ultrasound in seconds.

Massive pulmonary embolism presents with hypotension, hypoxia, and right ventricular dilatation, and requires reperfusion therapy. Chapter 14 develops the decision.

A crucial physiological point applies to all three and to right ventricular infarction: **excessive fluid administration worsens the situation** by distending an already pressure-loaded right ventricle, shifting the interventricular septum, and impairing left ventricular filling. Cautious fluid, early vasopressor, and prompt mechanical treatment is the sequence.

13.6.4 Cardiogenic shock

Recognition requires hypotension or the need for support to maintain pressure, together with evidence of hypoperfusion, in the presence of cardiac dysfunction adequate to explain it. Staging classifications describing a progression from at-risk through beginning shock, classic shock, deteriorating shock, and extremis are used to communicate severity and to guide escalation.

Cause. Acute coronary syndrome remains the commonest cause, and **early revascularisation improves survival** in that setting. Other causes include acute decompensation of chronic cardiomyopathy, myocarditis, valvular catastrophe including acute mitral regurgitation from papillary muscle rupture and acute aortic regurgitation, mechanical complications of infarction including ventricular septal rupture and free wall rupture, arrhythmia, takotsubo syndrome, and right ventricular infarction.

Management principles. Identify and treat the cause urgently. Support perfusion with vasopressors, with noradrenaline generally preferred as a first-line agent, and inotropes where cardiac output is inadequate, using dobutamine, milrinone with attention to its renal clearance and longer half-life, or levosimendan according to availability and the clinical situation. Optimise volume carefully, recognising that some patients are congested and some are relatively underfilled. Correct arrhythmia, acidosis, and hypoxia. Involve cardiology and critical care immediately.

Mechanical circulatory support is an area where the evidence has developed substantially and where hospitalists should know the current position rather than the historical one. Intra-aortic balloon counterpulsation did not improve mortality in a large randomised trial in infarct-related cardiogenic shock and its routine use has fallen. Venoarterial extracorporeal membrane oxygenation likewise did not improve mortality in a randomised trial in that population and carried substantial complications. A trial of a microaxial transvalvular flow pump in patients with ST elevation infarction and cardiogenic shock did report a mortality benefit at the cost of more complications. The overall picture is that these devices have specific roles in selected patients within experienced systems, and are not a general answer to shock.

13.6.5 Vasopressor and inotrope principles

Noradrenaline is the first-line vasopressor for most shock states. Comparative trial evidence against dopamine found more arrhythmic events with dopamine and worse outcomes in the cardiogenic subgroup.

Vasopressin is used as a second agent to reduce catecholamine requirement and has a particular rationale in distributive shock, where endogenous vasopressin is depleted.

Adrenaline provides inotropy and vasoconstriction and is associated with more tachyarrhythmia and lactate elevation.

Angiotensin II is available in some settings for catecholamine-refractory vasodilatory shock.

Mean arterial pressure targets. A target of approximately 65 millimetres of mercury is the conventional starting point, with trial evidence finding no benefit from routinely higher targets, and with evidence in older patients supporting permissive lower targets. Patients with chronic hypertension may require higher targets to maintain renal perfusion, and the target should be individualised against markers of perfusion rather than fixed.

Access. Central venous access is preferred for prolonged vasopressor administration, and short-term peripheral administration of dilute noradrenaline through a well-sited proximal cannula with close monitoring is acceptable and increasingly practised, since delaying vasopressor support while obtaining central access causes harm.

Corticosteroids in septic shock are recommended in patients requiring ongoing vasopressor support, based on trial evidence showing faster shock resolution, with mortality findings varying between trials.

Chapter 18 develops the antimicrobial and source control management of sepsis.

13.7 In-Hospital Cardiac Arrest and Post-Arrest Care

13.7.1 How in-hospital arrest differs

In-hospital cardiac arrest differs from out-of-hospital arrest in ways that shape both prevention and management.

It is usually preceded by deterioration. A substantial proportion of in-hospital arrests are preceded by hours of abnormal physiology, which is the entire premise of the rapid response systems described in Chapter 4, section 4.5. The most effective intervention in in-hospital arrest is preventing it.

Non-shockable rhythms predominate. Pulseless electrical activity and asystole account for the majority, reflecting the underlying causes of hypoxia, hypovolaemia, and progressive illness rather than primary arrhythmia. This changes the prognosis and the emphasis, since the treatable element is the reversible cause rather than defibrillation.

Comorbidity is high, which is why the decision about whether resuscitation is appropriate at all should have been made in advance for many patients. Chapter 20 addresses this.

13.7.2 Delivering resuscitation

High-quality chest compressions are the intervention with the strongest evidence and the one most often degraded. The elements: a rate of approximately 100 to 120 per minute; a depth of approximately 5 to 6 centimetres in an adult; complete recoil between compressions; minimal interruption, with hands-off time kept as short as possible around rhythm checks and defibrillation; and rotation of the compressor every two minutes because quality falls with fatigue faster than the compressor perceives.

Defibrillation for ventricular fibrillation and pulseless ventricular tachycardia should be delivered as early as possible, with compressions resumed immediately afterwards without pausing for a rhythm check.

Reversible causes should be actively sought throughout, using the conventional framework of hypoxia, hypovolaemia, hypothermia, and metabolic derangements including hyperkalaemia, together with tension pneumothorax, tamponade, toxins, and thrombosis, both coronary and pulmonary. In hospitalised patients, hyperkalaemia, hypovolaemia from bleeding, and pulmonary embolism are particularly worth considering, and each has a specific treatment.

Adrenaline improves the rate of return of spontaneous circulation and survival, with the important nuance from large trial evidence that the improvement in survival with favourable neurological outcome was not clearly demonstrated. This is worth understanding when discussing outcomes with families.

Antiarrhythmic therapy with amiodarone or lidocaine is used for shock-refractory ventricular fibrillation, improving the rate of survival to admission with less clear effect on longer-term neurological outcome.

Airway management may be by bag-mask ventilation, supraglottic device, or tracheal intubation, and trial evidence has not established the superiority of any single approach. What matters is that ventilation is adequate, that hyperventilation is avoided because it raises intrathoracic pressure and reduces venous return, and that intubation, if performed, does not interrupt compressions.

Waveform capnography is highly useful: it confirms tracheal tube placement, provides a continuous indicator of compression quality, alerts to return of spontaneous circulation through an abrupt rise, and carries prognostic information, with persistently very low values after prolonged resuscitation being an adverse sign.

Focused ultrasound during rhythm check pauses can identify tamponade, right ventricular dilatation, and absence of cardiac motion, and must be performed by someone competent to do it within the pause without prolonging it.

Extracorporeal cardiopulmonary resuscitation is available in selected centres for selected patients with refractory arrest and a plausible reversible cause.

Duration is a judgement rather than a rule, informed by the initial rhythm, the presumed cause, the quality of resuscitation, the end-tidal carbon dioxide, and any features suggesting a reversible process. Prolonged resuscitation is appropriate in specific circumstances including hypothermia, toxicological arrest, and pulmonary embolism after thrombolysis.

13.7.3 Post-arrest care

Return of spontaneous circulation is the beginning of the treatment, not its conclusion. Post-cardiac arrest syndrome comprises brain injury, myocardial dysfunction, systemic ischaemia-reperfusion response, and persistence of the precipitating pathology.

Oxygenation and ventilation. Avoid both hypoxaemia and hyperoxaemia, targeting a normal oxygen saturation range. Avoid hypocapnia, which reduces cerebral blood flow, and target normocapnia.

Haemodynamics. Maintain an adequate mean arterial pressure to support cerebral perfusion, using fluid, vasopressors, and inotropes as required, and treat the underlying cardiac cause.

Coronary angiography. Immediate angiography is indicated where the electrocardiogram shows ST elevation. In patients without ST elevation and without shock, randomised trials have not demonstrated benefit from immediate compared with delayed angiography, so the decision should be individualised with cardiology input.

Temperature management. This area has changed and practice should reflect the current evidence rather than earlier protocols. A large randomised trial comparing a target of 33 degrees Celsius with normothermia and early treatment of fever found no difference in mortality or neurological outcome. Current guidance emphasises **active prevention of fever**, maintaining temperature at or below approximately 37.5 degrees Celsius for a defined period, rather than routine deep hypothermia. Some evidence suggests possible benefit of lower targets in non-shockable rhythms, and practice varies. Follow current local protocol.

Seizures should be treated, and nonconvulsive status epilepticus should be actively sought with electroencephalography, as Chapter 10, section 10.5.5, argued.

Glucose, electrolytes, and sedation managed to conventional targets, with sedation minimised to permit neurological assessment as soon as it is safe.

13.7.4 Neuroprognostication

This is among the most consequential judgements in hospital medicine and is subject to a specific and serious risk: the self-fulfilling prophecy, in which a pessimistic prediction leads to withdrawal of treatment which then confirms the prediction.

Principles that guard against this:

Do not prognosticate too early. Assessment should not be made before a defined interval, conventionally at least 72 hours after return of circulation, and later in patients who received sedation, neuromuscular blockade, or temperature management, since these confound the clinical examination.

Use multiple modalities rather than any single finding. The recommended approach combines clinical examination, principally bilaterally absent pupillary and corneal reflexes; electrophysiology, including bilaterally absent short-latency somatosensory evoked potential responses and highly malignant electroencephalographic patterns; biomarkers, principally neuron-specific enolase; and imaging, showing diffuse anoxic injury on computed tomography or magnetic resonance.

Require concordance. No single test should determine the decision, and a prediction of poor outcome should rest on two or more concordant findings in a patient who remains unresponsive at the appropriate time.

Communicate honestly with the family throughout, including about uncertainty, and separate the prognostic discussion from the goals-of-care discussion, which is developed in Chapter 20.

Consider organ donation where appropriate, according to local pathways, and involve the relevant specialist service early rather than at the point of withdrawal.

13.7.5 After the arrest

Two obligations follow every in-hospital arrest and are frequently neglected.

Debrief the team. A structured debrief improves subsequent performance and addresses the second victim phenomenon described in Chapter 4, section 4.6.2.

Review whether it was preventable. Chapter 4, section 4.5.2, provided the chain of rescue as an analytic framework. A meaningful proportion of in-hospital arrests are preceded by unrecognised or unescalated deterioration, and each is an opportunity to identify a system failure.

Chapter Summary

- **An elevated troponin is not a diagnosis of infarction.** Type 2 infarction and non-ischaemic injury predominate among hospitalised medical patients, carry high mortality that is largely non-cardiac, and are treated by correcting the supply and demand imbalance rather than by applying the type 1 antithrombotic and invasive pathway.
- **Classify acute heart failure by congestion and perfusion before treating.** Acute pulmonary oedema with hypertension is a redistribution phenomenon requiring vasodilation and non-invasive ventilation rather than large-dose diuresis. Right ventricular failure is worsened by aggressive diuresis and vasodilation.
- **Dose loop diuretics adequately and assess the response the same day**, using urine output and a spot urine sodium a couple of hours after the dose. A modest creatinine rise during effective decongestion is usually acceptable, because venous congestion rather than low output drives most cardiorenal dysfunction.
- **New atrial fibrillation in acute illness is usually secondary.** Treat the precipitant, correct magnesium and potassium, and avoid removing a compensatory tachycardia. Anticoagulate for four weeks after cardioversion regardless of the pre-cardioversion strategy, and do not reduce direct oral anticoagulant doses outside the licensed criteria.
- **Mobitz type II block does not reliably respond to atropine.** Confirm mechanical capture during transcutaneous pacing rather than trusting the monitor. Assume a broad complex regular tachycardia is ventricular, and never give verapamil to one.

- **A magnet suspends tachytherapy in a defibrillator and produces asynchronous pacing in a pacemaker**, and does not change the pacing mode of a defibrillator.
- **Asymptomatic severe hypertension should not be lowered acutely.** The organ damage defines the emergency, not the number. Aortic dissection requires rate control before vasodilation, and hydralazine and sublingual nifedipine should be avoided.
- **A normal blood pressure does not exclude shock.** Bedside ultrasound is the highest-yield investigation in undifferentiated shock. Obstructive shock requires a mechanical answer, and excessive fluid worsens it.
- **Prevention is the most effective intervention in in-hospital arrest**, most of which is preceded by unrecognised deterioration and most of which presents in a non-shockable rhythm. Adrenaline improves return of circulation with less clear effect on neurological outcome.
- **Post-arrest care emphasises fever prevention rather than deep hypothermia**, and **neuroprognostication must be delayed, multimodal, and concordant** to avoid a self-fulfilling prophecy.

Review Questions

1. A patient admitted with pneumonia and atrial fibrillation at 150 beats per minute has a troponin of 180 nanograms per litre with no chest pain and no dynamic electrocardiographic change. The medical registrar proposes dual antiplatelet therapy and anticoagulation. State your position, your reasoning, and your management.
2. A patient with known heart failure presents with a blood pressure of 200 over 110, severe dyspnoea developing over one hour, and diffuse crackles. Explain the likely mechanism, and state what you would give and what you would specifically avoid.
3. A patient on 80 milligrams of oral furosemide daily is admitted with congestion and given 40 milligrams intravenously. Six hours later the urine output is 200 millilitres. Explain what went wrong, what measurement you would obtain, and your next three steps.
4. A patient with a defibrillator has received four shocks in an hour. Set out your immediate management, including what a magnet would and would not do.
5. A patient is found unresponsive on the ward. After eight minutes of resuscitation there is return of spontaneous circulation. The electrocardiogram shows no ST elevation and the patient remains comatose. Set out your post-arrest management priorities and state when and how you would approach prognostication.

CHAPTER 14: Acute Respiratory Failure and Ventilatory Support

Learning Objectives

After studying this chapter, the reader should be able to:

1. Classify respiratory failure by physiological mechanism, and use the alveolar-arterial gradient and acid-base pattern to distinguish hypoventilation from parenchymal disease and acute from chronic derangement.
2. Select an appropriate oxygen delivery device, state target saturation ranges, and describe the mechanisms and monitoring of high-flow nasal oxygen.
3. Apply noninvasive ventilation to the conditions where it is supported, recognise its contraindications, and predict and act on failure.
4. Decide when to intubate, and prepare for and manage the peri-intubation period safely.
5. Understand the principal ventilator modes and settings, calculate lung-protective tidal volumes, and troubleshoot common alarms.
6. Recognise acute respiratory distress syndrome, apply lung-protective ventilation, and describe which adjuncts have evidence of benefit and which have caused harm.
7. Stratify pulmonary embolism by severity and make defensible reperfusion decisions.
8. Assess readiness for liberation from ventilation, and manage tracheostomy and the chronically ventilated patient safely.

Chapter Overview

Respiratory failure is the commonest reason for escalation from a general ward to critical care, and the hospitalist's role sits precisely at the boundary: recognising the deteriorating patient, initiating support, deciding whether that support is a bridge or a ceiling, and knowing when it has failed.

Four principles run through the chapter.

Oxygenation and ventilation are separate problems. They have different mechanisms, different monitoring, and different treatments. A patient can be profoundly hypoxaemic with a normal carbon dioxide, or dying of hypercapnia with a normal saturation. The habit of using oxygen saturation as a general index of respiratory status is the source of a large proportion of the errors in this chapter.

Work of breathing predicts failure better than gas exchange. A patient maintaining normal numbers through visible effort is compensating, and compensation ends abruptly. The physical signs of impending fatigue are more useful than the blood gas.

Every escalation decision should be accompanied by a ceiling decision. Before starting noninvasive ventilation, the question of what happens if it fails must be answered, because the answer determines whether the therapy is a bridge to intubation or the maximum treatment the patient will receive. Deciding this in advance, with the patient where possible, is a core hospitalist responsibility and is addressed further in Chapter 20.

Delay is the commonest lethal error. Late intubation after prolonged failing noninvasive support is consistently associated with worse outcomes than earlier intubation. The instinct to persist with a less invasive therapy is understandable and frequently harmful.

14.1 Classification of Respiratory Failure by Physiology

14.1.1 The two types

Type 1, hypoxaemic respiratory failure, is defined by arterial oxygen tension below approximately 8 kilopascals, or 60 millimetres of mercury, with a normal or reduced carbon dioxide tension. The problem is gas exchange.

Type 2, hypercapnic respiratory failure, is defined by arterial carbon dioxide tension above approximately 6.0 kilopascals, or 45 millimetres of mercury. The problem is alveolar ventilation, which is minute ventilation minus dead space ventilation.

Some texts add further categories for perioperative atelectasis and for respiratory failure accompanying shock. These are useful teaching devices rather than distinct physiology, and the two principal types with their mechanisms carry most of the clinical weight.

14.1.2 Mechanisms of hypoxaemia

Five mechanisms produce a low arterial oxygen tension, and distinguishing them changes management.

Ventilation-perfusion mismatch is by far the commonest and underlies pneumonia, pulmonary oedema, atelectasis, obstructive lung disease, and pulmonary embolism. Regions with low ventilation relative to perfusion contribute desaturated blood. **It responds well to supplemental oxygen**, because raising the inspired concentration raises the oxygen content of even poorly ventilated units.

Shunt is the extreme of mismatch, in which blood passes through regions with no ventilation at all. Consolidation, complete collapse, and intracardiac or intrapulmonary vascular shunts produce it. **It responds poorly to supplemental oxygen**, because the shunted blood never contacts alveolar gas. Persistent hypoxaemia despite a high inspired oxygen concentration is therefore a signature of significant shunt and suggests that recruitment, positive pressure, or treatment of the underlying consolidation is required rather than more oxygen.

Hypoventilation produces hypoxaemia by displacing alveolar oxygen with carbon dioxide. It is distinguished by a normal alveolar-arterial gradient and by the accompanying hypercapnia, and it responds to oxygen but the underlying problem is ventilation.

Diffusion limitation contributes in interstitial disease, particularly during exertion.

Reduced inspired oxygen tension, at altitude, and **low mixed venous oxygen content** in low cardiac output states, which amplifies the effect of any of the above.

14.1.3 The alveolar-arterial gradient

The gradient distinguishes hypoventilation, in which the lungs are normal, from parenchymal or vascular disease. It is calculated as the alveolar oxygen tension, derived from the alveolar gas equation using the inspired oxygen fraction, barometric pressure, water vapour pressure, and the arterial carbon dioxide tension corrected by the respiratory quotient, minus the measured arterial oxygen tension.

A normal gradient with hypoxaemia and hypercapnia indicates pure hypoventilation: opioid or sedative effect, neuromuscular weakness, chest wall restriction, or central hypoventilation. The lungs are functioning normally and the problem is that not enough air is moving.

A raised gradient indicates mismatch, shunt, or diffusion limitation, meaning the lung itself is abnormal.

The gradient rises with age, and normal values must be age-adjusted. It is also unreliable at high inspired oxygen concentrations, where the ratio of arterial oxygen tension to inspired fraction is more commonly used.

The ratio of arterial oxygen tension to inspired oxygen fraction is widely used to grade severity, particularly in acute respiratory distress syndrome. Its principal limitation on a general ward is that the inspired fraction is not known with any accuracy when variable-performance devices are used, so a ratio calculated from an estimated fraction on a face mask is a rough approximation.

14.1.4 Mechanisms of hypercapnia

Three questions identify the mechanism, and the framing is deliberately simple because it directs treatment.

Is the patient not breathing enough because of reduced drive? Opioids, sedatives, alcohol, brainstem pathology, severe metabolic alkalosis, and central hypoventilation syndromes. The treatment is reversal or removal of the cause and ventilatory support.

Is the patient unable to breathe enough despite adequate drive? Neuromuscular disease including Guillain-Barré syndrome and myasthenic crisis, cervical cord pathology, critical illness weakness, chest wall disease, severe kyphoscoliosis, and morbid obesity. Chapter 10, section 10.3.9, addressed the localisation, and the monitoring point from Chapter 9, section 9.2.5, bears repeating: **these patients are monitored by vital capacity, not by oxygen saturation**, because saturation is preserved until immediately before collapse.

Is dead space ventilation excessive? Chronic obstructive pulmonary disease, severe asthma, and pulmonary embolism increase the proportion of each breath that does not participate in gas exchange, so a normal or even elevated minute ventilation fails to clear carbon dioxide. Treatment is directed at the underlying process.

14.1.5 Acute, chronic, and acute-on-chronic

This distinction is made from the blood gas and is essential to management.

Using the compensation relationships from Chapter 12, section 12.5.3: **acute** carbon dioxide retention raises bicarbonate only slightly, so the pH falls substantially. **Chronic** retention permits renal compensation over days, so bicarbonate is markedly elevated and the pH is near normal.

Acute-on-chronic retention shows a markedly elevated bicarbonate with an acidotic pH, indicating a patient with established chronic retention who has deteriorated acutely.

The clinical consequence is that a carbon dioxide of 9 kilopascals with a normal pH in a patient with chronic obstructive pulmonary disease is their baseline and requires no acute ventilatory intervention, whereas the same figure with a pH of 7.25 indicates acute decompensation requiring urgent support.

14.1.6 Assessing work of breathing

The blood gas describes the current state. The examination predicts the next hour.

Signs of increased work and impending fatigue: a respiratory rate that is high, and particularly one that has been high for hours; use of accessory muscles including sternocleidomastoid and scalenes; nasal flaring; tracheal tug; intercostal and supraclavicular recession; inability to speak in full sentences; the patient sitting forward and refusing to lie flat; diaphoresis; and **paradoxical abdominal movement**, in which the abdomen moves inward on inspiration, indicating diaphragmatic fatigue and impending failure.

Two ominous findings deserve specific emphasis.

A falling respiratory rate in a patient who was tachypnoeic, without clinical improvement, indicates exhaustion rather than recovery.

A normal or rising carbon dioxide in a tachypnoeic hypoxaemic patient is a serious finding. A patient working hard should be hypocapnic. Normocapnia in that context means the patient can no longer sustain the minute ventilation required, and represents the transition to failure.

A silent chest in an asthmatic likewise indicates airflow too low to generate wheeze and is a pre-arrest finding.

14.2 Oxygen Delivery Devices and High-Flow Nasal Cannula

14.2.1 Variable and fixed performance devices

The delivered oxygen concentration depends on the flow supplied, the reservoir available, and, crucially, the patient's own inspiratory flow rate.

Variable performance devices deliver an oxygen concentration that changes with the patient's breathing pattern. A breathless patient with a high inspiratory flow entrains more room air and receives a lower concentration than the nominal figure. This category includes nasal cannulae, simple face masks, and reservoir masks. Quoted concentration ranges for these devices are approximations and become progressively less accurate as the patient's respiratory distress increases, which is precisely when accuracy matters.

Fixed performance devices, principally air-entrainment masks with interchangeable valves, deliver a defined concentration by entraining air at a fixed ratio at flows exceeding the patient's peak inspiratory demand. They are the appropriate choice when the delivered concentration must be known and controlled, particularly in patients at risk of hypercapnic respiratory failure.

Practical points. Nasal cannulae at very high flows dry and damage the nasal mucosa. Simple face masks require a minimum flow to prevent rebreathing of exhaled gas. A reservoir mask requires the reservoir to be inflated before application and requires a high flow to keep it filled; a partially collapsed reservoir means the patient is not receiving the intended concentration.

14.2.2 Target saturations

The evidence has moved decisively away from liberal oxygen administration.

For most acutely unwell adults, a target saturation range in the region of 94 to 98 per cent is appropriate. Systematic review of randomised trials of liberal compared with conservative oxygen therapy in acutely ill adults found increased mortality with liberal supplemental oxygen, and specific trials in myocardial infarction and stroke have found no benefit and possible harm from routine oxygen in non-hypoxaemic patients.

For patients at risk of hypercapnic respiratory failure, including those with chronic obstructive pulmonary disease, obesity hypoventilation, chest wall deformity, and neuromuscular disease, a lower target range in the region of 88 to 92 per cent is appropriate, delivered through a fixed performance device.

The mechanism of oxygen-induced hypercapnia is worth understanding rather than reciting, because the common explanation is incomplete. Reduced hypoxic respiratory drive contributes but is a minor factor. The dominant mechanisms are **release of hypoxic pulmonary vasoconstriction**, which redistributes perfusion to poorly ventilated units and increases dead space, and **the Haldane effect**, whereby oxygenated haemoglobin carries less carbon dioxide, raising the dissolved carbon dioxide tension.

The essential clinical caution is that this concern must not be used to justify withholding oxygen from a hypoxaemic patient. Hypoxia kills faster than hypercapnia. The correct approach is controlled oxygen delivered through a fixed performance device with a defined target and repeat blood gas measurement, not oxygen withheld.

14.2.3 High-flow nasal oxygen

High-flow nasal oxygen delivers heated, humidified gas at flows substantially exceeding the patient's inspiratory demand, at a precisely set oxygen fraction, through wide-bore nasal prongs.

Its mechanisms are several and are worth knowing because they explain the indications.

Accurate oxygen delivery, because the flow exceeds peak inspiratory flow so entrainment of room air is minimal. This alone distinguishes it from every device in section 14.2.1.

Anatomical dead space washout, in which continuous high flow flushes the nasopharynx of exhaled carbon dioxide, so each breath begins with fresh gas. This reduces the effective dead space and improves the efficiency of ventilation.

A modest positive airway pressure effect, on the order of a few centimetres of water, greater with the mouth closed, which contributes to alveolar recruitment.

Heated humidification, which improves mucociliary function and secretion clearance and permits high flows to be tolerated comfortably.

Reduced work of breathing, resulting from the combination of the above.

Evidence. A randomised trial in patients with acute hypoxaemic non-hypercapnic respiratory failure comparing high-flow nasal oxygen with standard oxygen and with noninvasive ventilation did not show a difference in the primary outcome of intubation rate, but found lower ninety-day mortality in the high-flow group. It also has established roles in preventing post-extubation failure in selected patients and in preoxygenation before intubation.

Monitoring for failure is essential, because high-flow oxygen can maintain acceptable saturations in a patient whose underlying condition is worsening, masking deterioration and delaying intubation. A composite index combining oxygen saturation, inspired oxygen fraction, and respiratory rate has been validated to predict failure, with low values at defined time points indicating a high probability that high-flow therapy will not succeed. **Whatever index is used, the principle is to define in advance the time points at which the response will be assessed and the criteria for escalation**, rather than continuing indefinitely because the saturation looks acceptable.

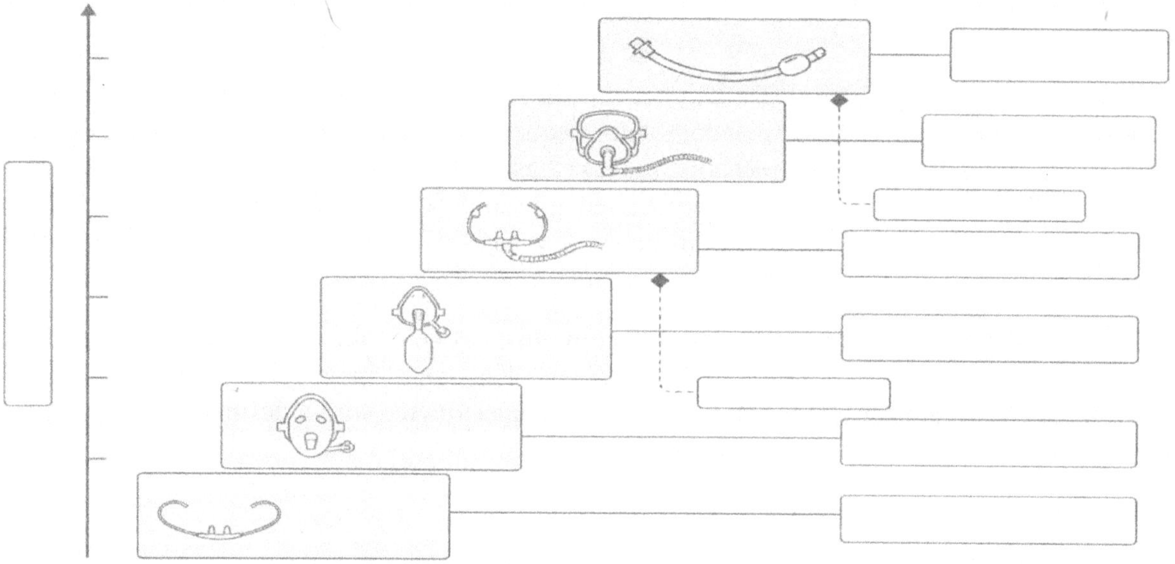

14.3 Noninvasive Ventilation: Indications, Contraindications, and Failure Prediction

14.3.1 The two modalities

Continuous positive airway pressure delivers a constant pressure throughout the respiratory cycle. It recruits collapsed alveoli, reduces shunt, and, in cardiogenic pulmonary oedema, reduces preload and afterload. It does not augment tidal volume and therefore does not directly assist ventilation.

Bilevel positive airway pressure, delivering a higher inspiratory and a lower expiratory pressure, augments tidal volume by the difference between the two, and therefore assists ventilation and clears carbon dioxide. The expiratory pressure performs the same functions as continuous positive pressure, including offsetting intrinsic positive end-expiratory pressure in obstructive disease and thereby reducing the effort required to trigger a breath.

The choice follows the physiology. A hypercapnic patient needs the ventilation assistance of bilevel support. A hypoxaemic patient with cardiogenic pulmonary oedema may be adequately treated with continuous positive pressure alone.

14.3.2 Where the evidence is strong

Exacerbation of chronic obstructive pulmonary disease with respiratory acidosis. This is the strongest indication in the field. In patients with a pH below approximately 7.35 and a raised carbon dioxide despite initial medical therapy and controlled oxygen, noninvasive ventilation reduces intubation rates, complications, length of stay, and mortality. It should be initiated early rather than after prolonged deterioration.

Acute cardiogenic pulmonary oedema. Both continuous positive pressure and bilevel support improve dyspnoea, oxygenation, and physiological parameters more rapidly than standard oxygen. Large trial evidence did not demonstrate a mortality difference against standard care, but the faster symptomatic and physiological improvement and reduced intubation rates justify use, and it is a mainstay of the presentation described in Chapter 13, section 13.2.2.

Chronic hypoventilation syndromes with acute decompensation, including obesity hypoventilation, chest wall disease, and neuromuscular disease, where the physiology is exactly what bilevel support addresses.

Prophylactic use after extubation in selected high-risk patients, addressed in section 14.8.3.

14.3.3 Where the evidence is weaker or the risks higher

De novo hypoxaemic respiratory failure, meaning pneumonia and acute respiratory distress syndrome in a patient without chronic lung disease, is the area of greatest caution. Failure rates are high, and failure is associated with worse outcomes than early intubation.

A specific mechanism explains part of this risk. A patient with a strong respiratory drive receiving pressure support generates large tidal volumes and large transpulmonary pressure swings, which can injure already inflamed lung in the same way that injurious mechanical ventilation does. This is termed patient self-inflicted lung injury, and it means that a patient who appears comfortable on noninvasive support with large tidal volumes may be sustaining ongoing injury. Monitoring the expired tidal volume, where the device permits, is therefore informative.

Helmet interfaces have shown promise in this population in comparison with face mask delivery, permitting higher pressures with better tolerance, though availability and familiarity vary.

Established post-extubation respiratory failure is a situation where noninvasive ventilation as a rescue therapy has been shown to be harmful, through delayed reintubation and increased mortality. This is different from prophylactic use immediately after extubation in high-risk patients, which is beneficial. The distinction between prevention and rescue is critical and frequently confused.

14.3.4 Contraindications

Absolute or near-absolute: respiratory or cardiac arrest; inability to protect the airway; severe encephalopathy such that the patient cannot cooperate or clear secretions; active vomiting or upper gastrointestinal bleeding with aspiration risk; facial trauma, burns, or recent upper airway or upper gastrointestinal surgery; and fixed upper airway obstruction.

Relative: haemodynamic instability requiring vasopressor support; undrained pneumothorax; copious secretions that the patient cannot clear; agitation or non-cooperation; and severe hypoxaemia in which any interruption would be catastrophic.

A note on reduced consciousness. Depressed conscious level due to hypercapnia in an exacerbation of chronic obstructive pulmonary disease is not an absolute contraindication and may improve rapidly with ventilation, provided the patient is in a monitored environment with immediate escalation available. Depressed consciousness from other causes generally is a contraindication.

14.3.5 Initiating, monitoring, and predicting failure

Before starting, answer the ceiling question. Is this a bridge to intubation if it fails, or is it the maximum therapy this patient will receive? The answer must be recorded, and it should be discussed with the patient while they can still participate, which means before the mask goes on rather than after. This is the single most important non-technical action in this section.

Setting up. Choose and fit the interface carefully, since leak and discomfort account for most early failures. Explain what will happen. Start at modest pressures and titrate upward as tolerated. Set the inspired oxygen fraction to achieve the appropriate target saturation, which for a hypercapnic patient is the lower range from section 14.2.2. Use humidification. Allow short breaks for the patient to drink and clear secretions if tolerated.

Monitoring. Continuous oximetry and observation of respiratory rate, work of breathing, and conscious level. **A blood gas at approximately one hour is mandatory**, with a further gas at around four hours and after any significant change in settings.

Predicting failure. The most useful indicators at one to two hours are: **failure of the pH to improve**, which is the single most informative variable in hypercapnic failure; failure of the respiratory rate to fall; persistently large tidal volumes; deteriorating conscious level; worsening or unchanged carbon dioxide; haemodynamic deterioration; inability to tolerate the interface; and copious secretions. Composite scoring systems combining these have been developed and validated.

Act on failure promptly. A patient not improving by one to two hours is unlikely to improve by six, and the decision made at that point, whether it is intubation or a change to a palliative approach, should be made then rather than deferred. The commonest lethal pattern in this chapter is a patient maintained on failing noninvasive ventilation overnight, intubated in the early morning in extremis.

14.4 Intubation Decisions and the Peri-Intubation Period

14.4.1 The indications

Four questions cover essentially all indications for tracheal intubation.

Is oxygenation failing despite maximal noninvasive support? Persistent hypoxaemia on high-flow oxygen or noninvasive ventilation, particularly with significant shunt physiology.

Is ventilation failing? Rising carbon dioxide with worsening acidosis despite noninvasive support, or the exhaustion described in section 14.1.6.

Is the airway unprotected or threatened? Reduced consciousness with loss of protective reflexes, expanding neck haematoma, airway burns, angioedema, or severe bulbar weakness. The commonly quoted rule about a specific coma score threshold is a heuristic rather than a rule, and the judgement should be based on the ability to protect and clear the airway rather than on a number.

Does the anticipated clinical course require it? A patient who will require transfer, a procedure, or is on a trajectory that will require intubation later is frequently better intubated in a controlled setting now than emergently in six hours. This is the indication most often missed.

14.4.2 Timing

Late intubation is worse than early intubation. Observational evidence consistently associates delayed intubation after failure of noninvasive support with higher mortality, and the physiological explanation is straightforward: a patient intubated after prolonged failure is exhausted, acidotic, catecholamine-depleted, and frequently hypovolaemic, which converts a controlled procedure into a high-risk one.

The counterweight is that intubation is not benign and that avoiding it where the patient will recover without it is a genuine good. The resolution is to define escalation criteria in advance and act on them, rather than making the decision under pressure in the middle of the night.

14.4.3 Preparing for a safe intubation

Intubation of a critically ill medical patient carries substantially higher complication rates than elective anaesthetic intubation, and the principal complications are hypoxaemia, hypotension, and cardiac arrest. Most are preventable by preparation.

Resuscitate before you intubate. Hypotension before induction predicts cardiovascular collapse after it, because induction agents vasodilate and positive pressure ventilation reduces venous return. Correct hypovolaemia, and have a vasopressor drawn up and ideally running before induction in any patient with marginal haemodynamics.

Preoxygenate properly. The aim is to denitrogenate the lungs and maximise the oxygen reservoir. Use a well-fitting reservoir mask at high flow, or noninvasive ventilation or high-flow nasal oxygen in patients who remain hypoxaemic on a mask. Apnoeic oxygenation, meaning nasal oxygen left in place during laryngoscopy, prolongs the safe apnoea time and costs nothing.

Position. Head elevation or a ramped position improves both preoxygenation and laryngoscopic view, and is particularly important in obesity and in pregnancy.

Assess the airway for predictors of difficulty, and have a plan for failure agreed and stated aloud before starting, including who will do what and what equipment is immediately available.

Choose induction agents with haemodynamics in mind. Ketamine and etomidate are relatively haemodynamically neutral. Propofol reliably causes vasodilation and myocardial depression and should be dose-reduced substantially or avoided in shock. Neuromuscular blockade improves intubating conditions and first-pass success; the choice between agents depends on duration requirements and on the contraindications to depolarising agents, which include hyperkalaemia, established denervation, prolonged immobility, significant burns beyond the acute phase, and a history of malignant hyperthermia.

Use videolaryngoscopy where available, since randomised evidence has shown improved first-attempt success compared with direct laryngoscopy in critically ill patients.

Confirm placement with waveform capnography. This is mandatory and not optional. A sustained capnograph trace confirms tracheal placement; auscultation, condensation in the tube, and chest movement do not. Unrecognised oesophageal intubation remains a cause of death and is entirely preventable by this single practice.

14.4.4 Immediately after intubation

Set the ventilator with lung-protective parameters from the first breath, as in section 14.5.2, rather than intending to adjust later.

Avoid over-ventilation. Vigorous manual ventilation after intubation causes hypotension by reducing venous return and, in patients with severe acidosis, an abrupt fall in carbon dioxide can precipitate arrhythmia. In a patient with a severe metabolic acidosis who was compensating with a high minute ventilation, that minute ventilation must be matched by the ventilator or the pH will fall abruptly.

Provide adequate analgesia and sedation, prioritising analgesia, and titrate to a defined target rather than to unresponsiveness.

Confirm position radiographically, insert a gastric tube, and reassess haemodynamics, since post-intubation hypotension is common and requires treatment rather than observation.

14.5 Mechanical Ventilation Basics for the Non-Intensivist

14.5.1 Modes

Modes differ in what the ventilator controls and what it allows to vary.

Volume control delivers a set tidal volume; the resulting airway pressure varies with the patient's compliance and resistance. Volume is guaranteed, pressure is not.

Pressure control delivers a set inspiratory pressure for a set time; the resulting tidal volume varies with compliance and resistance. Pressure is guaranteed, volume is not, which means that a deteriorating patient will silently receive smaller tidal volumes.

Pressure support is a spontaneous mode in which each patient-initiated breath is augmented to a set pressure. It requires an intact respiratory drive and is used during weaning.

Numerous hybrid and adaptive modes exist with manufacturer-specific names. For a non-intensivist, understanding the three principles above is sufficient to interpret most settings.

14.5.2 The settings that matter

Tidal volume should be set at approximately 6 to 8 millilitres per kilogram of **predicted body weight**, calculated from height and sex, not from actual weight. This is the single most important and most frequently mishandled setting. Predicted body weight in a short woman may be 45 kilograms while her actual weight is 90, and setting the tidal volume from the latter delivers double the intended volume. Charts and formulae for predicted body weight should be available at every ventilator.

Respiratory rate is set to achieve the required minute ventilation, guided by the carbon dioxide and pH and by the considerations in section 14.4.4.

Positive end-expiratory pressure recruits alveoli, prevents cyclical collapse and reopening, and improves oxygenation. Higher levels are used in acute respiratory distress syndrome, as in section 14.6.3.

Inspired oxygen fraction is titrated to the lowest value achieving the target saturation.

Inspiratory to expiratory ratio matters most in obstructive disease, where a longer expiratory time is required to permit complete exhalation.

14.5.3 Pressures and what they mean

Peak inspiratory pressure is the highest pressure during inspiration and reflects both airway resistance and lung compliance.

Plateau pressure, measured during an inspiratory pause with no flow, reflects lung and chest wall compliance alone, since the resistive component disappears when flow stops. **It should be kept below approximately 30 centimetres of water.**

The difference between the two is diagnostic. A high peak pressure with a normal plateau indicates a resistance problem: bronchospasm, secretions, a kinked or blocked tube, or biting. A high peak pressure with a high plateau indicates a compliance problem: pulmonary oedema, consolidation, pneumothorax, atelectasis, abdominal distension, or chest wall restriction. This single comparison resolves most high-pressure alarms.

Driving pressure, the plateau pressure minus the applied positive end-expiratory pressure, represents the pressure applied to the aerated lung, and lower values are associated with better outcomes in acute respiratory distress syndrome.

14.5.4 Troubleshooting

Acute deterioration in a ventilated patient should prompt disconnection from the ventilator and manual ventilation with a bag while a systematic assessment is made, since this immediately distinguishes patient problems from circuit problems.

The conventional structured approach considers: **displacement** of the tube, into a bronchus or out of the trachea; **obstruction** by secretions, blood, or kinking; **pneumothorax**, particularly tension; **equipment** failure anywhere in the circuit; and **breath stacking** with dynamic hyperinflation.

Dynamic hyperinflation, or intrinsic positive end-expiratory pressure, deserves specific attention because its management is counterintuitive. In severe airflow obstruction, incomplete exhalation causes progressive air trapping, which raises intrathoracic pressure, impedes venous return, and causes hypotension that may be mistaken for hypovolaemia or sepsis. **The treatment is to allow more time to exhale**: reduce the respiratory rate, reduce the tidal volume, shorten the inspiratory time, and treat the bronchospasm. In severe cases with haemodynamic collapse, briefly disconnecting the patient from the circuit and allowing passive exhalation with gentle chest compression produces immediate improvement and confirms the diagnosis.

Permissive hypercapnia, meaning acceptance of an elevated carbon dioxide and a degree of acidaemia in order to avoid injurious ventilation, is an established strategy in both severe obstruction and acute respiratory distress syndrome, with caution in raised intracranial pressure.

14.5.5 Care of the ventilated patient

Several interventions reduce complications and are within the hospitalist's scope where ventilated patients are cared for outside a closed intensive care model.

Elevation of the head of the bed; minimisation of sedation with daily assessment; structured oral care; subglottic secretion drainage where available; early mobilisation; venous thromboembolism and stress ulcer prophylaxis according to indication; nutrition; and delirium prevention as in Chapter 10, section 10.1.5.

14.5.6 Patient-ventilator asynchrony

Asynchrony, meaning a mismatch between the patient's respiratory effort and the ventilator's delivery, is common, uncomfortable, increases work of breathing, and is associated with prolonged ventilation. It is frequently treated by increasing sedation when the correct response is to adjust the ventilator.

The patterns worth recognising: **ineffective triggering**, in which the patient makes an effort that does not initiate a breath, most often caused by intrinsic positive end-expiratory pressure in obstructive disease or by an insensitive trigger setting; **double triggering**, in which a single prolonged effort initiates two consecutive breaths, usually because the set inspiratory time or tidal volume is too short for the patient's demand; **flow starvation**, in which the delivered inspiratory flow is inadequate for a patient with high drive, visible as a concave pressure waveform and as visible distress; and **delayed cycling**, in which the ventilator continues to deliver flow after the patient wishes to exhale.

The practical rule is to look at the patient and the waveforms together before reaching for sedation. Adding applied positive end-expiratory pressure to offset an intrinsic level, increasing inspiratory flow, adjusting the trigger sensitivity, or changing the cycling criterion resolves most asynchrony without additional sedative burden, and unnecessary sedation prolongs ventilation and contributes to the delirium described in Chapter 10.

14.6 Acute Respiratory Distress Syndrome: Recognition, Lung-Protective Strategy, and Adjuncts

14.6.1 Recognition

Acute respiratory distress syndrome is defined by an acute onset within approximately one week of a recognised insult, bilateral radiographic opacities not fully explained by effusion, collapse, or nodules, respiratory failure not fully explained by cardiac failure or fluid overload, and impaired oxygenation, graded by the ratio of arterial oxygen tension to inspired oxygen fraction in the presence of a minimum level of positive end-expiratory pressure.

More recent consensus definitions have extended the criteria to include patients receiving high-flow nasal oxygen at defined flows, to permit the use of pulse oximetry-derived ratios where arterial sampling is unavailable, and to accommodate resource-limited settings including the use of ultrasound for the radiographic criterion.

Two practical points. The syndrome is a description rather than a diagnosis, and **identifying and treating the precipitating cause is the principal therapeutic action**. Common causes are pneumonia, aspiration, sepsis of any source, trauma, pancreatitis, transfusion, and drug reactions. And distinguishing it from cardiogenic pulmonary oedema is essential; bedside echocardiography and clinical assessment as in Chapter 13, section 13.2.1, are usually sufficient.

14.6.2 Lung-protective ventilation

The foundation of management, and the intervention with the clearest mortality benefit, is limiting the mechanical injury caused by ventilation itself.

Tidal volume of approximately 6 millilitres per kilogram of predicted body weight, reduced further if plateau pressure remains high. The landmark trial comparing this with a higher tidal volume strategy demonstrated a mortality reduction and established the standard.

Plateau pressure limited to below approximately 30 centimetres of water.

Attention to driving pressure, keeping it as low as achievable.

Permissive hypercapnia accepted as the consequence, with attention to pH.

14.6.3 Adjuncts with evidence of benefit

Prone positioning. In moderate to severe disease, defined by an oxygenation ratio below a specified threshold, prolonged prone positioning for a substantial part of each day produced a marked mortality reduction in a randomised trial. It requires trained staff and careful attention to lines, tubes, pressure areas, and eyes, and it is the adjunct with the strongest evidence.

Higher positive end-expiratory pressure appears beneficial in moderate to severe disease, based on individual patient data meta-analysis, with the caveat that the method of titration matters.

Conservative fluid strategy after the resuscitation phase improved lung function and shortened ventilation without harming other organs.

Neuromuscular blockade in severe disease was beneficial in one trial and neutral in a later one conducted with a different sedation strategy. Current practice reserves it for severe disease with significant dyssynchrony rather than using it routinely.

Extracorporeal membrane oxygenation for very severe disease should prompt early discussion with a specialist centre. The principal randomised trial did not reach statistical significance for its primary outcome, and subsequent analyses have been interpreted as suggesting probable benefit, with the practical implication that referral criteria and early discussion matter more than a definitive verdict.

Corticosteroids remain an area of variable practice, with a positive randomised trial in a specific population and established benefit in particular aetiologies, and guidance should be followed for the underlying cause.

14.6.4 Interventions that have caused harm or shown no benefit

This list matters because each was widely adopted before being tested.

Aggressive recruitment manoeuvres with high-pressure positive end-expiratory pressure titration increased mortality in a large randomised trial and should not be applied routinely.

High-frequency oscillatory ventilation increased mortality in one large trial and showed no benefit in another.

Inhaled pulmonary vasodilators improve oxygenation without improving mortality, and are used as a temporising measure in refractory hypoxaemia rather than as therapy.

Routine use of higher tidal volumes to correct hypercapnia, which is the error the entire strategy exists to prevent.

14.7 Pulmonary Embolism: Severity Stratification and Reperfusion Decisions

14.7.1 Diagnosis in brief

Diagnostic pathways combine a clinical probability assessment with D-dimer testing and imaging. Validated approaches include structured probability scores, age-adjusted D-dimer thresholds which reduce unnecessary imaging in older patients, and algorithms that vary the D-dimer threshold according to the presence of specific clinical items.

Two settings where the standard algorithm does not apply have been noted earlier in this book. In the postoperative patient, D-dimer is uninterpretable and imaging should be obtained directly, as Chapter 8, section 8.5.2, described. In pregnancy, dedicated pathways apply.

Computed tomographic pulmonary angiography is the usual imaging modality, with ventilation-perfusion imaging as an alternative where contrast is contraindicated or in specific populations. Bedside echocardiography demonstrating right ventricular dilatation in a hypotensive patient may justify treatment before definitive imaging where the patient is too unstable to transfer.

14.7.2 Severity stratification

This is the central task, because it determines both the treatment and the location of care.

High-risk pulmonary embolism is defined by haemodynamic instability: cardiac arrest, obstructive shock, or persistent hypotension not explained by another cause. This category carries high short-term mortality and mandates consideration of reperfusion.

Intermediate-risk patients are haemodynamically stable but have evidence of right ventricular strain. The category is subdivided by whether both right ventricular dysfunction on imaging and elevated cardiac biomarkers are present, which defines the intermediate-high group, or only one or neither, which defines intermediate-low.

Low-risk patients are haemodynamically stable without right ventricular dysfunction or biomarker elevation, and with a low score on a validated clinical prognostic index. Selected low-risk patients can be managed as outpatients or with early discharge, using validated eligibility criteria, and this is an established and underused pathway.

14.7.3 Anticoagulation

Initiate promptly, including before imaging in patients with high clinical probability where imaging will be delayed, unless bleeding risk prohibits.

Direct oral anticoagulants are first-line for most patients. Two agents can be used as single-drug regimens from the outset with an initial higher-dose phase; two others require an initial period of parenteral anticoagulation before transition.

Low molecular weight heparin remains appropriate in pregnancy, in severe renal impairment with appropriate adjustment, and in specific situations where an oral agent is unsuitable.

Cancer-associated thrombosis was historically treated with low molecular weight heparin, and direct oral anticoagulants are now used widely, with attention to increased bleeding risk in gastrointestinal and genitourinary malignancy.

Unfractionated heparin is preferred where reperfusion is being considered, where haemodynamic instability is present, or where rapid reversibility is required.

14.7.4 Reperfusion decisions

High-risk pulmonary embolism. Systemic thrombolysis is indicated in the absence of absolute contraindications, and the evidence supports mortality benefit in this group. Where thrombolysis is contraindicated or has failed, catheter-directed therapy or surgical embolectomy should be considered where available, and extracorporeal support may be used as a bridge.

Intermediate-high risk. This is the difficult group and the most common source of uncertainty. A large randomised trial of systemic thrombolysis in normotensive patients with right ventricular dysfunction and biomarker elevation reduced haemodynamic decompensation but increased major bleeding and intracranial haemorrhage, with no mortality benefit. **Routine thrombolysis is therefore not indicated in this group.**

The accepted approach is close monitoring in an appropriate setting with **rescue reperfusion** if the patient deteriorates. Criteria for deterioration should be defined in advance and documented, since the decision is otherwise made late.

Catheter-directed therapies, including catheter-directed low-dose thrombolysis and mechanical thrombectomy, are used increasingly in this group with the rationale of achieving reperfusion at lower bleeding risk. The evidence base is developing rapidly and current trial results should be consulted.

Multidisciplinary pulmonary embolism response teams, bringing together respiratory, cardiology, interventional radiology, haematology, and critical care expertise rapidly, have been adopted in many institutions and are a reasonable model for making these decisions, given that no single specialty owns the pathway.

14.7.5 After the acute phase

Duration of anticoagulation depends on whether the event was provoked by a major transient risk factor, in which case a defined limited course is conventional; provoked by a persistent risk factor; or unprovoked, in which case extended anticoagulation is considered, weighing recurrence risk against bleeding risk, with the decision revisited periodically.

Follow-up should include assessment for persistent dyspnoea, since a proportion of patients develop chronic thromboembolic pulmonary hypertension, which is treatable and is missed when breathlessness after pulmonary embolism is attributed to deconditioning. A structured review at a defined interval should be arranged and communicated at discharge.

Investigation for occult malignancy should be limited to age-appropriate screening and directed evaluation of symptoms, since extensive routine screening has not been shown to improve outcomes.

14.8 Liberation, Tracheostomy, and the Chronically Ventilated Patient

14.8.1 Assessing readiness

Liberation from mechanical ventilation should be assessed daily rather than when it occurs to someone, because unnecessary additional days of ventilation carry cumulative risk.

Readiness criteria generally require that the precipitating condition is improving or resolved; that oxygenation is adequate at a modest inspired oxygen fraction and positive end-expiratory pressure; that the patient is haemodynamically stable without high-dose vasopressor support; that the patient can initiate spontaneous breaths; and that there is no immediate plan requiring continued ventilation.

A spontaneous breathing trial tests the patient's capacity to sustain ventilation with minimal support. Trials of shorter duration have been shown to be adequate compared with longer ones, and less supportive trial modes better identify patients who will succeed. Failure is indicated by tachypnoea, rising or falling respiratory rate, distress, tachycardia, hypertension or hypotension, desaturation, and deteriorating conscious level.

Coordinated interruption of sedation with the breathing trial improved outcomes in randomised evaluation compared with the breathing trial alone, and the pairing is standard practice.

14.8.2 Extubation and its complications

The cuff leak test, assessing for air movement around a deflated cuff, identifies patients at higher risk of post-extubation stridor from laryngeal oedema. Where the test is abnormal in a patient at risk, corticosteroids given several hours before extubation reduce that risk.

Post-extubation failure requiring reintubation occurs in a meaningful proportion of patients and is associated with worse outcomes, which is the reason to identify high-risk patients in advance rather than to delay extubation universally.

Prophylactic support immediately after extubation with high-flow nasal oxygen or noninvasive ventilation reduces reintubation in defined high-risk groups. As section 14.3.3 emphasised, this is different from using noninvasive ventilation as a rescue after failure has become established, which is harmful.

14.8.3 Tracheostomy

Indications include anticipated prolonged ventilation, facilitation of weaning by reducing dead space and resistance and permitting reduced sedation, secretion management, and upper airway obstruction or protection.

Timing. Randomised evidence comparing early with later tracheostomy in patients receiving mechanical ventilation did not demonstrate a mortality benefit from early placement, so the decision rests on the anticipated duration of ventilation and on individual factors including comfort, sedation requirements, and the plan for weaning.

Complications include early bleeding, tube displacement particularly before a tract has matured, obstruction, infection, and later stenosis, tracheomalacia, and rarely tracheo-oesophageal and tracheo-innominate artery fistula, the last of which presents with a sentinel bleed and is a surgical emergency.

Emergency management of tracheostomy problems deserves specific emphasis because ward staff encounter these patients and the correct sequence is not intuitive. National safety projects have published algorithms, and every institution caring for these patients should have them displayed at the bedside with the necessary equipment.

The single most important distinction is between a patient with a tracheostomy and a patient with a laryngectomy. A patient with a tracheostomy retains a connection between the upper airway and the trachea, so oxygenation and ventilation via the mouth and nose may be possible. A patient who has had a laryngectomy has no such connection, and **the stoma is the only airway**. Attempting to ventilate a laryngectomy patient through the face is futile and fatal. This must be identifiable at the bedside, and bed-head signage indicating which applies is a basic safety requirement.

14.8.4 The chronically ventilated patient

A proportion of patients cannot be liberated within the usual timeframe and enter a prolonged weaning course.

Management principles: transfer to a specialised weaning unit where these exist, since outcomes are better; systematic multidisciplinary rehabilitation addressing nutrition, mobility, muscle strength, and swallow; management of delirium and of the profound psychological burden, including sleep, communication, and depression, which are frequently untreated; and careful attention to communication with the patient, who is conscious, unable to speak, and frequently excluded from conversations about themselves.

Decisions about the ceiling of treatment must be revisited explicitly. A patient who has not weaned after a prolonged course is on a trajectory with a knowable prognosis, and the conversation about whether continued ventilation serves their goals should occur before a crisis forces it. Chapter 20 develops the structure of that conversation, and a point from it belongs here: the option of continuing indefinitely is not neutral, and presenting it as the default without discussion is itself a decision.

Home ventilation is appropriate and feasible for selected patients, particularly those with stable neuromuscular or chest wall disease, and requires specialist services, caregiver training, and equipment provision that must be arranged well in advance of discharge.

Chapter Summary

- **Oxygenation and ventilation are separate problems.** Type 1 failure is a gas exchange problem; type 2 is an alveolar ventilation problem. The alveolar-arterial gradient distinguishes pure hypoventilation from lung disease, and the bicarbonate distinguishes acute from chronic hypercapnia.
- **Work of breathing predicts failure better than gas exchange.** A falling respiratory rate without improvement, a normal carbon dioxide in a tachypnoeic hypoxaemic patient, paradoxical abdominal movement, and a silent chest are all pre-arrest findings.
- **Target 94 to 98 per cent for most patients and 88 to 92 per cent for those at risk of hypercapnic failure**, using a fixed performance device. Liberal oxygen increases mortality. Hypoxia kills faster than hypercapnia, so controlled oxygen is the answer, not withheld oxygen.
- **High-flow nasal oxygen** works through accurate delivery, dead space washout, modest positive pressure, and humidification. Define assessment time points and escalation criteria in advance, because it can mask deterioration.
- **Noninvasive ventilation has strong evidence in hypercapnic exacerbation of obstructive lung disease and in cardiogenic pulmonary oedema**, and is high-risk in de novo hypoxaemic failure. It is harmful as rescue for established post-extubation failure, though beneficial prophylactically. **Answer the ceiling question before the mask goes on**, and act on failure at one to two hours.
- **Late intubation is worse than early intubation.** Resuscitate before you intubate, preoxygenate properly, position the patient, and **confirm placement with waveform capnography**, which is mandatory.
- **Set tidal volume from predicted body weight calculated from height**, not actual weight. The comparison of peak with plateau pressure distinguishes resistance from compliance problems. Dynamic hyperinflation is treated by giving more time to exhale.

- **In acute respiratory distress syndrome, treat the cause and ventilate protectively.** Prone positioning has the strongest adjunct evidence. Aggressive recruitment with high-pressure titration and high-frequency oscillation have both caused harm.
- **Stratify pulmonary embolism by haemodynamics first.** Thrombolysis is indicated in high-risk disease and is not routine in intermediate-high risk, where the approach is monitoring with predefined criteria for rescue reperfusion.
- **A laryngectomy stoma is the only airway.** This distinction from tracheostomy must be identifiable at the bedside.

Review Questions

1. A patient with chronic obstructive pulmonary disease has a pH of 7.24, carbon dioxide of 9.5 kilopascals, and bicarbonate of 34 millimoles per litre. State what the pattern tells you about the time course, what it tells you about the acuity, and what you would do in the next hour.
2. A patient with pneumonia on high-flow nasal oxygen at 60 litres per minute and 80 per cent oxygen has a saturation of 93 per cent, a respiratory rate of 34, and is using accessory muscles. A colleague is reassured by the saturation. Explain why you are not, and state your plan.
3. A ventilated patient becomes acutely hypotensive with a high peak pressure. Describe your immediate actions and the single measurement that would most help you distinguish the likely causes.
4. A haemodynamically stable patient with confirmed pulmonary embolism has right ventricular dilatation on computed tomography and a raised troponin. A colleague proposes systemic thrombolysis. State your position, the evidence, and what you would do instead.
5. A patient on the ward with a tracheostomy becomes acutely hypoxic and distressed. Set out your assessment sequence, and state the single piece of information you must establish before attempting any airway manoeuvre.

CHAPTER 15: Gastrointestinal and Hepatic Emergencies

Learning Objectives

After studying this chapter, the reader should be able to:

1. Resuscitate and risk-stratify a patient with upper gastrointestinal bleeding, decide on the timing of endoscopy, and apply proton pump inhibitor therapy according to the evidence.
2. Manage lower gastrointestinal bleeding and describe the investigation of obscure bleeding.
3. Diagnose acute pancreatitis, predict severity, and apply a contemporary fluid and nutritional strategy.
4. Evaluate jaundice by pattern, recognise cholangitis, and determine the urgency of biliary drainage.
5. Recognise acute liver failure, initiate management, and identify when to contact a transplant centre.
6. Manage the decompensating cirrhotic patient, including ascites, spontaneous bacterial peritonitis, variceal bleeding, and hepatorenal syndrome.
7. Diagnose and treat *Clostridioides difficile* infection appropriately, and evaluate other causes of hospital-acquired diarrhoea.
8. Manage constipation, faecal impaction, and the neurogenic bowel, including recognition of autonomic dysreflexia.

Chapter Overview

Gastrointestinal and hepatic emergencies share a feature that shapes this chapter: the presenting sign is often a long way from the underlying problem, and the treatment frequently belongs to another specialty while the responsibility for recognition and resuscitation belongs to the hospitalist.

Four themes recur.

Resuscitation precedes diagnosis. In gastrointestinal bleeding and in cholangitis, restoring the circulation and, where relevant, achieving source control determine outcome more than any diagnostic refinement.

Several long-standing practices have been reversed by evidence, and all in the direction of doing less. Liberal transfusion in bleeding, aggressive fluid resuscitation in pancreatitis, routine early endoscopy, prophylactic antibiotics in pancreatitis, and routine correction of coagulopathy in liver disease were all standard and are now known to be unhelpful or harmful. Section 15.3 in particular describes a practice that has changed within recent memory.

The cirrhotic patient is a different physiological organism, and applying general medical reflexes to them causes harm. The coagulation tests do not mean what they appear to mean, the kidneys behave differently, the response to infection is blunted, and the margin for error in every direction is narrow. Section 15.6 is the longest in the chapter for this reason.

The unglamorous problems cause real harm. Constipation causes delirium, urinary retention, pain, and occasionally perforation, and is among the most neglected problems in inpatient medicine. Section 15.8 treats it seriously.

15.1 Upper Gastrointestinal Bleeding: Risk Scores, Timing of Endoscopy, and Proton Pump Inhibitor Logic

15.1.1 Initial assessment and resuscitation

Establish the severity from physiology, not from the appearance of the blood. Haemoglobin at presentation may be normal in acute bleeding before haemodilution occurs, and is therefore a poor early guide. Tachycardia, postural change, hypotension, and reduced peripheral perfusion are the relevant measurements.

Secure access and resuscitate with two large-bore cannulae, crystalloid initially, and blood products according to the loss. Activate a major haemorrhage protocol where bleeding is massive.

Transfusion threshold. A landmark randomised trial in acute upper gastrointestinal bleeding compared a restrictive threshold of approximately 70 grams per litre with a liberal threshold of approximately 90, and found improved survival and lower rebleeding with the restrictive strategy, including in patients with cirrhosis. The mechanism is thought to relate to the rise in portal pressure that accompanies volume expansion. **A restrictive strategy is therefore standard**, with exceptions for massive ongoing haemorrhage and for patients with acute coronary syndrome, where a higher threshold is generally applied. Chapter 7, section 7.5.3, addressed the general principles.

Assess for the features suggesting a variceal source, meaning known or suspected liver disease, stigmata of chronic liver disease, thrombocytopenia, and splenomegaly, because the initial pharmacological management differs.

Manage antithrombotic agents with a deliberate weighing rather than reflex cessation of everything, using the reasoning of Chapter 7, section 7.4. Reversal is appropriate in significant bleeding, and reversal agents for the direct oral anticoagulants and prothrombin complex concentrate for vitamin K antagonists should be available and their local availability known in advance.

15.1.2 Risk stratification

Validated scores serve two distinct purposes and should not be confused.

Pre-endoscopy scores identify patients at very low risk who may be managed without inpatient admission. The most widely used incorporates urea, haemoglobin, systolic pressure, pulse, and the presence of melaena, syncope, hepatic disease, and cardiac failure, and a score at the lowest end identifies a group with a very low probability of requiring intervention.

Post-endoscopy scores incorporate endoscopic findings and predict rebleeding and mortality.

A practically useful observation: a raised urea disproportionate to the creatinine suggests an upper gastrointestinal source, reflecting absorption of the protein load of digested blood, and is helpful when the source is uncertain.

15.1.3 Timing of endoscopy

The instinct that faster is better has been tested and does not hold.

For most patients, endoscopy within 24 hours of presentation is the standard, after adequate resuscitation.

Very early endoscopy is not superior. A randomised trial comparing endoscopy within six hours with endoscopy between six and twenty-four hours in patients predicted to be at high risk found no reduction in mortality, and the earlier group did not do better. Rushing a haemodynamically unstable, incompletely resuscitated patient to endoscopy is therefore not the correct response to concern.

The exception is the patient with ongoing haemodynamic instability despite resuscitation, in whom urgent endoscopy after or alongside continued resuscitation may be required, ideally with anaesthetic and airway support given the aspiration risk.

Erythromycin given before endoscopy acts as a prokinetic, improves gastric emptying of blood and clot, and improves visualisation, with attention to its effect on the QT interval.

15.1.4 Proton pump inhibitor logic

This is an area where practice frequently diverges from the evidence in a specific way.

Before endoscopy, proton pump inhibitor therapy reduces the proportion of patients found to have high-risk endoscopic stigmata and the need for endoscopic therapy, but has not been shown to reduce rebleeding, need for surgery, or mortality. It is therefore reasonable but not mandatory, and **it must never delay resuscitation or endoscopy**.

After endoscopy, the situation is different. In patients found to have high-risk stigmata, meaning active bleeding, a non-bleeding visible vessel, or an adherent clot, high-dose proton pump inhibitor therapy for a defined period following endoscopic haemostasis reduces rebleeding. This is the indication with the strongest support.

In patients with low-risk stigmata, meaning a clean-based ulcer or a flat pigmented spot, prolonged high-dose intravenous therapy is not required, oral therapy is adequate, and early feeding and discharge are appropriate.

15.1.5 Variceal bleeding

Suspected variceal bleeding requires several interventions that differ from non-variceal management and that should begin before endoscopy.

A vasoactive agent, either a vasopressin analogue or a somatostatin analogue, reduces portal pressure and should be started on suspicion.

Antibiotic prophylaxis is one of the most important interventions in this presentation and is frequently omitted. Prophylactic antibiotics in cirrhotic patients with gastrointestinal bleeding reduce bacterial infection, rebleeding, and **mortality**, and should be given to every such patient regardless of whether infection is apparent.

Endoscopic band ligation is the definitive therapy for oesophageal varices, performed within approximately 12 hours where the patient is stable enough. Gastric varices are managed differently, frequently with tissue adhesive injection.

Balloon tamponade is a temporising bridge for uncontrolled bleeding, requires airway protection, and carries significant complications, so it should be used with a defined plan for definitive therapy within hours.

Pre-emptive transjugular intrahepatic portosystemic shunt placement within a short window after endoscopic control, in patients meeting defined high-risk criteria based on liver disease severity and endoscopic findings, reduces rebleeding and improves survival. This is an important development and the decision requires early hepatology involvement rather than waiting for rebleeding to occur.

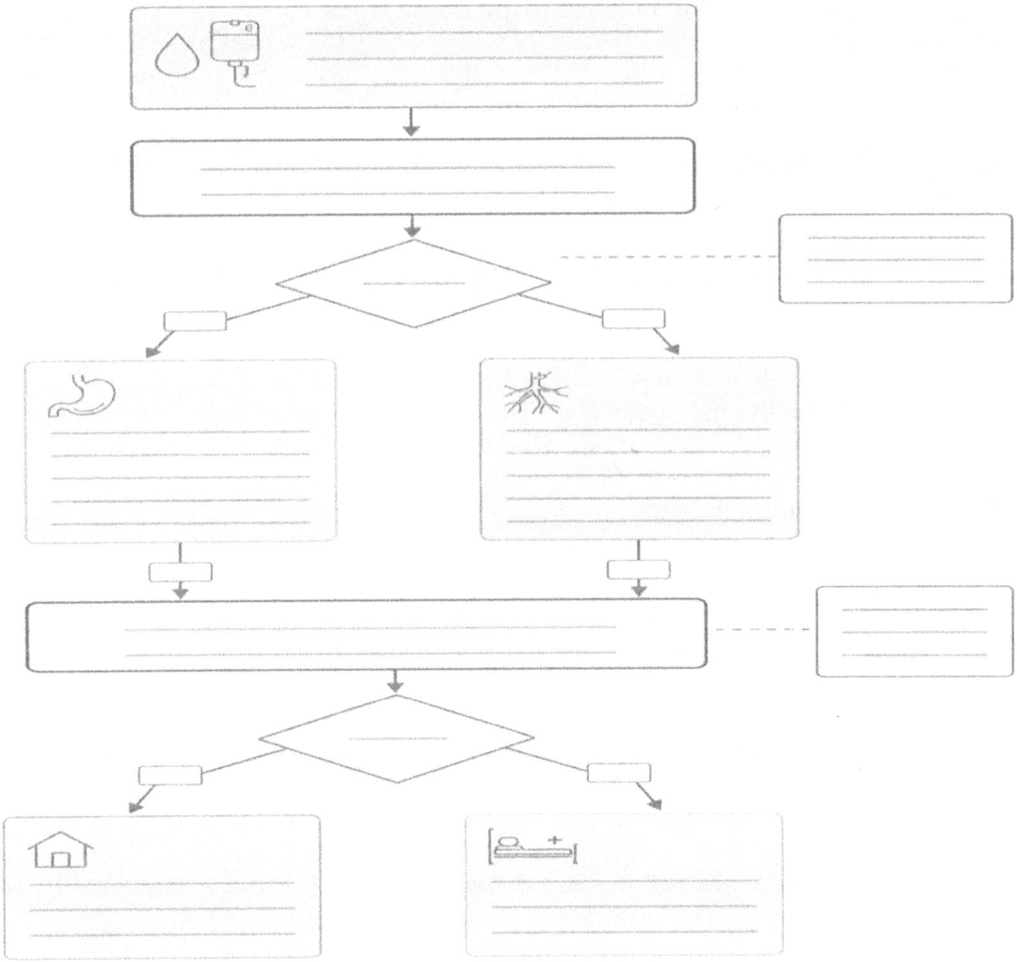

15.1.6 After the bleed

Test for *Helicobacter pylori* in peptic ulcer disease, recognising that testing during acute bleeding has reduced sensitivity, so a negative result during the acute episode should be repeated after recovery. Eradication substantially reduces recurrence.

Restart antithrombotic therapy deliberately. For patients taking aspirin for secondary cardiovascular prevention, early resumption after haemostasis is associated with lower mortality despite a modest increase in rebleeding, and prolonged interruption is harmful. The timing of anticoagulant resumption requires a weighing of thrombotic against rebleeding risk, ideally with gastroenterology and the relevant specialty.

Review the indication for any drug that contributed, including nonsteroidal anti-inflammatory agents and antiplatelet therapy without a clear indication.

15.2 Lower Gastrointestinal Bleeding and Obscure Bleeding

15.2.1 Initial approach

Lower gastrointestinal bleeding, meaning bleeding from a source distal to the ligament of Treitz, differs from upper bleeding in several practically important ways.

Most episodes stop spontaneously, with the great majority ceasing without intervention, which shapes the management toward observation and stratification rather than urgent intervention.

A brisk upper gastrointestinal source can present as apparent lower bleeding. A meaningful proportion of patients presenting with haematochezia and haemodynamic instability have an upper source, and this possibility should be actively excluded in the unstable patient, generally by upper endoscopy first. The urea to creatinine relationship noted in section 15.1.2 is helpful.

Causes in approximate order of frequency: diverticular bleeding, which is characteristically painless and brisk; angioectasia; ischaemic colitis; haemorrhoids and anorectal disease; post-polypectomy bleeding; colorectal neoplasia; inflammatory bowel disease; and radiation proctopathy.

15.2.2 Investigation and management

Risk stratification using a validated score incorporating age, sex, previous admission with bleeding, examination findings, haemodynamics, and haemoglobin identifies patients suitable for discharge and outpatient investigation, and this pathway is underused.

Colonoscopy is the principal diagnostic and therapeutic modality. Randomised evidence has not demonstrated benefit from urgent colonoscopy within 24 hours compared with a later elective procedure, so the timing should be driven by clinical stability and bowel preparation quality rather than by protocol.

Computed tomographic angiography is the investigation of choice in the patient with ongoing brisk bleeding, since it localises the source and can be followed immediately by transcatheter embolisation. It requires active bleeding at a sufficient rate to be visible.

Surgery is reserved for uncontrolled bleeding after failure of endoscopic and radiological therapy, and localisation before surgery substantially improves outcomes.

15.2.3 Obscure and occult bleeding

Occult bleeding presents as iron deficiency anaemia or positive faecal occult blood testing without visible blood. **Overt obscure bleeding** presents with visible bleeding whose source is not identified after upper and lower endoscopy.

The small bowel is the usual site, and the principal causes are angioectasia, particularly in older patients and those with aortic stenosis or renal failure, small bowel tumours, ulceration including that related to nonsteroidal anti-inflammatory drugs, and Meckel diverticulum in younger patients.

Investigation proceeds through repeat upper and lower endoscopy, since a proportion of missed lesions are within reach of standard endoscopy, then capsule endoscopy, then device-assisted enteroscopy which permits therapy, with computed tomographic or magnetic resonance enterography where a structural lesion is suspected.

In any older patient with iron deficiency anaemia, gastrointestinal investigation is mandatory rather than optional, and Chapter 7, section 7.5.2, and Chapter 12 both made this point in other contexts. Attributing iron deficiency to diet or to aspirin without investigation misses malignancy.

15.3 Acute Pancreatitis: Severity Prediction and Fluid Strategy

15.3.1 Diagnosis

Diagnosis requires two of three features: characteristic abdominal pain, typically epigastric and radiating to the back; serum lipase or amylase elevated to at least three times the upper limit of normal; and characteristic findings on cross-sectional imaging.

Lipase is preferred to amylase, having better sensitivity and specificity and remaining elevated longer. **The degree of enzyme elevation does not correlate with severity** and should not be used to grade it, and serial measurement adds nothing.

Computed tomography is not required for diagnosis in a patient with typical pain and enzyme elevation, and early imaging underestimates necrosis, which takes several days to declare. It is indicated where the diagnosis is uncertain, where the patient deteriorates, or to assess complications after the first several days.

Establish the cause, since this determines subsequent management. Gallstones and alcohol account for the majority. Also consider hypertriglyceridaemia, which requires a markedly elevated level to be causative; hypercalcaemia; drugs; endoscopic retrograde cholangiopancreatography; trauma; autoimmune pancreatitis; and, in older patients without an obvious cause, pancreatic or periampullary malignancy. **Every patient requires abdominal ultrasound** to assess for gallstones.

15.3.2 Severity prediction

Severity is classified by the presence and persistence of organ failure and of local complications.

Mild disease has no organ failure and no local or systemic complications. **Moderately severe** disease has transient organ failure resolving within a defined period, or local or systemic complications. **Severe** disease has persistent organ failure.

Prediction at admission is imperfect. Numerous scoring systems exist and none performs outstandingly. The variables most useful in practice are: a **persistently elevated or rising urea over the first day**, which is among the better single predictors; a rising haematocrit indicating haemoconcentration; **persistence of the systemic inflammatory response beyond the first day**; and a substantially elevated C-reactive protein at around 48 hours. Simple bedside scoring systems combining a small number of variables perform comparably to more complex ones.

The most useful practical approach is repeated assessment rather than a single score, since severity declares itself over the first days, and a patient whose organ dysfunction persists beyond 48 hours has severe disease regardless of the admission score.

15.3.3 Fluid strategy: a practice that has changed

This deserves specific emphasis because the teaching has reversed.

The former standard was aggressive early fluid resuscitation, on the reasoning that third-space losses and pancreatic microcirculatory failure required large volumes, with recommendations for high infusion rates in the first day.

A randomised trial comparing aggressive with moderate fluid resuscitation in acute pancreatitis was stopped early because the aggressive strategy produced significantly more fluid overload without any improvement in the development of moderately severe or severe pancreatitis. The finding is consistent with the general principles of fluid stewardship in Chapter 12, section 12.2.5.

Current practice is therefore a moderate, goal-directed approach: a modest bolus in patients with evidence of hypovolaemia, followed by a maintenance-level infusion, with regular reassessment against clinical markers of perfusion and with active de-escalation once the patient is stable. **Balanced crystalloid is preferred to saline**, with evidence suggesting less systemic inflammation.

Reassess frequently, and treat fluid as the drug it is, with a defined endpoint rather than a fixed rate continued for days.

15.3.4 Nutrition, antibiotics, and intervention

Feed early. Oral feeding should be started as soon as the patient can tolerate it, which for mild disease is frequently within the first day, without waiting for pain to resolve completely or enzymes to normalise. Where oral intake is not possible, enteral feeding is preferred to parenteral. Trial evidence has not shown benefit from routine early nasoenteric tube feeding compared with on-demand oral feeding in predicted severe disease.

Do not give prophylactic antibiotics. Antimicrobial prophylaxis in acute pancreatitis, including in necrotising disease, has not been shown to reduce infected necrosis or mortality, and it contributes to resistance and fungal superinfection. This is a specific instance of the argument in Chapter 11, section 11.7.2. Antibiotics are indicated for proven or strongly suspected infected necrosis and for concurrent infection such as cholangitis.

Infected necrosis is suspected in a patient with necrosis who deteriorates or fails to improve after the first week or two, with gas in the collection on imaging being suggestive. **The management**

principle is delay and step up: intervention should be deferred where possible until the collection has walled off, conventionally around four weeks, and should proceed through the least invasive effective route, beginning with percutaneous or endoscopic drainage and escalating to necrosectomy only if required. A step-up approach reduces major complications compared with primary open necrosectomy, and endoscopic approaches compare favourably with surgical ones.

Endoscopic retrograde cholangiopancreatography in gallstone pancreatitis is indicated for concurrent cholangitis and for persistent biliary obstruction. **It is not indicated routinely** in gallstone pancreatitis without these features.

Cholecystectomy for mild gallstone pancreatitis should be performed during the index admission rather than deferred, since deferral is associated with a substantial rate of recurrent biliary events before the delayed operation.

15.4 Jaundice, Biliary Obstruction, and Cholangitis

15.4.1 Classifying jaundice

The first division is by the bilirubin fraction.

Unconjugated hyperbilirubinaemia arises from increased production, as in haemolysis and resorption of a large haematoma, or from impaired conjugation, of which Gilbert syndrome is the common benign cause, characteristically producing mild isolated unconjugated hyperbilirubinaemia that rises with fasting or illness and requires no investigation once recognised.

Conjugated hyperbilirubinaemia indicates hepatocellular dysfunction or impaired biliary excretion, and is the category requiring investigation.

The second division is by the **pattern of liver enzyme derangement**, which directs the imaging and the differential.

Hepatocellular injury, with transaminase elevation disproportionate to alkaline phosphatase, points to viral hepatitis, drug-induced liver injury, alcohol-related hepatitis, autoimmune hepatitis, ischaemic hepatitis, and Wilson disease. Very marked transaminase elevation, into the thousands, has a short differential comprising ischaemic hepatitis, paracetamol and other toxins, acute viral hepatitis, and acute biliary obstruction from a passing stone, which can transiently produce a hepatitic pattern.

Cholestatic injury, with alkaline phosphatase and gamma-glutamyl transferase elevation disproportionate to transaminases, points to biliary obstruction, drug-induced cholestasis, primary biliary cholangitis, primary sclerosing cholangitis, and infiltrative disease.

A ratio comparing the relative elevation of transaminase and alkaline phosphatase is used to formalise this classification and is helpful when the picture is mixed.

Confirm that alkaline phosphatase is hepatic in origin by checking gamma-glutamyl transferase, since bone is the other major source.

15.4.2 Imaging

Ultrasound is the first investigation, assessing for biliary dilatation, gallstones, liver parenchymal appearance, and vascular patency. Its principal limitation is that the distal common bile duct is frequently obscured by bowel gas, and that ducts may not be dilated in early or intermittent obstruction.

Magnetic resonance cholangiopancreatography provides detailed non-invasive biliary imaging and is the next step where obstruction is suspected but not confirmed.

Endoscopic ultrasound is highly sensitive for small distal stones and for periampullary lesions.

Endoscopic retrograde cholangiopancreatography should be reserved as a therapeutic rather than a diagnostic procedure, given its complication rate including post-procedure pancreatitis.

15.4.3 Acute cholangitis

Cholangitis is infection of an obstructed biliary tree and is a surgical and endoscopic emergency, not a medical one, because the antibiotic cannot reach an obstructed system in adequate concentration.

Presentation. The classical triad of fever, jaundice, and right upper quadrant pain is present in only a proportion of cases, and the addition of hypotension and confusion defines a more severe presentation. As Chapter 9, section 9.3.1, noted, presentation is blunted in older and immunosuppressed patients, and cholangitis in an older patient may present as confusion and hypotension without pain.

Diagnosis follows structured criteria combining systemic inflammation, cholestasis, and imaging evidence of biliary obstruction or aetiology, with a graded severity classification.

Management has three components delivered concurrently: resuscitation and organ support; **antimicrobial therapy** with agents covering enteric Gram-negative organisms and anaerobes, adjusted for local resistance patterns and for healthcare association; and **biliary drainage**, which is the definitive treatment.

Timing of drainage is determined by severity. Severe disease with organ dysfunction requires urgent drainage, conventionally within hours. Moderate disease requires early drainage. Mild disease that responds to antimicrobial therapy may proceed to drainage on a semi-elective basis.

Route of drainage is usually endoscopic. Where endoscopic access is impossible, percutaneous transhepatic drainage or endoscopic ultrasound-guided approaches are alternatives, and the decision should involve gastroenterology and interventional radiology early rather than after failure.

15.4.4 Acute cholecystitis and drug-induced liver injury

Acute cholecystitis is distinguished from cholangitis by the absence of biliary obstruction and jaundice in most cases. Management is antimicrobial therapy with early cholecystectomy where the patient is fit, since early surgery is superior to delayed surgery, and percutaneous cholecystostomy for patients unfit for operation.

Drug-induced liver injury deserves specific mention because it is a diagnosis of exclusion that is frequently not considered. It can produce hepatocellular, cholestatic, or mixed patterns, may begin weeks after the drug was started and occasionally after it was stopped, and the culprit list is long, including antimicrobials, antiseizure medications, herbal and dietary supplements which patients do not report as drugs, and immune checkpoint inhibitors.

A prognostic observation of practical importance: hepatocellular drug-induced injury accompanied by significant jaundice, in the absence of biliary obstruction, carries a substantial mortality, and identifies a patient requiring close observation and hepatology involvement rather than reassurance.

Management is withdrawal of the agent, supportive care, and consideration of specific antidotes where they exist. Rechallenge is generally contraindicated, and the reaction must be documented and communicated as in Chapter 11, section 11.5.1.

15.5 Acute Liver Failure and Hepatic Encephalopathy

15.5.1 Acute liver failure

Acute liver failure is defined by the development of coagulopathy and hepatic encephalopathy in a patient without pre-existing liver disease, within a defined interval from the onset of illness. The interval from jaundice to encephalopathy is used to subclassify the presentation, with shorter intervals paradoxically associated with better spontaneous survival but a higher risk of cerebral oedema.

Causes vary geographically. Paracetamol toxicity is the commonest cause in several high-income countries. Others include viral hepatitis, drug-induced injury, autoimmune hepatitis, Budd-Chiari syndrome, Wilson disease, ischaemic hepatitis, pregnancy-related liver disease, and mushroom poisoning.

The single most important management action is early contact with a transplant centre. This should occur when the diagnosis is suspected, not when the patient deteriorates, because transfer of an encephalopathic coagulopathic patient becomes progressively more hazardous and because assessment for transplantation requires time. Established criteria exist for identifying patients unlikely to survive without transplantation, and these should be applied by, or in discussion with, the specialist centre.

Specific management points:

Acetylcysteine is the antidote in paracetamol toxicity and should be given without waiting for confirmatory levels where the history is suggestive. It is also used in some non-paracetamol acute liver failure.

Do not correct the coagulopathy routinely. The prolonged international normalised ratio is a prognostic marker and its correction removes the ability to track the trajectory. As Chapter 7, section 7.3.5, described, the haemostatic state in liver disease is rebalanced rather than simply deficient. Products are given for active bleeding or before invasive procedures, not to normalise a number.

Monitor and treat hypoglycaemia, which is common and easily missed in an encephalopathic patient.

Maintain a high index of suspicion for infection, which is frequent, poorly signalled, and a common cause of deterioration and of transplant ineligibility.

Cerebral oedema is the leading cause of death in hyperacute presentations. Management includes head elevation, avoidance of hypotonic fluids, treatment of fever and seizures, maintenance of adequate cerebral perfusion pressure, and hyperosmolar therapy. Markedly elevated arterial ammonia is associated with the risk of intracranial hypertension, and this is one of the few settings in which ammonia measurement has genuine utility.

Avoid sedatives where possible, since serial neurological assessment is the principal monitor.

Renal failure is common and may require renal replacement therapy, which also assists ammonia clearance.

15.5.2 Hepatic encephalopathy in chronic liver disease

This is a different entity from the encephalopathy of acute liver failure and is managed differently.

Grading uses a standard scale ranging from subtle changes detectable only on testing, through disorientation and drowsiness, to coma. **Covert encephalopathy**, the mildest form, is common, impairs driving and daily function, and is not detected without specific testing.

The dominant principle is that hepatic encephalopathy is almost always precipitated, and that identifying the precipitant is the treatment. The list to work through in every case:

Infection, and particularly spontaneous bacterial peritonitis, which is the reason every such patient requires a diagnostic paracentesis; gastrointestinal bleeding, which delivers a large protein load; constipation; dehydration and over-diuresis; electrolyte disturbance, particularly hypokalaemia, which increases renal ammoniagenesis, and hyponatraemia; sedatives and opioids; renal impairment; a recently placed portosystemic shunt; non-adherence to lactulose; and, less commonly, hepatocellular carcinoma or portal vein thrombosis.

Ammonia measurement should not be used to diagnose, exclude, or monitor hepatic encephalopathy in cirrhosis. The correlation with clinical grade is poor, sampling and handling errors are common, and a normal value in a compatible clinical picture does not exclude the diagnosis while an elevated value in a well patient does not establish it. Chapter 10, section 10.6.2, made this point and it is repeated here because the practice is entrenched.

Treatment. Lactulose titrated to produce two to three soft stools daily is first-line, administered orally or by nasogastric tube, or by enema in a patient unable to take it enterally. Rifaximin added to lactulose reduces recurrence and is used for secondary prophylaxis after an episode.

Do not restrict dietary protein. This is an outdated practice which worsens the sarcopenia that is itself associated with encephalopathy and with mortality. Adequate protein intake is recommended.

Exclude other causes of altered mental state rather than attributing all confusion in a cirrhotic patient to encephalopathy. Chapter 10 lists the differential, and the specific traps here are subdural haematoma in a patient with coagulopathy and falls, hyponatraemia, alcohol withdrawal, Wernicke encephalopathy, and sepsis.

15.6 Cirrhosis Decompensation: Ascites, Spontaneous Bacterial Peritonitis, Varices, and Hepatorenal Syndrome

15.6.1 The unifying physiology

The complications in this section share a mechanism, and understanding it makes the management coherent rather than a list.

Portal hypertension produces splanchnic arterial vasodilation, mediated principally by nitric oxide. This reduces effective arterial blood volume despite total body sodium and water excess, which activates the renin-angiotensin-aldosterone system, the sympathetic nervous system, and antidiuretic hormone. The consequences are sodium and water retention producing ascites, dilutional hyponatraemia, renal vasoconstriction predisposing to hepatorenal physiology, and a hyperdynamic circulation with limited reserve.

Simultaneously, portal hypertension produces portosystemic collaterals, of which varices are the clinically important form, and impaired hepatic clearance and reticuloendothelial function with bacterial translocation, producing susceptibility to infection.

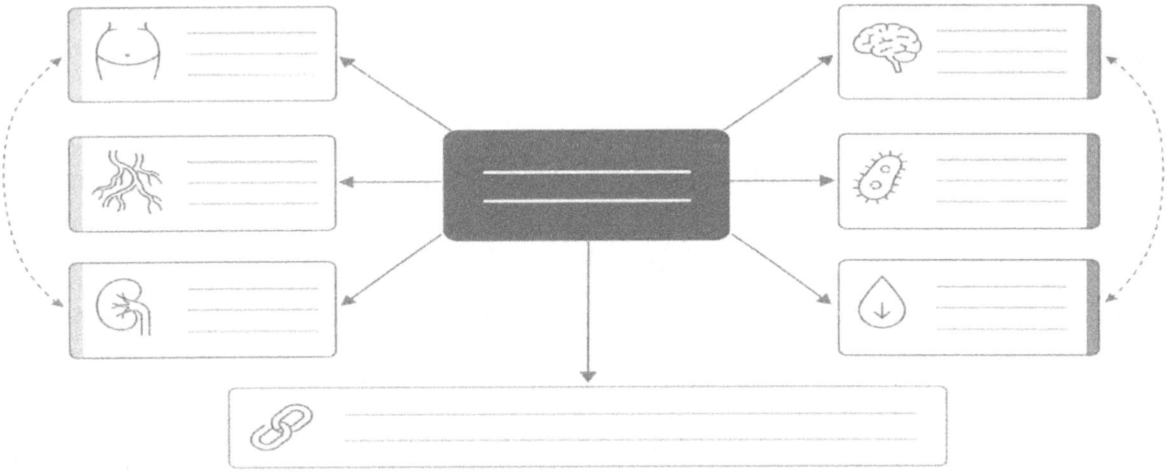

15.6.2 Ascites

Diagnostic paracentesis should be performed in every cirrhotic patient admitted with ascites, regardless of whether infection is suspected. This is the single most important rule in this section and the one most often broken.

Interpretation. The serum-ascites albumin gradient, calculated as serum albumin minus ascitic albumin, distinguishes portal hypertensive ascites, indicated by a high gradient, from other causes including peritoneal malignancy, tuberculosis, and pancreatic ascites, indicated by a low gradient.

Send the fluid for cell count and differential, albumin, protein, and culture in blood culture bottles inoculated at the bedside, which substantially improves yield.

Management of uncomplicated ascites rests on sodium restriction and diuretics. Dietary sodium restriction to a moderate level is the foundation and is more effective than fluid restriction, which is reserved for significant hyponatraemia. Diuresis uses a combination of an aldosterone antagonist with a loop diuretic in a maintained ratio, titrated together. Weight loss targets are modest and differ depending on whether peripheral oedema is present, since oedema can be mobilised faster than ascites without depleting the intravascular space.

Large-volume paracentesis is appropriate for tense or symptomatic ascites and provides more rapid relief than diuresis. **Albumin replacement is required for large volumes removed**, at a defined dose per litre above a threshold, to prevent post-paracentesis circulatory dysfunction, which precipitates renal impairment and hyponatraemia.

Refractory ascites, meaning ascites that does not respond to maximal tolerated diuretic therapy or that recurs rapidly, is managed by repeated large-volume paracentesis with albumin, by transjugular intrahepatic portosystemic shunt in selected patients, and by referral for transplant assessment, since refractory ascites is a marker of poor prognosis.

Drugs to avoid in ascites and advanced cirrhosis: nonsteroidal anti-inflammatory agents, which precipitate renal failure and diuretic resistance; aminoglycosides; and, in refractory ascites with hypotension, angiotensin system inhibitors and, in some circumstances, non-selective beta-blockers, the last being an area of ongoing debate where dose reduction rather than cessation is often appropriate.

15.6.3 Spontaneous bacterial peritonitis

Diagnosis rests on an ascitic polymorphonuclear cell count at or above a defined threshold, conventionally 250 cells per cubic millimetre, regardless of culture result. Culture is negative in a substantial proportion and a negative culture does not exclude the diagnosis.

Presentation is frequently subtle. Fever, abdominal pain, and tenderness may all be absent. The presentation may be encephalopathy, renal impairment, hypotension, or simply a patient who is not right. This is why the rule in section 15.6.2 exists.

Treatment is a third-generation cephalosporin or an alternative guided by local resistance and by whether the infection is healthcare-associated, with a defined course length.

Albumin infusion reduces renal impairment and mortality in spontaneous bacterial peritonitis, given at a defined dose on the day of diagnosis and again a couple of days later. This is a strong recommendation based on randomised evidence and is frequently omitted.

Prophylaxis is indicated after an episode of spontaneous bacterial peritonitis, during gastrointestinal bleeding as noted in section 15.1.5, and in patients with low ascitic protein and advanced disease, using an oral quinolone or an alternative according to local guidance and resistance.

15.6.4 Varices

Screening for varices is part of the assessment of every patient with cirrhosis, with contemporary guidance permitting non-invasive stratification using liver stiffness and platelet count to identify patients in whom endoscopy can be deferred.

Primary prophylaxis for patients with varices at risk of bleeding uses a non-selective beta-blocker, with carvedilol favoured in current guidance for its additional effect on intrahepatic resistance, or endoscopic band ligation where beta-blockade is contraindicated or not tolerated.

Acute bleeding is managed as in section 15.1.5.

Secondary prophylaxis after a bleed combines a non-selective beta-blocker with repeated band ligation until eradication.

15.6.5 Hepatorenal syndrome and acute kidney injury

Acute kidney injury in cirrhosis is common, carries high mortality, and has a broad differential that must be worked through before the diagnosis of hepatorenal syndrome is made.

The differential: prerenal from hypovolaemia, over-diuresis, bleeding, or large-volume paracentesis without albumin; acute tubular injury from sepsis, hypotension, or nephrotoxins; intrinsic renal disease, particularly the glomerulonephritides associated with viral hepatitis; obstruction; and hepatorenal syndrome.

Hepatorenal syndrome is a diagnosis of exclusion, requiring the presence of cirrhosis with ascites, an acute rise in creatinine meeting defined criteria, **no improvement after withdrawal of diuretics and a volume challenge with albumin over two days**, absence of shock, absence of recent nephrotoxin exposure, and absence of structural renal disease indicated by proteinuria, haematuria, or abnormal renal ultrasound. The former division into two types has been replaced by classification within the acute kidney injury framework.

Management comprises withdrawal of diuretics and nephrotoxins, treatment of any precipitating infection, and a vasoconstrictor combined with albumin. A vasopressin analogue with albumin is the established treatment and has randomised evidence of improved renal function, with careful attention to the risk of respiratory failure and volume overload, particularly in patients with existing pulmonary compromise. Noradrenaline with albumin is an alternative in a monitored setting.

Transjugular intrahepatic portosystemic shunt and renal replacement therapy have defined roles, and **liver transplantation is the definitive treatment**, which is why early transplant assessment matters.

15.6.6 Acute-on-chronic liver failure

This is a distinct syndrome in which acute decompensation is accompanied by organ failure beyond the liver, and it carries a very high short-term mortality that rises with the number of failing organs.

Recognising it matters because it changes the trajectory and the urgency: a cirrhotic patient with two or more organ failures has a prognosis measured in weeks without intervention, and requires either intensive support with transplant assessment or an early and honest conversation about goals, as Chapter 20 develops. Deciding which of these applies, and doing so early, is a core hospitalist responsibility in this population.

15.7 *Clostridioides difficile* and Hospital-Acquired Diarrhoea

15.7.1 The testing problem

Clostridioides difficile is the archetypal diagnostic stewardship problem, introduced in Chapter 2, section 2.7.3, and it is worth restating precisely why.

Colonisation is common in hospitalised patients, particularly those who have received antibiotics. Highly sensitive molecular assays detect the organism or its toxin gene in colonised patients who do not have disease. A positive result in a patient whose diarrhoea has another explanation therefore leads to treatment of a non-disease, unnecessary antimicrobial exposure, isolation, and, importantly, failure to identify the actual cause of the diarrhoea.

The rules that follow:

Test only unformed stool, in a patient with clinically significant diarrhoea. Testing formed stool detects colonisation by definition.

Do not test if the patient has received laxatives within the preceding period, or where enteral feeding or another clear cause explains the stool.

Use a two-stage algorithm rather than a single molecular test where possible, since a molecular test detects the presence of a toxigenic organism while a toxin immunoassay detects active toxin production, and discordant results identify probable colonisation.

Do not test for cure. Tests remain positive for weeks after clinical resolution, and a repeat positive in a recovered patient generates unnecessary treatment.

Do not repeat testing within a short interval after a negative result unless the clinical picture has changed materially.

15.7.2 Assessment and severity

Risk factors include recent antimicrobial exposure, particularly to fluoroquinolones, clindamycin, broad-spectrum cephalosporins, and carbapenems; advanced age; hospitalisation and long-term care residence; immunosuppression; and gastric acid suppression, whose contribution is debated but which is a reason to review the indication for a proton pump inhibitor in every affected patient.

Severity assessment uses combinations of white cell count, renal function, temperature, albumin, lactate, and clinical and radiological evidence of colitis. Definitions vary between guidelines, and local criteria should be used.

Fulminant disease is defined by hypotension or shock, ileus, or megacolon, and carries high mortality.

Assess for complications: toxic megacolon, indicated by colonic dilatation with systemic toxicity, which may present with paradoxically reduced diarrhoea as the colon becomes atonic; perforation; and ileus, which similarly may mask the diarrhoea.

15.7.3 Treatment

Stop the inciting antimicrobial wherever clinically possible, since this alone resolves a proportion of cases and substantially improves the response to treatment.

First-line therapy in current major guidance is an oral non-absorbed macrocyclic antibiotic, which has lower recurrence rates than oral vancomycin, or oral vancomycin as an alternative. **Metronidazole has been demoted** and is now recommended only where the preferred agents are unavailable, since it is less effective.

Fulminant disease requires higher-dose oral or nasogastric vancomycin, intravenous metronidazole as an adjunct given that oral delivery to the colon may be impaired by ileus, and consideration of rectal vancomycin instillation where ileus is present.

Surgical involvement should be early rather than at the point of collapse in fulminant disease, with options including subtotal colectomy and a diverting loop ileostomy with colonic lavage.

Recurrent disease, which affects a substantial minority, is managed with a different agent from the initial course, a tapering and pulsed vancomycin regimen, or the macrocyclic agent. A monoclonal antibody against toxin B reduces recurrence when given alongside standard therapy in selected patients.

Faecal microbiota transplantation is highly effective for multiply recurrent disease and is an established therapy, with standardised live biotherapeutic products now available in some settings. Referral for this should not be delayed until the patient has had many recurrences.

Infection control requires contact precautions, single-room isolation, **hand hygiene with soap and water rather than alcohol-based gel**, since spores are not killed by alcohol, and sporicidal environmental cleaning.

Do not use antimotility agents in acute severe disease.

15.7.4 Other causes of hospital-acquired diarrhoea

A structured differential prevents the diagnostic anchoring that a positive *Clostridioides difficile* test produces.

Medications are the commonest cause overall and the most frequently overlooked: laxatives, whether prescribed or given as part of a bowel regimen; magnesium-containing preparations and antacids; proton pump inhibitors; metformin; colchicine; several antimicrobials through non-infective mechanisms; chemotherapy and immune checkpoint inhibitors, the latter producing an immune-mediated colitis requiring corticosteroids rather than antimicrobials; and sorbitol-containing liquid preparations.

Enteral feeding, through osmotic load, rate, and formulation.

Overflow diarrhoea from faecal impaction, which is common, is treated in the exactly opposite way to infective diarrhoea, and is identified by examination as in section 15.8.

Ischaemic colitis, particularly after a hypotensive episode, as noted in Chapter 9, section 9.3.2.

Inflammatory bowel disease, either a first presentation or a flare, and recognising that *Clostridioides difficile* frequently complicates it.

Other infective causes including norovirus, which causes ward outbreaks and requires specific infection control, and, in the immunocompromised, cytomegalovirus colitis and parasitic infection.

Malabsorption, including bile acid malabsorption and pancreatic insufficiency, in the appropriate context.

15.8 Constipation and the Neurogenic Bowel

15.8.1 Why this matters more than it appears to

Constipation in hospitalised patients is common, is treated as a nursing inconvenience, and causes a series of consequences that are attributed to other things: abdominal pain, nausea and reduced oral intake, urinary retention, delirium, agitation, overflow diarrhoea that is then investigated as infection, and in the extreme, stercoral ulceration and perforation, which carries a high mortality. Vagal responses to straining and to disimpaction cause bradycardia and hypotension.

The causes in hospital are predictable and largely iatrogenic: opioids, which act directly on enteric receptors and to which tolerance does not develop; immobility; dehydration and reduced oral intake; anticholinergic burden; iron supplements; calcium channel blockers; ondansetron; hypercalcaemia, hypokalaemia, and hypothyroidism; and the practical realities of using a bedpan or a commode without privacy, at the wrong height, in an unfamiliar environment, with the wrong posture and inadequate time.

15.8.2 Assessment

Take a history that establishes the baseline, since normal frequency varies widely and the change matters more than the interval.

Examine the abdomen and, where clinically indicated and with consent, perform a rectal examination. This distinguishes an empty rectum, suggesting slow transit or proximal obstruction, from a loaded rectum with hard stool, indicating impaction, and identifies overflow. It is also the examination that identifies the anorectal pathology that plain films cannot.

Exclude obstruction before treating aggressively. Complete constipation with vomiting and distension, particularly in a patient with malignancy or previous surgery, requires imaging rather than a stimulant laxative.

Plain abdominal radiography has limited value for assessing faecal loading and should not be used routinely for this purpose, though it retains a role in suspected obstruction and in assessing colonic dilatation.

15.8.3 Treatment

Prevention is the correct approach, and the single most important rule is that **every patient prescribed an opioid should be prescribed a laxative at the same time**, unless there is a specific reason not to.

Laxative classes and their appropriate use:

Osmotic agents, including macrogol preparations and lactulose, draw water into the lumen and are the general first-line choice. Macrogol preparations are generally better tolerated than lactulose, which causes bloating and flatulence and whose principal alternative use is in hepatic encephalopathy.

Stimulants, including senna and bisacodyl, increase motility and are appropriate in combination with an osmotic agent, particularly in opioid-induced constipation where the mechanism is reduced motility.

Bulk-forming agents require adequate fluid intake and mobility and are generally inappropriate for immobile, dehydrated, or opioid-treated inpatients, in whom they can worsen impaction.

Softeners have weak supporting evidence and are frequently used as monotherapy where a combination would be more effective.

Rectal preparations, including suppositories and enemas, are appropriate for rectal loading and for impaction. Phosphate enemas require caution in older patients and in renal impairment because of the risk of significant electrolyte disturbance.

Peripherally acting mu-opioid receptor antagonists are effective in opioid-induced constipation refractory to conventional laxatives, and act without reversing analgesia.

Faecal impaction requires rectal clearance, which may need manual evacuation with appropriate analgesia and consent, followed by a maintenance regimen to prevent recurrence. Treating impaction with oral laxatives alone worsens the overflow without clearing the obstruction.

15.8.4 The neurogenic bowel

Patients with spinal cord injury, multiple sclerosis, spina bifida, and advanced Parkinson disease have neurogenic bowel dysfunction, and the management depends on the level of the lesion.

Upper motor neurone, or reflexic, bowel results from lesions above the conus medullaris. The reflex arc is intact but voluntary control is lost, producing a hyperreflexic bowel with a spastic external sphincter and retained stool. **Management uses the intact reflex**: a scheduled programme with a suppository or a mini-enema followed by digital rectal stimulation, performed at a consistent time, usually after a meal to exploit the gastrocolic response.

Lower motor neurone, or areflexic, bowel results from lesions of the conus, cauda equina, or peripheral nerves. The reflex arc is lost, producing a flaccid bowel with a lax sphincter and a high risk of incontinence. **Management relies on manual evacuation** at scheduled intervals with a firmer stool consistency deliberately maintained.

General principles for both: a consistent daily or alternate-day schedule; positioning upright where possible, since supine evacuation is mechanically disadvantageous; adequate time and privacy; consistent stool consistency achieved with diet and titrated laxatives; and, for patients in whom conservative management fails, transanal irrigation, which is effective and underused.

Involve the patient's own established regimen. Patients with long-standing spinal cord injury usually have a bowel programme that works, and the commonest error on admission is to disrupt it by substituting a generic ward laxative regimen. Ask, and continue what they do at home.

15.8.5 Autonomic dysreflexia

This deserves specific emphasis because it is a life-threatening emergency, it is triggered by exactly the problems discussed in this section, and it is frequently unrecognised by clinicians who do not work with spinal cord injury.

It occurs in patients with spinal cord lesions at or above approximately the sixth thoracic level. A noxious stimulus below the level of the lesion, most commonly bladder distension or bowel distension and impaction, triggers unopposed sympathetic outflow below the lesion, producing severe vasoconstriction and hypertension, which cannot be modulated by descending inhibition.

Presentation: a sudden severe rise in blood pressure, frequently far above the patient's usual level, which in these patients may be low at baseline so that an apparently normal reading is dangerously elevated; pounding headache; flushing and sweating above the level of the lesion; pallor and piloerection below it; nasal congestion; anxiety; and reflex bradycardia. Complications include intracranial haemorrhage, seizures, and death.

Management, in order: sit the patient upright and lower the legs to promote venous pooling; loosen constrictive clothing and appliances; **identify and remove the stimulus**, checking first for bladder distension and catheter blockage, then for bowel loading, using topical anaesthetic before any rectal intervention since the intervention itself is a further stimulus; and give a rapid-acting, short-duration antihypertensive if the pressure remains dangerously elevated after the stimulus is addressed. Monitor for a subsequent fall in pressure once the stimulus is relieved.

Every institution caring for these patients should have this pathway available, and patients frequently know their own triggers and management better than the admitting team.

Chapter Summary

- **Resuscitate first.** In upper gastrointestinal bleeding, use a **restrictive transfusion threshold**, which improves survival including in cirrhosis. Very early endoscopy is not superior to endoscopy within twenty-four hours.
- **Proton pump inhibitors have their clearest role after endoscopy** in patients with high-risk stigmata. In suspected variceal bleeding, a vasoactive agent and **antibiotic prophylaxis**, which reduces mortality, should be given before endoscopy.
- **Most lower gastrointestinal bleeding stops spontaneously**, urgent colonoscopy confers no benefit, and a brisk upper source must be excluded in the unstable patient. Iron deficiency anaemia in an older patient always requires investigation.

- **Aggressive fluid resuscitation in acute pancreatitis has been shown to cause harm**, and a moderate goal-directed approach with balanced crystalloid is now standard. Feed early, do not give prophylactic antibiotics, and delay intervention for necrosis until it has walled off, using a step-up approach.
- **Cholangitis is an obstruction problem, not an antibiotic problem.** Severity determines the urgency of drainage, and presentation is blunted in older patients.
- **In acute liver failure, contact a transplant centre early**, do not routinely correct the coagulopathy, and watch for hypoglycaemia, infection, and cerebral oedema.
- **Hepatic encephalopathy is almost always precipitated**, and finding the precipitant is the treatment. **Ammonia should not be used to diagnose or monitor it**, and protein should not be restricted.
- **Every cirrhotic patient admitted with ascites requires a diagnostic paracentesis**, because spontaneous bacterial peritonitis presents without abdominal signs. **Albumin reduces renal failure and mortality** in that condition and is frequently omitted.
- **Hepatorenal syndrome is a diagnosis of exclusion** requiring failure to respond to albumin challenge and withdrawal of diuretics. Acute-on-chronic liver failure with multiple organ failures carries a prognosis measured in weeks and requires an early decision between intensive support with transplant assessment and a change in goals.
- **Do not test formed stool for *Clostridioides difficile*, do not test after laxatives, and do not test for cure.** Metronidazole has been demoted to a third-line agent, and faecal microbiota transplantation should be considered early in recurrent disease.
- **Prescribe a laxative with every opioid.** Constipation causes delirium, retention, and overflow diarrhoea, and **autonomic dysreflexia** triggered by bowel or bladder distension is a life-threatening emergency in patients with high spinal cord lesions.

Review Questions

1. A patient with known cirrhosis presents with haematemesis, a heart rate of 118, and a haemoglobin of 82 grams per litre. State your transfusion threshold and justify it, and list the three interventions you would deliver before endoscopy.
2. A patient with acute pancreatitis and a raised urea is prescribed 250 millilitres per hour of crystalloid for the first 24 hours by a colleague citing standard teaching. State your position, the evidence, and what you would prescribe instead.
3. A cirrhotic patient is admitted with confusion, no fever, and a soft abdomen. The team requests an ammonia level and starts lactulose. State what is wrong with this approach and what you would do.
4. A patient with a *Clostridioides difficile* positive molecular test has one loose stool per day and received lactulose yesterday. Explain how you would interpret this and what you would do.
5. A patient with a T4 spinal cord injury develops a severe headache, flushing above the chest, and a blood pressure of 170 over 100, when their usual systolic is 95. State your diagnosis, your immediate actions in order, and the two commonest triggers.

CHAPTER 16: Acute Kidney Injury and Renal Replacement Decisions

Learning Objectives

After studying this chapter, the reader should be able to:

1. Apply the consensus definition of acute kidney injury, describe the limitations of creatinine as a marker, and explain the emerging distinction between functional and structural injury.
2. Evaluate the prerenal and tubular injury framework critically, use urinary indices and microscopy appropriately, and recognise the limitations of both.
3. Exclude obstruction reliably and recognise the glomerular and interstitial causes that require urgent specialist involvement.
4. Practise nephrotoxin stewardship and adjust drug dosing safely in unstable renal function.
5. State the indications for renal replacement therapy and describe the current evidence on timing and modality.
6. Manage the dialysis-dependent inpatient safely, including access protection and the specific complications of each modality.
7. Describe cardiorenal and hepatorenal physiology and their management implications.

Chapter Overview

Acute kidney injury complicates a large proportion of medical admissions, is independently associated with mortality, and is frequently the result of care rather than of disease. It is also the organ failure most often managed badly by non-specialists, and the reasons are identifiable.

Acute kidney injury is a syndrome, not a diagnosis. Recording it as the problem and moving on is equivalent to recording "anaemia" and stopping. It has a cause, and the cause determines the treatment.

Creatinine is a poor and late marker. By the time it has risen, substantial injury has occurred. It is affected by muscle mass, by the volume in which it is distributed, and by drugs that alter its secretion without affecting glomerular filtration. Section 16.1 develops this because most of the errors in this chapter follow from treating creatinine as though it were a direct measurement of renal function.

The treatment is usually to stop something rather than to start something. Nephrotoxin withdrawal, correction of volume state, and relief of obstruction account for the majority of reversible acute kidney injury. Section 16.4 is therefore among the most practically valuable in the chapter.

Both hypovolaemia and fluid overload cause harm, and the reflex to give fluid to any patient whose creatinine has risen is responsible for a great deal of iatrogenic pulmonary oedema. Chapter 12, sections 12.1 and 12.2, established the framework.

16.1 Definitions, Biomarkers, and Phenotyping

16.1.1 The consensus definition

Acute kidney injury is defined by any of three criteria: a rise in serum creatinine of at least a defined small absolute amount within 48 hours; a rise to at least one and a half times a known or presumed baseline within seven days; or a urine output below a defined threshold per kilogram per hour sustained over six hours.

Severity is staged in three grades by the magnitude of the creatinine rise and the duration and severity of oliguria, with the highest stage additionally defined by the initiation of renal replacement therapy.

The urine output criterion is more sensitive and earlier than the creatinine criterion and is routinely ignored because it requires accurate hourly measurement, which requires either a catheter or diligent nursing measurement. A patient meeting the urine output criterion alone has acute kidney injury, and the omission of this criterion means that a substantial proportion of cases are identified late.

16.1.2 The limitations of creatinine

Creatinine is a convenient and imperfect surrogate, and understanding its failure modes prevents specific errors.

It is a late marker. Glomerular filtration must fall substantially before creatinine rises detectably, and the rise lags the injury by a day or more. A patient whose creatinine is normal this morning may have sustained significant injury yesterday.

It is not at steady state during acute illness. The relationships between creatinine and glomerular filtration rate that underpin estimating equations assume a stable state. In a patient whose function is actively changing, an estimated filtration rate calculated from a single creatinine is meaningless and may be dangerously misleading for drug dosing, as section 16.4.4 develops.

It depends on production, which depends on muscle mass. A frail, sarcopenic, elderly patient, a patient with cirrhosis, an amputee, and a patient with a spinal cord injury all produce less creatinine, so a value within the reference range may represent markedly reduced filtration. Conversely a muscular young person may have a creatinine above the range with entirely normal function.

It is diluted by volume expansion. In a fluid-overloaded patient, the creatinine concentration underestimates the degree of injury because the same amount is distributed in a larger volume. This is a recognised phenomenon and means that acute kidney injury is under-detected in exactly the patients who have received large volumes of fluid.

Some drugs raise creatinine without reducing filtration by inhibiting its tubular secretion. Trimethoprim, cimetidine, and several other agents do this, producing an apparent deterioration that is not a change in glomerular function.

Baseline is frequently unknown. Where no prior value exists, back-calculation from an assumed normal filtration rate is commonly used and introduces substantial error, systematically misclassifying patients with unrecognised chronic kidney disease.

16.1.3 Alternative and emerging markers

Cystatin C is produced at a more constant rate across body compositions and is less affected by muscle mass, making it useful where creatinine is unreliable, particularly in sarcopenia, cirrhosis, and amputation. It is affected by thyroid dysfunction, corticosteroids, and inflammation, and is more expensive and less widely available. Equations combining creatinine and cystatin C perform better than either alone.

Tubular damage biomarkers, including cell cycle arrest markers and markers of tubular injury measured in urine, rise before creatinine and identify tubular stress or damage. Their role in ward practice remains limited by availability, cost, and uncertainty about how the result should change management, which is the reasoning of Chapter 2, section 2.7.2, applied to a novel test.

The conceptual contribution of these markers is greater than their current practical use, because they permit a distinction that creatinine cannot make. A patient may have a raised creatinine with no evidence of tubular damage, representing purely functional or haemodynamic impairment; a patient may have tubular damage markers elevated with a normal creatinine, representing subclinical injury; and a patient may have both, representing established injury with functional consequence. This framework explains why the traditional dichotomy in section 16.2 is unsatisfactory.

16.1.4 Phenotyping and why it matters

Community-acquired and hospital-acquired acute kidney injury differ. The former is more often single-cause, volume-related, and reversible. The latter is more often multifactorial, associated with sepsis, surgery, and nephrotoxins, and occurs in sicker patients.

Sepsis-associated acute kidney injury is the commonest form in hospitalised patients and is discussed in section 16.2.4.

Recognising that acute kidney injury is a syndrome with subtypes matters because the interventions differ. Volume repletion helps the hypovolaemic patient and harms the congested one. Nephrotoxin withdrawal helps where a nephrotoxin is present. Immunosuppression is required for glomerulonephritis and harmful otherwise.

16.1.5 The long-term consequences and the follow-up gap

Acute kidney injury is not an episode from which patients simply recover. It is associated with an increased subsequent risk of chronic kidney disease, of end-stage kidney disease, of cardiovascular events, and of death, and the risk rises with severity and with recurrence.

The practical consequence for the hospitalist is a follow-up obligation that is routinely unmet. Every patient who has had acute kidney injury requires: a documented record of the episode, its severity, and its likely cause; a plan for repeat renal function measurement after discharge; a clear statement of which medications were stopped, which should be restarted, and by whom; and, where function has not returned to baseline or where the episode was severe, referral for nephrology follow-up.

Chapter 3, section 3.4.2, described the discharge summary requirements, and acute kidney injury is one of the findings most often lost at that transition, with a specific and common consequence: a patient whose renin-angiotensin system inhibitor was appropriately held during the acute illness and never restarted, losing a disease-modifying therapy permanently.

16.1.6 Distinguishing acute injury from chronic disease

A patient presenting with an elevated creatinine and no prior results poses a common problem: is this new, longstanding, or acute on chronic? The distinction changes the urgency, the investigation, and the prognosis entirely.

Features favouring chronic disease: small kidneys with increased echogenicity and loss of corticomedullary differentiation on ultrasound, with the important exception that kidneys remain normal or enlarged in diabetic nephropathy, amyloidosis, polycystic disease, myeloma, and human immunodeficiency virus-associated nephropathy; normochromic anaemia; secondary hyperparathyroidism with hyperphosphataemia and hypocalcaemia; and the absence of any acute precipitant.

Features favouring acute injury: a documented recent normal value, which resolves the question immediately and is why retrieving prior results is the first step; an identifiable precipitant; normal-sized kidneys with normal echotexture; and the absence of the chronic markers above.

Acute on chronic is the commonest pattern in older hospitalised patients and carries the worst prognosis, since reduced renal reserve means a smaller insult produces a larger deterioration and recovery is less complete.

Two practical cautions. Anaemia and mineral bone markers are unreliable discriminators in acutely unwell patients, since anaemia has many acute causes and phosphate rises acutely with tissue breakdown. And a patient with chronic kidney disease who develops acute injury requires the same systematic search for a cause as anyone else; attributing a rise to progression of known chronic disease without investigation misses reversible causes in a population where they are common.

16.2 Prerenal Physiology Against Acute Tubular Injury

16.2.1 The traditional framework and its limitations

The classical division into prerenal, intrinsic renal, and postrenal causes remains a useful first sort and should be applied to every case, principally because it prompts exclusion of obstruction, which is the reversible cause that must not be missed.

The subdivision of the prerenal and tubular categories into a clean dichotomy is more problematic, and clinicians should understand why.

They exist on a continuum rather than as separate entities. Sustained hypoperfusion produces tubular injury, so the same patient moves from one category to the other without a discrete transition.

"Prerenal" implies reversibility that is not guaranteed. The term suggests that volume repletion will correct the problem, which is true in straightforward hypovolaemia and false in the many patients whose reduced renal perfusion arises from heart failure, cirrhosis, or sepsis.

"Acute tubular necrosis" is a histological term that frequently does not describe the histology. Biopsy studies in clinical acute kidney injury attributed to this mechanism show variable and often minimal necrosis, with a picture better described as tubular injury or stress.

The clinically useful reframing is to ask what the mechanism of reduced function is, and whether it is correctable, rather than to place the patient in a category.

16.2.2 Urinary indices

Urinary sodium handling was traditionally used to distinguish avid sodium retention, indicating a kidney responding appropriately to perceived hypovolaemia, from failure of sodium reabsorption, indicating tubular injury.

The fractional excretion of sodium is the conventional measure, with low values interpreted as prerenal and higher values as tubular injury.

Its confounders are numerous and clinically common:

Diuretics invalidate it entirely, since they cause sodium excretion regardless of the underlying state. In a diuretic-treated patient, the fractional excretion of urea is used instead, which is less affected because urea handling is proximal.

Chronic kidney disease raises the baseline fractional excretion.

Contrast-associated injury, rhabdomyolysis, and early sepsis may all produce a low fractional excretion despite tubular injury.

Glomerulonephritis and obstruction may produce a low value.

The practical position is that a low fractional excretion of sodium in a patient not on diuretics supports a haemodynamic mechanism, that a high value supports tubular injury, and that neither result should override the clinical assessment. The measurement is a contributor rather than an arbiter.

16.2.3 Urine microscopy

Examination of the urine sediment is inexpensive, informative, and almost entirely neglected in contemporary ward practice, in part because the skill has been lost.

A bland sediment with few cells and no casts supports a haemodynamic mechanism or obstruction.

Muddy brown granular casts and renal tubular epithelial cells support tubular injury, and the quantity correlates with severity.

Red cell casts and dysmorphic red cells indicate glomerular bleeding and are effectively diagnostic of glomerulonephritis. This finding mandates urgent nephrology involvement, as section 16.3.3 describes.

White cell casts suggest interstitial nephritis or pyelonephritis.

Crystals may indicate a crystalline nephropathy from drugs, from tumour lysis, or from ethylene glycol poisoning.

Even where formal microscopy is unavailable, a dipstick and a laboratory report identifying blood and protein in a patient with acute kidney injury should prompt the same question: is this glomerular?

16.2.4 Sepsis-associated acute kidney injury

This deserves separate treatment because the traditional model is wrong in an important way.

The intuitive account is that sepsis causes hypotension, which causes renal ischaemia, which causes tubular necrosis. Experimental and clinical evidence indicates that renal blood flow in sepsis is frequently normal or even increased, and that the mechanisms are considerably more complex, involving microcirculatory heterogeneity with shunting, inflammatory injury mediated by circulating mediators, and an apparently adaptive downregulation of tubular cell metabolism.

The practical implications:

Restoring blood pressure does not necessarily restore renal function, and continuing to give fluid in pursuit of a urine output response after the patient is adequately filled causes overload without benefit.

Fluid overload is independently associated with worse renal outcomes in sepsis, which reverses the intuition that more fluid protects the kidney.

Treating the infection and achieving source control are the renal interventions, as much as any haemodynamic manoeuvre.

16.2.5 Other specific mechanisms worth knowing

Rhabdomyolysis. Suspect it after prolonged immobility including a long lie as in Chapter 9, section 9.6.4, after seizures, after compartment syndrome, with certain drugs including statins and stimulants, and in severe exertion. Creatine kinase is the diagnostic test. Management is volume repletion, which is the intervention with the clearest benefit, together with monitoring for and treatment of hyperkalaemia, hypocalcaemia which should generally not be corrected unless symptomatic because calcium deposits in injured muscle, hyperphosphataemia, and compartment syndrome. Evidence for urinary alkalinisation and for mannitol is weak and neither is established.

Tumour lysis syndrome, addressed in Chapter 17, producing crystalline nephropathy from uric acid and calcium phosphate.

Abdominal compartment syndrome, in which raised intra-abdominal pressure impairs renal venous drainage and perfusion, occurring after massive resuscitation, in pancreatitis, and with tense ascites, and relieved by decompression.

Contrast-associated injury, whose revised evidential status was described in Chapter 7, section 7.2.4.

Cholesterol embolisation, occurring days to weeks after arterial instrumentation, with livedo reticularis, digital ischaemia with preserved pulses, eosinophilia, and low complement.

16.3 Obstructive and Glomerular Causes on the Ward

16.3.1 Exclude obstruction first

This is the first action in every case of acute kidney injury, for three reasons: obstruction is entirely reversible if relieved promptly and produces permanent damage if not; it is easy to exclude; and it is asymptomatic in a substantial proportion of cases, particularly when it develops gradually.

Perform a bladder scan. This takes seconds, requires no ordering, and identifies retention immediately. A patient with a distended bladder needs a catheter, not an ultrasound request.

Then arrange renal tract ultrasound where obstruction remains possible.

Two limitations of ultrasound matter. Dilatation may be absent in early obstruction before the collecting system has distended, and in obstruction where the ureter is encased rather than compressed, as in retroperitoneal fibrosis and malignant infiltration. **Where clinical suspicion is high and ultrasound is negative, cross-sectional imaging is indicated.**

Causes to consider: prostatic enlargement; a blocked or malpositioned urinary catheter, which is a common and immediately correctable cause in hospitalised patients and should be checked physically rather than assumed patent; pelvic and retroperitoneal malignancy; stones, which cause acute kidney injury when bilateral or in a single functioning kidney; retroperitoneal fibrosis; clot; papillary necrosis; and neurogenic bladder.

Post-obstructive diuresis follows relief of significant obstruction, and can be substantial. It requires monitoring of urine output, electrolytes, and volume state, with replacement of a proportion of the losses. The important caution is not to replace millilitre for millilitre indefinitely, since doing so perpetuates the diuresis; replacement should be partial and tapered against the clinical state.

16.3.2 Interstitial nephritis

Acute interstitial nephritis is a drug reaction in the great majority of cases and is important because it is treatable and because recognising it depends entirely on considering it.

Drugs implicated include proton pump inhibitors, which are the commonest current cause in many series and are prescribed to a large proportion of inpatients; nonsteroidal anti-inflammatory agents; beta-lactams and several other antimicrobial classes; allopurinol; and immune checkpoint inhibitors, which produce it with some frequency.

The classical triad of fever, rash, and eosinophilia is present in only a small minority and its absence must not be used to exclude the diagnosis. Peripheral eosinophilia is inconsistent, and urinary eosinophils have poor test characteristics and should not be relied upon.

Suggestive findings are sterile pyuria, white cell casts, modest proteinuria, and a temporal relationship to a new drug, typically over days to weeks.

Management is withdrawal of the offending agent, which is the definitive treatment, with corticosteroids used in some cases where recovery is delayed or injury is severe, generally after biopsy confirmation and with nephrology involvement.

16.3.3 Glomerular disease and the diagnosis that must not be missed

Rapidly progressive glomerulonephritis is the nephrological emergency. It produces irreversible loss of renal function over days to weeks, it is treatable, and the outcome depends heavily on how quickly treatment begins.

The finding that identifies it is acute kidney injury accompanied by an active urinary sediment: haematuria, particularly with dysmorphic red cells or red cell casts, together with proteinuria. **A patient with acute kidney injury, blood, and protein on urinalysis requires urgent nephrology discussion the same day.**

Causes include anti-neutrophil cytoplasmic antibody-associated vasculitis; anti-glomerular basement membrane disease, which is the most time-critical and which may present with pulmonary haemorrhage as a pulmonary-renal syndrome; lupus nephritis; immunoglobulin A nephropathy and post-infectious glomerulonephritis; and cryoglobulinaemic disease.

Initial investigation, sent urgently and in parallel rather than sequentially: anti-neutrophil cytoplasmic antibodies, anti-glomerular basement membrane antibodies, antinuclear and anti-double-stranded DNA antibodies, complement components, cryoglobulins, hepatitis B and C and human immunodeficiency virus serology, a paraprotein screen with serum free light chains, and urine protein quantification. Chest imaging is indicated where pulmonary involvement is suspected.

Renal biopsy establishes the diagnosis and is arranged by nephrology, and treatment is frequently begun before the result in a rapidly deteriorating patient.

16.3.4 Other intrinsic causes worth recognising

Myeloma-related kidney disease. Cast nephropathy from monoclonal free light chains is a common presentation of myeloma and is reversible if treated early. **Any unexplained acute kidney injury in an older patient warrants a paraprotein screen including serum free light chains**, particularly where there is anaemia, hypercalcaemia, or bone pain. Serum and urine electrophoresis alone may miss light chain only disease, so free light chain assay is required.

Thrombotic microangiopathy presents with acute kidney injury, microangiopathic haemolytic anaemia with fragmented red cells, and thrombocytopenia. The differential includes thrombotic thrombocytopenic purpura, which is a haematological emergency requiring plasma exchange, haemolytic uraemic syndrome, drug-induced microangiopathy, malignant hypertension, and pregnancy-associated disease. Chapter 17 develops the haematological management, and the essential point here is that this triad requires urgent recognition and haematology involvement.

Hypercalcaemia causes acute kidney injury through volume depletion and vasoconstriction, and is addressed in Chapter 12, section 12.4.4.

Crystalline nephropathies from drugs including aciclovir at high intravenous doses, methotrexate, sulfonamides, and from tumour lysis.

16.4 Nephrotoxin Stewardship and Drug Dosing in Acute Kidney Injury

16.4.1 Why this is the highest-yield section

Medication review is the intervention most likely to change the course of acute kidney injury in a hospitalised patient, because a substantial proportion of hospital-acquired acute kidney injury is drug-related, and because withdrawal is immediate, free, and reversible.

The discipline is to perform a complete medication review at the moment acute kidney injury is identified, not at some later point, and to document the result.

16.4.2 The principal nephrotoxins

Nonsteroidal anti-inflammatory drugs are the most important and the most avoidable. They impair the prostaglandin-mediated afferent arteriolar vasodilation that maintains glomerular filtration when perfusion pressure falls, so they are most dangerous in exactly the states where that mechanism is most needed: hypovolaemia, heart failure, cirrhosis, chronic kidney disease, and advanced age. The combination of a nonsteroidal agent, a renin-angiotensin system inhibitor, and a diuretic is a recognised high-risk triad, and it is prescribed routinely.

Aminoglycosides, which cause dose and duration dependent tubular injury, requiring careful dosing, level monitoring, and the shortest possible course.

Vancomycin, whose nephrotoxicity is dose related and which is best dosed by area under the curve where the service supports it. Its combination with a particular antipseudomonal penicillin has been associated with increased creatinine rise, and there is an ongoing argument about how much of this represents true injury as against an effect on creatinine measurement or secretion, which is a good example of why an isolated creatinine rise requires interpretation.

Amphotericin B, with liposomal formulations substantially less nephrotoxic.

Calcineurin inhibitors, which cause dose-dependent vasoconstriction and chronic interstitial injury, and which interact extensively.

Iodinated contrast, with the caveats of Chapter 7, section 7.2.4.

Proton pump inhibitors, principally through interstitial nephritis, and prescribed extremely widely without ongoing indication.

Chemotherapeutic and immunological agents, including platinum agents, high-dose methotrexate, and immune checkpoint inhibitors.

16.4.3 The agents that are not nephrotoxins but require decisions

This category causes confusion and deserves precision.

Renin-angiotensin system inhibitors do not damage the kidney. They reduce glomerular filtration pressure by dilating the efferent arteriole, which is beneficial in the long term for proteinuric kidney disease and heart failure, and which becomes problematic during acute illness when perfusion is already compromised.

The conventional practice is temporary withholding during acute illness, particularly with volume depletion, sepsis, or hypotension. The evidence for benefit from withholding is weaker than the confidence with which it is done, and the practice should be applied with judgement rather than reflexively.

The critical point is restarting. Permanent discontinuation of an agent that was providing cardiac or renal protection, because nobody restarted it after the acute episode, is a common and serious harm. The decision to hold must be accompanied by a documented plan to reassess, with a named owner, as Chapter 3, section 3.4.2, requires.

Metformin is not nephrotoxic. It accumulates in renal impairment and contributes to lactic acidosis, so it is held during acute kidney injury and restarted when function recovers.

Sodium-glucose cotransporter-2 inhibitors produce a small early fall in filtration rate that is haemodynamic and expected, and confer long-term renal protection. They are generally held during significant acute illness, partly because of the ketoacidosis risk described in Chapter 7, section 7.1.3, and should be restarted, since permanent discontinuation removes a disease-modifying therapy.

Diuretics do not treat acute kidney injury and do not improve renal outcomes. They treat fluid overload, which is a separate and legitimate indication. Giving a loop diuretic in an attempt to convert oliguric to non-oliguric injury does not improve renal recovery or survival, and in a volume-depleted patient it causes harm.

16.4.4 Dosing in unstable renal function

The central problem is that estimating equations assume a steady state that does not exist during acute kidney injury. A creatinine that is rising rapidly reflects a filtration rate substantially lower than the calculated estimate, and a creatinine that is falling during recovery reflects a filtration rate higher than the estimate. Dosing from a calculated estimate in an unstable patient therefore systematically errs, and in the rising phase it errs toward overdosing.

Practical principles:

Loading doses generally do not require adjustment, since they are determined by volume of distribution rather than by clearance. Underloading an antimicrobial in a septic patient because their creatinine is high is a specific and harmful error.

Maintenance doses require adjustment for renally cleared drugs, by dose reduction, interval extension, or both.

Know which estimate the drug licence uses. Many dosing recommendations were derived using a creatinine clearance estimate that incorporates weight, rather than the body-surface-area-indexed estimated filtration rate reported by laboratories, and the two diverge substantially at the extremes of body size.

Involve pharmacy, which is the single most effective practical step and is underused.

Drugs requiring particular attention in acute kidney injury include direct oral anticoagulants and low molecular weight heparins, with bleeding risk from accumulation; gabapentinoids, which accumulate and cause sedation and delirium; opioids with renally cleared active metabolites, notably morphine and codeine, for which alternatives are preferred; digoxin; lithium; sulfonylureas; and several antimicrobials, some of which cause neurotoxicity and seizures at accumulated concentrations, as Chapter 10, section 10.6.5, noted.

Consider what will change when function recovers, since a dose appropriate for severe impairment becomes subtherapeutic as the kidney recovers, and this transition is frequently missed.

16.4.5 A structured response when acute kidney injury is identified

Care bundles for acute kidney injury have been widely implemented, with variable evidence of effect, and the value of the approach lies less in any single element than in ensuring that a defined set of actions occurs rather than being assumed. A workable sequence, performed at the moment the injury is recognised:

Establish the baseline. Retrieve prior creatinine values, because the same value means entirely different things in a patient whose baseline was 70 and one whose baseline was 160, and because unrecognised chronic kidney disease changes the interpretation and the prognosis.

Assess volume state properly, using the multiple imperfect measures of Chapter 12, section 12.1, rather than assuming depletion. State explicitly whether the patient is hypovolaemic, euvolaemic, or overloaded, because the treatment diverges completely.

Perform a bladder scan and arrange imaging where obstruction is possible.

Send urinalysis, and look at the result rather than filing it.

Review every medication, and document what was stopped, what was continued, and why.

Identify the precipitant explicitly and record it. "Acute kidney injury" without a mechanism is an incomplete problem statement, and the next clinician cannot build on it.

Set a monitoring plan: how often creatinine will be checked, whether urine output will be measured hourly and how, and what change would prompt escalation.

Define the escalation trigger and the person to contact, so that deterioration overnight produces action rather than a note.

Record the follow-up requirement as in section 16.1.5, at the time rather than at discharge, since by discharge the episode has frequently been forgotten.

16.5 Indications and Timing of Renal Replacement Therapy

16.5.1 The urgent indications

A small number of situations require renal replacement therapy without further deliberation.

Refractory hyperkalaemia, meaning a significant elevation not controlled by medical measures or recurring rapidly after them. Chapter 12, section 12.4.1, described the medical management, and the point that bears repeating is that stabilising and shifting measures buy time but do not remove potassium.

Refractory metabolic acidosis with haemodynamic or respiratory consequences.

Refractory fluid overload, particularly with pulmonary oedema in an oliguric patient not responding to diuresis.

Uraemic complications, meaning encephalopathy, pericarditis, or bleeding attributable to uraemia. These are late findings and should ideally be anticipated rather than awaited.

Certain poisonings, where the toxin is dialysable and the exposure is significant. Agents removed effectively include lithium, salicylates, methanol, ethylene glycol, metformin in severe lactic acidosis, valproate, theophylline, and barbiturates. Toxicology advice should be sought early, since the decision depends on the agent, the concentration, and the clinical state rather than on renal function.

16.5.2 Timing in the absence of an urgent indication

This is the question that generates most uncertainty, and the evidence has become clearer.

The intuition was that starting earlier, before complications develop, would improve outcomes by controlling volume, acid-base, and uraemic toxins sooner.

The trial evidence does not support routine early initiation. Several large randomised trials comparing accelerated with standard or delayed strategies in critically ill patients with acute kidney injury have not demonstrated a mortality benefit from early initiation. One large trial found **more dependence on renal replacement therapy at 90 days in the accelerated group**, and delayed strategies consistently avoid the therapy entirely in a substantial proportion of patients whose function recovers.

The practical position is therefore that in the absence of an urgent indication, a watchful strategy with close monitoring, defined trigger criteria, and prompt initiation when those triggers are reached is appropriate, and that starting because the creatinine has reached a particular value is not.

This is a decision to make with nephrology or critical care rather than alone, and the value of an early discussion is to agree the trigger criteria in advance so that initiation, when it becomes necessary, is not delayed by a conversation that could have happened yesterday.

16.5.3 Modality

Intermittent haemodialysis provides efficient solute clearance in short sessions, requires haemodynamic tolerance of rapid fluid and solute shifts, and permits time off the machine.

Continuous renal replacement therapy provides slower clearance over 24 hours, is better tolerated haemodynamically, and permits precise fluid management. It requires continuous anticoagulation of the circuit and immobilises the patient.

Prolonged intermittent or hybrid therapies occupy a middle position.

Peritoneal dialysis is used for acute indications in some settings, particularly where resources are constrained.

Comparative evidence has not demonstrated a mortality difference between modalities. The choice is therefore made on practical grounds: continuous therapy is generally preferred in haemodynamic instability and where cerebral oedema or raised intracranial pressure makes rapid osmotic shifts dangerous, and intermittent therapy is preferred where the patient is stable and mobilisation is a priority.

Circuit anticoagulation with regional citrate is preferred in current guidance for continuous therapy where it is available, with careful monitoring for citrate accumulation in liver failure.

Dose. Higher-intensity therapy has been compared with conventional intensity in large trials without demonstrating benefit, so conventional targets are used.

16.5.4 Complications and discontinuation

Complications include hypotension during treatment, particularly with intermittent therapy; vascular access complications including infection, thrombosis, and bleeding; electrolyte disturbances from the prescription; hypothermia; loss of nutrients and of therapeutic drugs, which requires dose adjustment in the opposite direction from section 16.4.4; and dialysis disequilibrium syndrome in patients with severe uraemia undergoing rapid initial clearance, which is prevented by limiting the first session's intensity.

Discontinuation should be considered actively rather than by default. **Recovering urine output is the best available predictor** of successful liberation, and a patient producing increasing volumes of urine without diuretics is a candidate for a trial off therapy.

16.5.5 Practical points that recur on the ward

Several questions arise repeatedly when a ward patient is being considered for renal replacement therapy, and brief answers prevent delay.

Vascular access for acute therapy is a temporary non-tunnelled dialysis catheter, placed under ultrasound guidance, with site selection balancing infection risk against the requirement to preserve future access options, and with the subclavian route avoided for the reasons in section 16.6.2.

Nutrition should not be restricted in anticipation of dialysis. Patients with acute kidney injury are catabolic and protein restriction worsens outcomes; the requirement rises further once renal replacement therapy is established because amino acids are lost in the effluent.

Drug dosing changes again once therapy starts, in the opposite direction from section 16.4.4, because dialysis clears many agents. Antimicrobial underdosing in patients on continuous therapy is a recognised and serious problem, and doses should be reviewed with pharmacy at initiation rather than left at the impaired-function dose.

Electrolyte prescriptions within the therapy matter. Potassium, phosphate, and magnesium are removed continuously, and hypophosphataemia in particular is common with prolonged continuous therapy and causes the respiratory muscle weakness described in Chapter 12, section 12.7.1.

Anticoagulation of the circuit must be considered alongside the patient's own bleeding risk and any systemic anticoagulation, and the two are frequently prescribed by different teams without reference to each other.

16.5.6 The decision not to dialyse

This is a legitimate and frequently appropriate decision that is often avoided rather than made.

For a frail, multimorbid, elderly patient, the survival advantage of dialysis over conservative kidney management is substantially attenuated, and dialysis carries considerable burden: repeated hospital attendance, vascular access procedures and their complications, symptomatic dialysis sessions, dietary and fluid restriction, and loss of independence. For some patients, conservative management with symptom control and preservation of function is the better option.

The decision requires a structured conversation about what the patient values and what each course would involve in practice, and it should occur before a crisis. Chapter 20 develops the structure of these conversations. The point that belongs here is that offering dialysis as though it were the default and non-treatment as a failure to treat misrepresents the choice.

16.6 Managing the Dialysis-Dependent Inpatient

16.6.1 The information to establish on admission

A patient established on dialysis who is admitted for an unrelated problem requires a specific set of information, and obtaining it in the first hour prevents most of the errors that follow.

Modality and schedule, including which days and which unit.

Access type and location: arteriovenous fistula, graft, tunnelled central catheter, or peritoneal catheter.

Dry weight and the current weight, which together indicate fluid state more reliably than examination.

Residual urine output, which determines whether the patient has any capacity to excrete fluid, potassium, or drugs.

Usual medications, including phosphate binders, which must be given with meals, erythropoiesis-stimulating agents, vitamin D analogues, calcimimetics, and any agent dosed around dialysis sessions.

Transplant status and any relevant immunosuppression.

Contact the patient's dialysis unit, which holds the recent trajectory and can advise on the schedule.

16.6.2 Access protection

This was introduced in Chapter 7, section 7.2.1, and is repeated because the consequences of failure are permanent.

In a patient with an arteriovenous fistula or graft, that arm must not be used for blood pressure measurement, venepuncture, cannulation, or peripherally inserted central catheters. This should be signposted at the bedside and written in the orders rather than assumed to be known.

Examine the access daily for a palpable thrill and audible bruit. Loss of either indicates thrombosis and requires urgent vascular access referral, since salvage is time-dependent.

Preserve the non-dominant arm veins in any patient with advanced chronic kidney disease who may require future access, and avoid subclavian catheters entirely where possible because subclavian stenosis can render an entire limb unusable.

Tunnelled catheters should not be used for routine blood sampling or drug administration by ward staff except under agreed protocol, given the infection risk.

16.6.3 Specific management issues

Fluid. Dialysis patients with minimal residual urine output cannot excrete administered fluid. **Maintenance intravenous fluid is contraindicated in an anuric dialysis patient** unless there is a specific reason and a plan for removal. This is a common and avoidable cause of pulmonary oedema.

Hyperkalaemia is managed medically as in Chapter 12, section 12.4.1, with the recognition that dialysis is the definitive treatment and should be arranged promptly. Stabilising and shifting measures remain necessary while it is being arranged.

Missed dialysis is an emergency, not an inconvenience. A patient who has missed sessions may present with hyperkalaemia, pulmonary oedema, or uraemia, and arranging dialysis takes priority.

Infection. Dialysis patients have high rates of bacteraemia, particularly catheter-related, with *Staphylococcus aureus* prominent, and a high rate of metastatic complication including endocarditis, discitis, and epidural abscess. A dialysis patient with unexplained fever or bacteraemia requires a thorough search for a deep focus and a low threshold for echocardiography. Chapter 18 develops this.

Peritoneal dialysis peritonitis presents with cloudy effluent, abdominal pain, and sometimes systemic features. Diagnosis rests on the effluent cell count and differential with culture, and treatment is usually with intraperitoneal antibiotics in conjunction with the renal unit. Any dialysis patient with abdominal symptoms should have the effluent examined.

Cardiovascular disease is highly prevalent and presents atypically. Troponin is frequently chronically elevated, so the trend rather than the absolute value carries the information, as Chapter 13, section 13.1.1, described.

Bleeding. Uraemic platelet dysfunction is not reflected in the platelet count or standard coagulation tests, and desmopressin has a role in acute bleeding, alongside correction of anaemia and dialysis itself.

Anaemia and mineral bone disease management should continue and should not be disrupted by admission.

16.6.4 Procedures and discharge

Coordinate procedures with the dialysis schedule, generally performing them the day after a session to allow correction of volume and electrolytes while avoiding the immediate post-dialysis period of intravascular depletion and residual anticoagulation. Chapter 7, section 7.2.2, addressed this.

On discharge, confirm that the next dialysis session is arranged, that the unit knows the patient has been admitted and what changed, and that the medication list reflects any adjustments made. Communication with the dialysis unit is the equivalent of the primary care handover described in Chapter 3, and it is more often omitted.

16.6.5 The kidney transplant recipient

A patient with a functioning transplant admitted for any reason requires specific care, and the general principle is that **the graft is the patient's most valuable possession and immunosuppression should not be interrupted**, as Chapter 7, section 7.7.2, argued for transplant recipients generally.

Continue immunosuppression, converting to intravenous equivalents while fasting, with pharmacy input on conversion ratios which differ by agent, and monitor drug levels, since absorption and clearance change during acute illness.

A rising creatinine in a transplant recipient is graft dysfunction until proven otherwise and requires urgent transplant unit involvement. The differential is broad and includes rejection, calcineurin inhibitor toxicity, infection including BK virus, obstruction at the ureteric anastomosis, vascular complications including renal artery stenosis, recurrence of the original disease, and the ordinary causes of acute kidney injury described throughout this chapter.

Volume depletion is poorly tolerated by a denervated single graft, and nonsteroidal anti-inflammatory drugs should be avoided absolutely.

Infection risk follows the timeline in Chapter 11, section 11.3.5, and opportunistic infection must be considered in any febrile transplant recipient.

Drug interactions are extensive and clinically important, particularly with azole antifungals, macrolides, rifamycins, and several anticonvulsants, all of which alter calcineurin inhibitor concentrations substantially.

Contact the transplant centre early. They hold the graft history, the immunological risk profile, and the drug level trajectory, and their involvement changes management in a way that generic renal advice does not.

16.7 Cardiorenal and Hepatorenal Physiology

16.7.1 The cardiorenal syndromes

The interaction between cardiac and renal dysfunction is bidirectional and is conventionally classified into five types by which organ fails first and whether the process is acute or chronic, together with a fifth type in which a systemic process affects both.

The classification is a communication device rather than a management tool. The physiological insight beneath it is more useful.

16.7.2 Venous congestion is the dominant mechanism

The intuitive model holds that a failing heart reduces cardiac output, which reduces renal perfusion, which reduces filtration. This is true in low output states and is not the dominant mechanism in most decompensated heart failure.

The evidence points to venous congestion as the principal driver. Elevated central venous pressure is transmitted to the renal veins, which reduces the pressure gradient across the kidney, since filtration depends on the difference between arterial inflow pressure and venous outflow pressure. Raised renal venous pressure also increases renal interstitial pressure within the encapsulated kidney, compressing tubules and further reducing filtration. Raised intra-abdominal pressure from ascites and bowel oedema contributes by the same mechanism.

The clinical consequences are important and counterintuitive:

Decongestion frequently improves renal function, and a modest rise in creatinine during effective decongestion in a patient who is becoming less congested is usually acceptable, as Chapter 13, section 13.2.5, argued.

Giving fluid to a congested patient with a rising creatinine worsens both problems. The instinct to fluid-challenge any patient whose creatinine has risen is precisely wrong in this population, and requires the volume assessment discipline of Chapter 12, section 12.1.

A patient whose creatinine rises while congestion is unchanged or worsening is not being over-diuresed, and requires assessment for a different problem: hypoperfusion, obstruction, a nephrotoxin, or intrinsic renal disease.

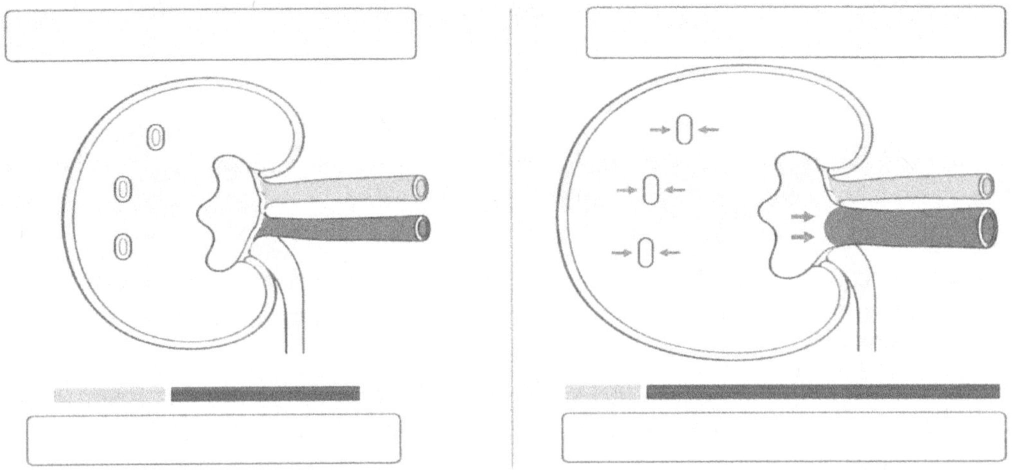

16.7.3 Hepatorenal physiology

The mechanism was described in Chapter 15, section 15.6.1, and is repeated here from the renal perspective because it is a genuinely distinct form of acute kidney injury.

The sequence is portal hypertension producing splanchnic arterial vasodilation, which reduces effective arterial blood volume despite total body fluid excess, which activates the renin-angiotensin-aldosterone and sympathetic systems, producing intense renal vasoconstriction. The kidney is structurally normal, which is why the condition is reversible with liver transplantation and why the urinary sediment is bland.

The management implications are that the treatment is vasoconstriction of the splanchnic bed combined with albumin to expand the effective volume, rather than the fluid loading and diuretic withdrawal that would treat a conventional prerenal state, and that Chapter 15, section 15.6.5, sets out the diagnostic criteria and therapy in full.

The practical trap for the hospitalist is that the diagnosis is made too readily. Acute kidney injury in a cirrhotic patient is far more often due to hypovolaemia, over-diuresis, bleeding, sepsis, or a nephrotoxin than to hepatorenal syndrome, and each of those has a different and simpler treatment. The diagnostic criteria require exclusion of those causes and failure to respond to albumin challenge for a defined period, and applying that discipline is what prevents both under-treatment of a reversible cause and over-treatment with a vasoconstrictor.

16.7.4 Other systemic interactions

Abdominal compartment syndrome, as in section 16.2.5, operating through the same venous and interstitial pressure mechanism.

Pulmonary-renal syndromes, in which a single systemic process affects both organs, principally the small vessel vasculitides and anti-glomerular basement membrane disease, as in section 16.3.3.

Thrombotic microangiopathy, in which endothelial injury affects multiple organs simultaneously.

Sepsis, which is the commonest systemic process producing simultaneous cardiac and renal dysfunction, as in section 16.2.4.

Chapter Summary

- **Acute kidney injury is a syndrome, not a diagnosis**, and recording it without a cause is an incomplete assessment. The urine output criterion is more sensitive and earlier than creatinine and is routinely ignored.
- **Creatinine is a late marker that is not at steady state during acute illness**, is affected by muscle mass, is diluted by volume expansion, and is raised by some drugs without any change in filtration.
- **Exclude obstruction first**, starting with a bladder scan, and remember that ultrasound may be negative in early obstruction and in encasing retroperitoneal disease.
- **Urinary indices are contributors rather than arbiters**, and are invalidated by diuretics. **Sediment examination identifies the glomerular causes**, and acute kidney injury with blood and protein on urinalysis requires same-day nephrology discussion.
- **Sepsis-associated injury is not simply ischaemic.** Renal blood flow is frequently preserved, and fluid overload worsens renal outcomes. Treating the infection is the renal intervention.
- **Medication review is the highest-yield action.** Nonsteroidal anti-inflammatory drugs are the most avoidable nephrotoxin, and the triad with a renin-angiotensin system inhibitor and a diuretic is prescribed routinely.
- **Renin-angiotensin system inhibitors and sodium-glucose cotransporter-2 inhibitors are not nephrotoxins.** Withholding them acutely is reasonable; failing to restart them is a serious and common harm.
- **Loading doses generally need no adjustment**; underloading an antimicrobial in a septic patient because the creatinine is high is a specific error. Estimating equations are invalid in unstable function.
- **Diuretics do not treat acute kidney injury.** They treat fluid overload.
- **Early initiation of renal replacement therapy confers no mortality benefit** in the absence of an urgent indication, and may increase long-term dialysis dependence. Agree trigger criteria in advance rather than deferring the conversation.
- **Maintenance intravenous fluid is contraindicated in an anuric dialysis patient**, and the fistula arm must not be used for anything.
- **Venous congestion, not low output, is the dominant mechanism in cardiorenal dysfunction**, which is why decongestion improves renal function and why fluid loading a congested patient worsens both problems.

Review Questions

1. A frail 84-year-old woman weighing 45 kilograms has a creatinine of 90 micromoles per litre, described as normal by the admitting team. Explain why this may not be reassuring, and state what you would do to clarify the picture.
2. A patient with heart failure has a creatinine that has risen from 110 to 165 micromoles per litre over two days of intravenous diuresis. She is less breathless, her jugular venous pressure has fallen, and her weight is down three kilograms. A colleague proposes stopping the diuretic and giving fluid. State your position and the physiological reasoning.

3. A patient develops acute kidney injury on day five of an admission. Urinalysis shows blood and protein. Set out your immediate actions, the investigations you would send, and the timeframe in which you would act.
4. A septic patient with a creatinine of 280 micromoles per litre requires gentamicin. The junior doctor proposes reducing the first dose because of renal impairment. Explain why this is wrong and what you would do instead.
5. A patient on maintenance haemodialysis is admitted with pneumonia. List the six pieces of information you would establish in the first hour, and state the single fluid prescribing error you would specifically avoid.

CHAPTER 17: Endocrine, Haematologic, and Oncologic Emergencies

Learning Objectives

After studying this chapter, the reader should be able to:

1. Distinguish and manage diabetic ketoacidosis and the hyperosmolar hyperglycaemic state, including their different fluid and insulin strategies.
2. Prescribe inpatient glycaemic therapy safely and prevent hypoglycaemia.
3. Recognise and treat thyroid storm and myxoedema coma, and interpret thyroid function tests during acute illness.
4. Manage adrenal crisis and recognise pituitary apoplexy.
5. Evaluate thrombocytopenia systematically and manage heparin-induced thrombocytopenia, thrombotic thrombocytopenic purpura, immune thrombocytopenia, and disseminated intravascular coagulation.
6. Reverse anticoagulation appropriately and manage massive haemorrhage.
7. Recognise and treat the principal oncologic emergencies.
8. Identify and manage immune-related adverse events from checkpoint inhibitor therapy.

Chapter Overview

This chapter collects emergencies from three specialties that share a practical feature: each contains conditions where the correct action must be taken within hours, where the diagnosis rests on recognising a pattern rather than on a confirmatory test, and where the natural instinct is frequently wrong.

Four ideas recur.

Sequence matters. In thyroid storm, iodine given before a thionamide fuels hormone synthesis. In myxoedema coma, thyroid hormone given before corticosteroid can precipitate adrenal crisis. In hyperosmolar states, insulin given before adequate fluid causes circulatory collapse. In each case the drugs are correct and the order determines the outcome.

The reflex response is sometimes the harmful one. Platelets in thrombotic thrombocytopenic purpura and in heparin-induced thrombocytopenia, warfarin alone in heparin-induced thrombocytopenia, and calcium in tumour lysis are all interventions that appear to address the abnormal number and that worsen the disease.

Treat before confirming. Adrenal crisis, spinal cord compression, and thrombotic thrombocytopenic purpura all require action on suspicion, because the confirmatory test is slower than the disease.

Iatrogenic disease is prominent. Insulin, heparin, corticosteroids, and checkpoint inhibitors are all treatments whose complications occupy substantial parts of this chapter. Section 17.8 addresses a class of adverse events that did not exist a decade ago and that hospitalists now encounter regularly.

17.1 Diabetic Ketoacidosis and the Hyperosmolar Hyperglycaemic State

17.1.1 Diagnosis of diabetic ketoacidosis

Three components define the diagnosis, and all three should be documented.

Ketonaemia, measured as beta-hydroxybutyrate at the bedside where available, which is preferable to urinary ketone testing because urinary strips detect acetoacetate rather than the dominant ketone body and become misleadingly positive during recovery.

Acidosis, with a reduced bicarbonate and pH.

Hyperglycaemia, which is present in most cases and **is not required for the diagnosis**. Euglycaemic ketoacidosis occurs with sodium-glucose cotransporter-2 inhibitors as described in Chapter 7, section 7.1.3, and also in pregnancy, in starvation, with heavy alcohol use, and in patients who have taken some insulin. The consequence is direct: **check ketones in any unwell diabetic patient regardless of the glucose**, and in any patient on one of these agents who is acidotic.

Severity markers identifying a patient requiring higher-level care include marked ketonaemia, a very low bicarbonate or pH, an admission potassium below the reference range, reduced conscious level, hypoxia, hypotension, tachycardia or bradycardia, and a wide anion gap.

Establish the precipitant in every case: infection, which may be occult; omitted insulin, whether through non-adherence, pump failure, or inability to afford supplies; new presentation of diabetes; myocardial infarction; pancreatitis; and drugs including corticosteroids, sodium-glucose cotransporter-2 inhibitors, and some antipsychotics.

17.1.2 Management of ketoacidosis

Fluid first. Volume depletion is substantial, and restoring the circulation lowers glucose, improves renal perfusion and ketone clearance, and improves the response to insulin. Isotonic crystalloid is used, with balanced solutions increasingly preferred over saline given the chloride load discussed in Chapter 12, section 12.2.2. The rate should reflect the degree of depletion and the patient's cardiac status, with more caution in older patients and those with heart failure.

Insulin as a fixed-rate weight-based intravenous infusion, titrated against the fall in ketones rather than against the glucose. The purpose of insulin here is to switch off ketogenesis, not primarily to lower glucose.

Continue the patient's usual long-acting basal insulin alongside the infusion. This is a change from older practice and prevents rebound ketosis when the infusion is stopped, and it makes the eventual transition considerably safer.

Potassium is the element that kills. Total body potassium is markedly depleted despite a serum concentration that is frequently normal or high on presentation, because acidosis and insulin deficiency have shifted potassium extracellularly. Insulin drives it back into cells rapidly. **Insulin should not be started if the potassium is below a defined threshold** until replacement has begun, and potassium must be added to the fluids and monitored at least hourly to two-hourly during treatment. Hypokalaemia during treatment is a leading cause of death in this condition.

Add glucose to the regimen when the blood glucose falls below a defined threshold, while continuing the insulin infusion at the same rate, because the acidosis and ketosis take longer to resolve than the hyperglycaemia and stopping insulin to prevent hypoglycaemia halts the treatment of the actual disease.

Monitor against defined targets: an hourly fall in ketones, a rise in bicarbonate, and a fall in glucose, all at specified rates. Failure to meet these targets usually means either inadequate insulin delivery, most often a problem with the line or the pump, or an untreated precipitant such as sepsis.

Do not give bicarbonate except in exceptional circumstances, since it has not been shown to improve outcomes and is associated with hypokalaemia, paradoxical central acidosis, and delayed ketone clearance.

Resolution is defined biochemically by clearance of ketosis and normalisation of bicarbonate and pH, not by normalisation of glucose. **The transition to subcutaneous insulin requires an overlap**, with the subcutaneous short-acting dose given with a meal and the infusion continued for a defined period afterwards. Stopping the infusion at the moment of the subcutaneous injection produces a gap in insulin delivery and relapse, as Chapter 7, section 7.1.4, described.

Other considerations: thromboprophylaxis, since these patients are prothrombotic; a nasogastric tube in the patient with reduced consciousness and gastric stasis, given aspiration risk; and identification and treatment of the precipitant, which is the intervention most often forgotten in the focus on the biochemistry.

17.1.3 The hyperosmolar hyperglycaemic state

This is a different condition requiring different treatment, and applying a ketoacidosis protocol to it causes harm.

The differences. Glucose is typically much higher. Osmolality is markedly raised and defines the condition. Ketosis and acidosis are absent or mild, because residual insulin is sufficient to suppress ketogenesis though not to control glucose. Dehydration is far more profound, with fluid deficits that may reach many litres. The patients are older, frequently have significant comorbidity, and mortality is substantially higher than in ketoacidosis. Onset is over days rather than hours.

Management principles that differ:

Fluid alone is the initial treatment. Glucose falls substantially with rehydration, and insulin given before adequate volume replacement shifts both glucose and water intracellularly, which can precipitate circulatory collapse. Insulin is added later, at a low rate, if the glucose is not falling adequately with fluid alone or if significant ketonaemia is present.

Correct slowly. Targets are expressed as a controlled rate of fall in osmolality and glucose, with the reasoning of Chapter 12, section 12.3.7, applying directly: an adapted brain shrinks when the extracellular osmolality falls too quickly. Both cerebral oedema and osmotic demyelination are described complications of overly rapid correction.

Anticipate a rise in sodium as glucose falls, which is expected and is not by itself an indication to change the fluid, and calculate the corrected sodium to judge the true osmolar trajectory.

Thromboprophylaxis is particularly important, since the risk of venous thromboembolism in this condition is high.

Mixed pictures are common, with features of both conditions, and are managed by attending to the dominant physiology while respecting the correction limits of the hyperosmolar state.

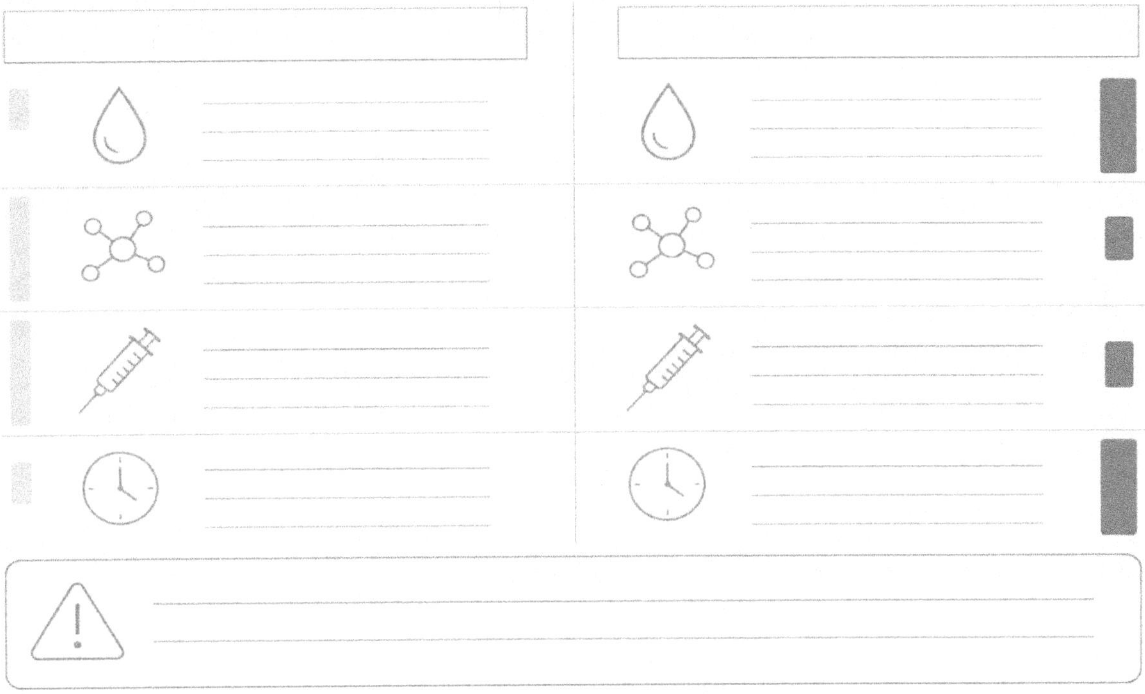

17.2 Inpatient Glycaemic Management and Hypoglycaemia Prevention

17.2.1 Targets and regimen

Target range for most hospitalised patients is approximately 6 to 10 millimoles per litre, with a somewhat wider acceptable range in patients at high risk from hypoglycaemia, including the frail, those with limited life expectancy, and those with impaired awareness. Tight control confers no inpatient benefit and increases hypoglycaemia.

Basal-bolus regimens outperform correction-scale-only prescribing, producing better control without excess hypoglycaemia, as Chapter 7, section 7.1.4, described. A correction scale is a supplement to a scheduled regimen, not a substitute for one, and prescribing correction insulin alone in a patient with type 1 diabetes is unsafe.

Never omit basal insulin in type 1 diabetes, including when the patient is fasting.

Match the regimen to the nutritional situation. A patient eating normally needs basal and prandial insulin. A patient not eating needs basal insulin with correction doses. A patient on continuous enteral feed needs a regimen matched to the feed schedule, and interruption of the feed without adjustment of insulin is a common cause of hypoglycaemia.

17.2.2 Steroid-induced hyperglycaemia

This is common, predictable, and frequently unmanaged.

The pattern is characteristic. Once-daily morning prednisolone produces a rise in glucose during the afternoon and evening with relative normalisation overnight and in the early morning. Testing only fasting glucose therefore misses it entirely, and the correct monitoring includes a pre-evening-meal measurement.

Treatment follows the pattern. An intermediate-acting insulin given in the morning matches the profile of once-daily prednisolone better than a long-acting basal insulin, which produces overnight hypoglycaemia. Dexamethasone, with its longer duration, produces a more sustained effect requiring a different approach.

Anticipate the fall. When the corticosteroid dose is reduced or stopped, insulin requirements fall rapidly, and a regimen that was correct yesterday will cause hypoglycaemia today. This transition should be planned rather than discovered.

17.2.3 Hypoglycaemia

Insulin is a high-alert medication and is among the drugs most commonly involved in serious inpatient medication errors. The recurring error types are: abbreviation of the word units, which has been misread as a zero or a four; confusion between insulin preparations with similar names; administration at the wrong time relative to meals; and continuation of a dose when the patient has not eaten.

Causes of inpatient hypoglycaemia include reduced or interrupted nutritional intake, including for procedures; interruption of enteral feed; renal impairment reducing insulin and sulfonylurea clearance; sepsis; adrenal insufficiency; malnutrition and liver disease; alcohol; and prescribing errors.

Sulfonylurea-induced hypoglycaemia is prolonged and relapsing, particularly with longer-acting agents and in renal impairment, and requires observation well beyond the initial correction. Refractory cases may require specific treatment beyond glucose administration, and toxicology advice should be sought.

After every hypoglycaemic episode, change something. Treating the episode and leaving the regimen unaltered guarantees recurrence, and the review should identify which dose or which circumstance was responsible.

17.2.4 Practical safeguards

Several measures reduce inpatient glycaemic harm and are within the hospitalist's control.

Write insulin prescriptions in full. The word units should be written out rather than abbreviated, since the abbreviation has been misread as an additional digit with fatal consequences. Specify the preparation by its full name, since several have similar names and different durations of action.

Match timing to meals rather than to drug rounds. Rapid-acting insulin given an hour after the meal arrives, or before a meal that then does not arrive, is a common and avoidable cause of both hyperglycaemia and hypoglycaemia. Where the patient is fasting for a procedure, the prandial dose should be withheld explicitly rather than by omission.

Involve the patient. Many people with long-standing diabetes manage their own insulin more accurately than a ward team can, and self-administration policies exist in many institutions for exactly this reason. Removing an experienced patient's control of their own regimen without a clinical reason worsens their glycaemic outcomes and is a common source of complaint.

Do not stop a patient's usual regimen without a plan to replace it. An admission clerking that lists insulin under withheld medications, with no substitute prescribed, is a recognised cause of ketoacidosis developing in hospital.

Continuous glucose monitoring is used increasingly by patients and is being evaluated for inpatient use. Where a patient uses their own device, it provides valuable trend information, and the practical points from Chapter 7, section 7.1.4, apply: it should not be relied upon for critical decisions, and it may require removal or shielding for some imaging and procedures.

17.3 Thyroid Storm, Myxoedema Coma, and Non-Thyroidal Illness

17.3.1 Thyroid storm

Thyroid storm is decompensated thyrotoxicosis with organ dysfunction, and it is a clinical diagnosis. **The degree of thyroid hormone elevation does not distinguish storm from uncomplicated thyrotoxicosis**, so waiting for a result to decide whether to treat is a mistake.

Precipitants include infection, surgery, trauma, parturition, ketoacidosis, radioiodine therapy, withdrawal of antithyroid medication, and **iodine load, including from radiographic contrast**, which is a genuinely under-recognised precipitant in hospitalised patients.

Features comprise fever, often marked; tachyarrhythmia, frequently atrial fibrillation, and high-output cardiac failure; central nervous system disturbance ranging from agitation and delirium to seizures and coma; and gastrointestinal features including vomiting, diarrhoea, and jaundice, the last being an adverse prognostic sign. Structured scoring systems exist to support the diagnosis and should be used to prompt rather than to gate treatment.

Treatment, in a sequence that matters:

A beta-blocker, conventionally propranolol, which controls the adrenergic manifestations and, at higher doses, inhibits peripheral conversion of thyroxine to the more active triiodothyronine. Caution is required in the presence of severe cardiac failure, where a shorter-acting agent permits titration.

A thionamide to block hormone synthesis. Propylthiouracil is generally preferred in storm because it additionally inhibits peripheral conversion.

Iodine, given at least an hour after the thionamide. Iodine blocks release of preformed hormone, but administered before synthesis has been blocked it supplies substrate and worsens the condition. This ordering is the most commonly misremembered element of the regimen.

A glucocorticoid, which inhibits peripheral conversion and treats the relative adrenal insufficiency of the hypermetabolic state.

Supportive care: cooling, with the specific caution that **aspirin should be avoided** because it displaces thyroid hormone from binding proteins and raises the free fraction; fluid and electrolyte management, recognising very high requirements; treatment of arrhythmia and cardiac failure; and identification and treatment of the precipitant.

Refractory cases may require bile acid sequestrants to interrupt enterohepatic recirculation, or plasma exchange, and warrant endocrine and critical care involvement.

17.3.2 Myxoedema coma

Decompensated hypothyroidism carries high mortality and presents in a way that is easily attributed to other causes.

Features: hypothermia, sometimes profound and sometimes with an apparently normal temperature that is inappropriate for concurrent infection; bradycardia; hypoventilation with carbon dioxide retention; hyponatraemia; hypoglycaemia; reduced conscious level; non-pitting oedema; and hypotension.

Precipitants include infection, cold exposure, sedatives and opioids, myocardial infarction, stroke, and non-adherence or interruption of thyroid replacement.

Treatment:

Give intravenous hydrocortisone before thyroid hormone. Coexisting adrenal insufficiency, whether primary as part of an autoimmune polyglandular process or secondary from pituitary disease, is common, and administering thyroid hormone first accelerates cortisol metabolism and can precipitate adrenal crisis.

Then thyroid hormone replacement, intravenously, with regimens varying between guidance in whether thyroxine alone or combined with triiodothyronine is used, and with dose reduction in older patients and those with cardiac disease because of the risk of precipitating ischaemia and arrhythmia.

Supportive care: passive rewarming rather than aggressive external warming, which causes vasodilation and cardiovascular collapse; ventilatory support for hypercapnic respiratory failure; careful fluid management given the hyponatraemia, which is generally managed by treating the hypothyroidism and by fluid restriction rather than by saline; glucose; and treatment of the precipitant, with a low threshold for empirical antimicrobial therapy since infection may be present without fever or leucocytosis.

17.3.3 Non-thyroidal illness

Thyroid function tests are frequently abnormal in acutely unwell patients without thyroid disease, in a pattern that evolves through the illness: an early fall in triiodothyronine, then a fall in thyroxine in more severe illness, with thyroid-stimulating hormone typically normal or low and rising transiently above the reference range during recovery.

The practical consequences are two.

Do not test thyroid function routinely in acutely unwell patients unless thyroid disease is genuinely suspected, since the result will frequently be abnormal and will generate confusion rather than information. This is a specific application of the stewardship reasoning in Chapter 2, section 2.7.2.

Do not treat the abnormality. Thyroid hormone replacement in non-thyroidal illness has not been shown to improve outcomes. Where the picture is ambiguous and the question matters, repeat testing after recovery resolves it.

17.4 Adrenal Crisis and Pituitary Apoplexy

17.4.1 Adrenal crisis

Chapter 7, section 7.6, addressed perioperative corticosteroid management. This section addresses the acute emergency.

Recognition is the entire problem, because the presentation is non-specific and the diagnosis is made by considering it. The features are **hypotension disproportionate to the apparent clinical situation and refractory to fluid and vasopressors**, together with nausea, vomiting, abdominal pain that may mimic an acute abdomen, weakness, fever, and confusion. Biochemically, hyponatraemia is usual, hyperkalaemia occurs in primary adrenal insufficiency but not in secondary, and hypoglycaemia may be present.

Who is at risk: patients with known primary or secondary adrenal insufficiency; patients on long-term corticosteroid therapy, whose risk was set out in Chapter 7, section 7.6.2, including those on inhaled, topical, and injected preparations which patients do not report as steroids; patients who have recently stopped prolonged corticosteroid therapy; patients with pituitary disease; and patients receiving checkpoint inhibitors, as section 17.8 describes.

Precipitants include infection, particularly gastrointestinal illness which prevents absorption of oral replacement, surgery, trauma, and missed doses.

Treatment is given on suspicion and must not wait for confirmation. Intravenous hydrocortisone immediately, followed by continued replacement either as an infusion or as divided doses; fluid resuscitation with saline containing glucose; and treatment of the precipitant.

If diagnostic testing is planned, a random cortisol and adrenocorticotropic hormone sample may be taken before the first dose provided this causes no delay, and dexamethasone may be used initially since it does not interfere with the cortisol assay. Neither consideration justifies withholding treatment.

Prevention is the more important intervention and belongs in the discharge plan: every patient with adrenal insufficiency requires sick day rules, meaning instruction to double the oral dose during febrile illness and to use an emergency injection when vomiting; an emergency injection kit with training for the patient and a family member; and a steroid emergency card. Chapter 3, section 3.4.2, applies.

17.4.2 Pituitary apoplexy

Haemorrhage or infarction of the pituitary gland, usually into a pre-existing adenoma, produces a syndrome that is frequently mistaken for subarachnoid haemorrhage or meningitis.

Features: sudden severe headache; visual field loss, classically bitemporal from chiasmal compression; ophthalmoplegia from involvement of the cranial nerves in the cavernous sinus, with the third nerve most commonly affected; nausea and vomiting; meningism; reduced conscious level; and features of acute hypopituitarism, of which adrenal insufficiency is the immediately dangerous component.

Precipitants include anticoagulation, major surgery particularly cardiac surgery, dynamic pituitary testing, head injury, and pregnancy and postpartum haemorrhage, the last producing the related syndrome of postpartum pituitary necrosis.

Management: **immediate hydrocortisone**, which treats the adrenal insufficiency and may reduce oedema; urgent magnetic resonance imaging of the pituitary, since computed tomography may be unremarkable; formal assessment of visual fields and acuity; measurement of the full pituitary hormone profile before replacement where this does not cause delay; and urgent joint endocrine and neurosurgical involvement. Surgical decompression is indicated for significant or deteriorating visual compromise and for reduced consciousness, and conservative management is appropriate for stable patients without visual deficit.

17.4.3 A note on the patient on long-term corticosteroids

Because this group is large and is encountered constantly, the practical rules deserve collecting in one place.

Identify them. Ask specifically about steroid tablets, inhalers, creams, eye drops, nasal sprays, and injections, since patients do not classify several of these as medication, as Chapter 3, section 3.2.3, described.

Never stop long-term corticosteroids abruptly on admission. This is a recognised cause of iatrogenic adrenal crisis and occurs when a medication list is rationalised without attention to why each agent is present.

Increase the dose during acute illness, following local sick day guidance, and give the equivalent dose intravenously if the patient cannot absorb enterally, which is the situation in vomiting and in ileus.

Anticipate the associated problems: hyperglycaemia as in section 17.2.2; infection risk including opportunistic organisms as in Chapter 11, section 11.3.5; gastrointestinal and bone effects; and the neuropsychiatric effects described in Chapter 10, section 10.6.5.

Plan the taper and communicate it. A patient discharged on a corticosteroid course requires a written plan stating the dose, the reduction schedule, and who will supervise it, and Chapter 3, section 3.4.2, applies.

17.5 Thrombocytopenia: Heparin-Induced, Thrombotic Microangiopathic, Immune, and Consumptive

17.5.1 A systematic approach

First, confirm it is real. Pseudothrombocytopenia from platelet clumping in the anticoagulant used for the sample is common, harmless, and produces unnecessary investigation. It is identified by examining the blood film and confirmed by repeating the count in a different anticoagulant.

Second, examine the blood film. This is the single most informative investigation and is frequently not requested. It identifies clumping, red cell fragments indicating microangiopathy, blasts indicating marrow infiltration, and dysplastic changes.

Third, classify by mechanism: reduced production, from marrow disease, drugs, infection, alcohol, or nutritional deficiency of vitamin B12 or folate; increased destruction, whether immune or consumptive; sequestration in an enlarged spleen; and dilution after massive transfusion.

Fourth, ask three questions that direct urgency:

Is the patient bleeding? Bleeding severity correlates poorly with the count, and other haemostatic defects frequently coexist.

Is there evidence of microangiopathy? Fragments on the film with anaemia and a raised lactate dehydrogenase change the situation entirely and require emergency action.

Is the patient thrombosing? Thrombosis with thrombocytopenia is a specific and dangerous combination pointing toward heparin-induced thrombocytopenia, antiphospholipid syndrome, disseminated intravascular coagulation, or paroxysmal nocturnal haemoglobinuria.

17.5.2 Heparin-induced thrombocytopenia

This condition is characterised by antibodies against a complex of platelet factor 4 and heparin, which activate platelets and produce a **prothrombotic** state despite the low count.

Recognition uses a structured clinical scoring system incorporating the magnitude of the platelet fall, its timing, the presence of thrombosis or other sequelae, and the presence of other causes. The characteristic timing is a fall beginning around five to ten days after heparin exposure, or earlier where there has been recent prior exposure.

Testing is two-stage: an immunoassay with high sensitivity and poor specificity, followed by a functional assay with high specificity. A positive immunoassay alone does not establish the diagnosis. Testing should not delay management in a patient with a high clinical probability.

Management, where the four rules matter more than anything else:

Stop all heparin, including low molecular weight heparin, line flushes, and heparin-bonded catheters. This is necessary and by itself insufficient.

Start an alternative non-heparin anticoagulant at therapeutic dose, because the thrombotic risk persists and is high for weeks. Options include direct thrombin inhibitors, fondaparinux, and direct oral anticoagulants, with the choice depending on the clinical situation, renal and hepatic function, and local availability.

Do not give platelet transfusions except for life-threatening bleeding, since they fuel the thrombotic process.

Do not start a vitamin K antagonist alone or early, because the initial fall in protein C produces a transient hypercoagulable state that can cause venous limb gangrene and skin necrosis. A vitamin K antagonist may be introduced later once the platelet count has recovered, with overlap.

Document the diagnosis prominently and communicate it, since future heparin exposure must be avoided.

17.5.3 Thrombotic thrombocytopenic purpura

This is a haematological emergency with high untreated mortality and an effective treatment, and the diagnosis rests on recognising a pattern rather than on a test that returns in time.

The pattern is microangiopathic haemolytic anaemia with fragments on the film, thrombocytopenia, and evidence of organ involvement, most often neurological or renal. The classical pentad including fever and renal failure is incomplete in the great majority and **waiting for it guarantees delay**.

Mechanism is severe deficiency of the von Willebrand factor cleaving protease, congenital or, more commonly, acquired through autoantibodies, producing ultra-large multimers that cause platelet aggregation in the microcirculation.

Diagnosis is supported by a validated clinical prediction score using readily available parameters, and confirmed by protease activity assay, which should be sent before treatment but must not delay it.

Treatment is urgent plasma exchange, with corticosteroids, and with an anti-von Willebrand factor agent and rituximab according to current protocols. **Involve haematology immediately**, since plasma exchange requires arrangement that takes hours.

Do not transfuse platelets except for life-threatening haemorrhage.

The differential includes haemolytic uraemic syndrome, complement-mediated microangiopathy, drug-induced microangiopathy, malignant hypertension, disseminated intravascular coagulation, pregnancy-associated syndromes, and disseminated malignancy, and distinguishing these requires haematology input.

17.5.4 Immune thrombocytopenia

A diagnosis of exclusion characterised by isolated thrombocytopenia with an otherwise normal blood count and film, and no alternative cause.

Investigation excludes secondary causes: drugs, of which the list is long and includes several antimicrobials, anticonvulsants, and heparin; infection including human immunodeficiency virus, hepatitis C, and *Helicobacter pylori*; autoimmune disease; lymphoproliferative disorders; and common variable immunodeficiency.

Treatment is indicated by bleeding or by a count below a threshold, rather than by the count alone in an asymptomatic patient. First-line therapy is corticosteroids, with immunoglobulin used where a rapid rise is required, as in active bleeding or before an urgent procedure. Second-line options include thrombopoietin receptor agonists, rituximab, and splenectomy.

17.5.5 Disseminated intravascular coagulation

This is always secondary, and the treatment is treatment of the cause.

Triggers include sepsis, which is the commonest; malignancy, particularly acute promyelocytic leukaemia and mucin-secreting adenocarcinomas; obstetric catastrophes; major trauma and burns; severe pancreatitis; and severe immune reactions.

Diagnosis rests on the combination of thrombocytopenia, prolonged clotting times, a falling fibrinogen, and raised fibrin degradation products in an appropriate clinical context, with scoring systems available to formalise it. **A falling trend is more informative than a single value**, and fibrinogen may be within the reference range early because it is an acute phase reactant.

Management principles: treat the underlying cause, which is the only intervention that reverses the process; **transfuse according to bleeding rather than to numbers**, since correcting laboratory values in a non-bleeding patient confers no benefit; give fibrinogen replacement where the concentration is low and the patient is bleeding, since fibrinogen is frequently the limiting factor; and consider anticoagulation in the predominantly thrombotic phenotype, which is a haematology decision.

17.5.6 Other causes worth recognising

Several further causes recur in hospitalised patients and are missed when the differential stops at the four conditions above.

Drug-induced immune thrombocytopenia occurs with a long list of agents, of which the ones most often implicated in inpatients are several antimicrobials including vancomycin, linezolid, and beta-lactams, quinine and quinidine, some anticonvulsants, and checkpoint inhibitors. The characteristic timing is around a week after first exposure or within hours on re-exposure, and the count typically recovers within days of withdrawal. **The practical rule is to review every drug started in the preceding fortnight**, including those regarded as innocuous.

Sepsis causes thrombocytopenia through several mechanisms and is by far the commonest cause in acutely unwell inpatients. The count falls early and recovers with the infection, and a failure to recover should prompt reconsideration.

Dilutional thrombocytopenia after massive transfusion, as in section 17.6.3.

Hypersplenism, in which sequestration produces a moderate stable thrombocytopenia, most often in the context of portal hypertension as described in Chapter 15, section 15.6.1.

Nutritional deficiency of vitamin B12 or folate, which produces a macrocytic picture with abnormalities in more than one lineage.

Marrow infiltration or failure, suggested by abnormalities in other lineages, by blasts or leucoerythroblastic changes on the film, and by systemic features, and requiring haematological assessment.

Antiphospholipid syndrome, which combines thrombocytopenia with thrombosis and is easily confused with heparin-induced thrombocytopenia.

Pregnancy-associated syndromes, including gestational thrombocytopenia, pre-eclampsia and its haemolytic variant, and the microangiopathies of pregnancy, which require obstetric and haematological input.

17.6 Anticoagulant Reversal and Massive Transfusion

17.6.1 Principles of reversal

Establish what the patient is taking, when the last dose was given, and the renal function, since for the direct oral anticoagulants the time since the last dose and the clearance determine how much drug is present and whether reversal is needed at all.

Establish whether the bleeding is major, meaning bleeding into a critical site, bleeding causing haemodynamic compromise, or bleeding requiring transfusion. Reversal is indicated for major bleeding and before emergency surgery that cannot be delayed, and is not indicated for minor bleeding that can be managed by local measures and by withholding the drug.

17.6.2 Agent-specific reversal

Vitamin K antagonists. Intravenous vitamin K, which takes hours to act and is essential for sustained correction, together with **four-factor prothrombin complex concentrate**, which acts within minutes and is preferred to fresh frozen plasma because it corrects faster, in a much smaller volume, and without the transfusion-associated risks. Dosing is guided by the international normalised ratio and body weight.

Unfractionated heparin. Protamine sulphate, dosed against the amount of heparin administered in the preceding period.

Low molecular weight heparin. Protamine provides partial reversal only.

Dabigatran. A specific monoclonal antibody fragment provides rapid and complete reversal. Dabigatran is also dialysable, which is relevant where the antidote is unavailable.

Factor Xa inhibitors. A specific reversal agent exists, with prothrombin complex concentrate used where it is unavailable or where local protocol directs, recognising that the latter use is not supported by the same level of evidence.

Activated charcoal may be considered where ingestion was very recent.

Antiplatelet agents. Platelet transfusion is generally not beneficial and randomised evidence in intracerebral haemorrhage associated with antiplatelet therapy found worse outcomes with platelet transfusion. Desmopressin has a possible role. The main intervention is discontinuation and supportive care.

Know what your institution stocks and where it is before you need it, since several of these agents are expensive, are held in limited quantity, and require pharmacy authorisation.

17.6.3 Massive haemorrhage

Activate the protocol early. Massive haemorrhage protocols exist to deliver products rapidly in defined ratios without individual requests, and the commonest failure is late activation.

Ratio-based resuscitation. Trial evidence supports early balanced administration of red cells, plasma, and platelets in approximately equal ratios in trauma, rather than red cells alone with later correction. The principle extends to non-traumatic massive haemorrhage with local adaptation.

Tranexamic acid early. Antifibrinolytic therapy reduces mortality in trauma and in obstetric haemorrhage when given early, and the benefit falls with delay, so it should be given as soon as major haemorrhage is recognised rather than after the products arrive.

Avoid the lethal triad of hypothermia, acidosis, and coagulopathy, which are mutually reinforcing. Warm the patient and the fluids actively.

Give calcium. This is the element most often forgotten. Citrate in blood products chelates calcium, and ionised hypocalcaemia during massive transfusion impairs coagulation and myocardial contractility. Ionised calcium should be measured and replaced during any large transfusion.

Replace fibrinogen, which falls earliest and is frequently the limiting factor, using cryoprecipitate or fibrinogen concentrate according to local availability.

Use viscoelastic testing where available to guide targeted product replacement rather than fixed ratios once the initial phase has passed.

Achieve haemostasis. Products buy time; the definitive intervention is surgical, endoscopic, or radiological control, and the resuscitation should not delay it.

17.6.4 Practical points on product use

Three points cause repeated difficulty on the ward.

Fresh frozen plasma is a poor haemostatic agent in most situations for which it is prescribed. It contains coagulation factors at physiological rather than concentrated levels, so correcting a significantly deranged clotting profile requires large volumes, which causes circulatory overload and, in liver disease, raises portal pressure. Its legitimate uses are narrower than its prescribing pattern suggests, and factor concentrates are preferable where available and indicated.

Do not correct laboratory abnormalities in a non-bleeding patient simply because they are abnormal. This applies to the international normalised ratio in liver disease as Chapter 15, section 15.5.1, described, to disseminated intravascular coagulation as section 17.5.5 described, and to mild thrombocytopenia. Transfusion carries real risk and confers benefit only where there is bleeding or a planned procedure with meaningful bleeding risk.

Know the local pathway before the emergency. Which reversal agents are stocked, where they are held, who authorises them, how long the massive haemorrhage pack takes to arrive, and who to telephone are all questions that should be answered during a quiet afternoon rather than during a haemorrhage. This is systems work of the kind described in Chapter 1, section 1.2.2, and it is the difference between a protocol that exists and one that functions.

17.7 Oncologic Emergencies

17.7.1 Malignant spinal cord compression

The single most important fact is that outcome depends on neurological status at the time treatment begins. A patient who is ambulant when treated usually remains ambulant; a patient who is paraplegic when treated usually remains paraplegic. This makes the condition a time-critical emergency and makes the recognition of its early features the intervention that matters.

The early feature is back pain, which typically precedes neurological signs by weeks. Pain that is progressive, worse on lying flat or at night, band-like, or radicular, in a patient with known malignancy or with risk factors for it, should prompt investigation before weakness develops.

Later features are weakness, sensory disturbance with a level, gait difficulty, and sphincter dysfunction, the last being a late and adverse finding.

Investigation is whole-spine magnetic resonance imaging, urgently, and whole-spine rather than the symptomatic level because multiple levels are involved in a substantial proportion.

Immediate treatment is high-dose corticosteroid given on suspicion while imaging is arranged, unless lymphoma is suspected and tissue diagnosis is required, in which case oncological advice should be sought first.

Definitive treatment is radiotherapy, surgical decompression with stabilisation, or both, with surgery favoured in selected patients with a single level of compression, good performance status, spinal instability, or radioresistant tumour. The decision requires urgent oncology and spinal surgical input.

Nursing management while the spine is unstable or unassessed requires flat bed rest with log rolling until instability is excluded.

17.7.2 Superior vena cava obstruction

Presentation: facial and upper limb swelling, distended neck and chest wall veins, plethora, dyspnoea, cough, and headache that is worse on bending forward or lying flat.

Cause is most often lung cancer or lymphoma, and in a substantial proportion it is the presenting feature of an undiagnosed malignancy. Thrombosis around an indwelling central catheter is an increasingly common non-malignant cause.

The key clinical judgement is whether this is a true emergency. Airway compromise from laryngeal or tracheal oedema, and cerebral oedema with reduced consciousness, are emergencies requiring immediate intervention. Most presentations are subacute and permit time.

This matters because tissue diagnosis should generally precede treatment. Corticosteroids and radiotherapy can render a lymphoma undiagnosable, and lymphoma is highly treatable when correctly identified. In a stable patient, obtaining a diagnosis first is the correct sequence.

Treatment comprises endovascular stenting, which provides rapid symptomatic relief and is increasingly first-line; radiotherapy or chemotherapy according to tumour type; anticoagulation for catheter-associated thrombosis; and corticosteroids, whose evidence base is weaker than their use suggests.

17.7.3 Tumour lysis syndrome

Massive cell death releases intracellular contents, producing hyperkalaemia, hyperphosphataemia, hyperuricaemia, and secondary hypocalcaemia from calcium phosphate precipitation, with acute kidney injury from urate and calcium phosphate crystal deposition.

Risk is highest in high-grade lymphomas and acute leukaemias, in bulky disease with a high tumour burden, with a high white cell count and high lactate dehydrogenase, and in patients with pre-existing renal impairment or volume depletion. It occurs most often after initiation of therapy but can occur spontaneously in highly proliferative disease.

Prevention is the principal intervention: identify risk before treatment, give vigorous hydration, and give urate-lowering therapy, with a xanthine oxidase inhibitor for lower-risk patients and a recombinant urate oxidase for high-risk patients, the latter acting on existing urate rather than only preventing its formation. **The urate oxidase is contraindicated in glucose-6-phosphate dehydrogenase deficiency** because it causes haemolysis, and samples for urate measurement after its administration require specific handling on ice to prevent ex vivo degradation.

Two management cautions:

Do not give calcium for asymptomatic hypocalcaemia, since it promotes calcium phosphate precipitation in tissues and in the kidney. Treat only symptomatic hypocalcaemia or that causing arrhythmia.

Do not alkalinise the urine routinely. Although it increases urate solubility, it decreases calcium phosphate solubility and is no longer recommended.

Monitoring requires frequent measurement of potassium, phosphate, calcium, urate, and renal function during the risk period, and renal replacement therapy should be discussed early where the biochemistry is progressing.

17.7.4 Other oncologic emergencies

Hypercalcaemia of malignancy, addressed in Chapter 12, section 12.4.4, and worth noting here as frequently the presenting feature of advanced disease and an adverse prognostic marker warranting a goals-of-care discussion alongside treatment.

Neutropenic sepsis, addressed in Chapter 11, section 11.3.

Raised intracranial pressure from brain metastases, presenting with headache, vomiting, focal deficit, seizures, and reduced consciousness, treated with corticosteroid, seizure control, and urgent oncological and neurosurgical assessment.

Leukostasis in acute leukaemia with a very high blast count, producing respiratory and neurological compromise, and requiring urgent haematological intervention.

Malignant pericardial effusion with tamponade, addressed in Chapter 13, section 13.6.3.

Malignant bowel obstruction, requiring a decision between surgical, endoscopic, and medical management, the last using antisecretory and antiemetic therapy, and frequently occurring in patients for whom the goals of care require explicit discussion.

17.7.5 Recognising the goals-of-care question

Several conditions in this section carry a particular feature that deserves explicit statement: they are frequently the presenting manifestation of advanced or progressive malignancy, and treating the emergency without addressing what it signifies serves the patient poorly.

Hypercalcaemia of malignancy, malignant bowel obstruction, malignant pericardial effusion, and spinal cord compression in a patient with widely disseminated disease are all associated with limited remaining survival. The emergency treatment is frequently appropriate and should be given, and it should be accompanied by a conversation.

The practical approach is to treat the emergency and, in parallel, to establish three things: what the patient understands about their disease and its trajectory; what the treating oncology team's assessment of prognosis and remaining treatment options is, which requires contacting them rather than inferring; and what the patient's own priorities are.

Two specific errors recur. The first is delivering a sequence of increasingly burdensome emergency interventions without anyone stepping back to ask whether the trajectory has changed, which is how patients come to die in hospital after a fourth admission that no one anticipated would be the last. The second is the opposite, withholding effective and appropriate treatment on an assumption about prognosis that has not been checked with the people who hold the information.

Chapter 20 develops the structure of these conversations, and the point that belongs here is that an oncologic emergency is one of the more reliable prompts that the conversation is due.

17.8 Immune-Related Adverse Events from Checkpoint Inhibitors

17.8.1 Why hospitalists must know this

Immune checkpoint inhibitors are now used across many tumour types, including in adjuvant settings, and patients receiving them present to general medical services with complications that are unfamiliar, that mimic commoner conditions, and whose management is frequently the opposite of what the mimicked condition would require.

The mechanism is removal of the brakes on T cell activation, which produces antitumour immunity and, in a proportion of patients, autoimmunity against normal tissue in any organ.

Timing. Events occur at any point, typically within the first months but including after treatment has been completed, sometimes many months later. A patient who stopped therapy six months ago remains at risk, and the drug history must extend beyond current medications.

17.8.2 The organising principle

Any new symptom in a patient who has received a checkpoint inhibitor is an immune-related adverse event until proven otherwise. This framing is deliberately strong because the alternative, treating the diarrhoea as gastroenteritis, the breathlessness as infection, and the fatigue as cancer progression, is the source of most of the harm.

Infection must be excluded concurrently, not sequentially, since the treatment for the adverse event is immunosuppression and giving it to a patient with untreated infection is dangerous.

17.8.3 The principal events

Colitis, presenting with diarrhoea, abdominal pain, and occasionally perforation. It is distinguished from infective causes by testing and, where necessary, by endoscopy. Antimotility agents should be avoided in significant disease.

Hepatitis, usually detected on blood testing rather than symptomatically.

Dermatological events, from rash and pruritus to the severe cutaneous adverse reactions described in Chapter 11, section 11.6.3.

Endocrinopathies, which are common and which are managed differently from other events. **Thyroiditis** produces a thyrotoxic phase followed by hypothyroidism. **Hypophysitis** produces secondary adrenal insufficiency, which is the dangerous component, together with other pituitary hormone deficiencies. **Primary adrenal insufficiency** and **fulminant type 1 diabetes presenting as ketoacidosis** also occur.

Pneumonitis, presenting with dyspnoea and cough with radiological infiltrates, which mimics infection and pulmonary progression of malignancy.

Myocarditis, which is uncommon and carries very high mortality. **Any new cardiac symptom, arrhythmia, or troponin elevation in a patient on a checkpoint inhibitor should prompt consideration of myocarditis** and urgent cardiology involvement. It frequently coexists with myositis and myasthenic syndromes.

Neurological events, including a myasthenia-like syndrome, an inflammatory neuropathy resembling Guillain-Barré syndrome, and encephalitis, all of which require the monitoring described in Chapter 14, section 14.1.4, where respiratory muscles may be involved.

Haematological and renal events, the latter usually interstitial nephritis as in Chapter 16, section 16.3.2.

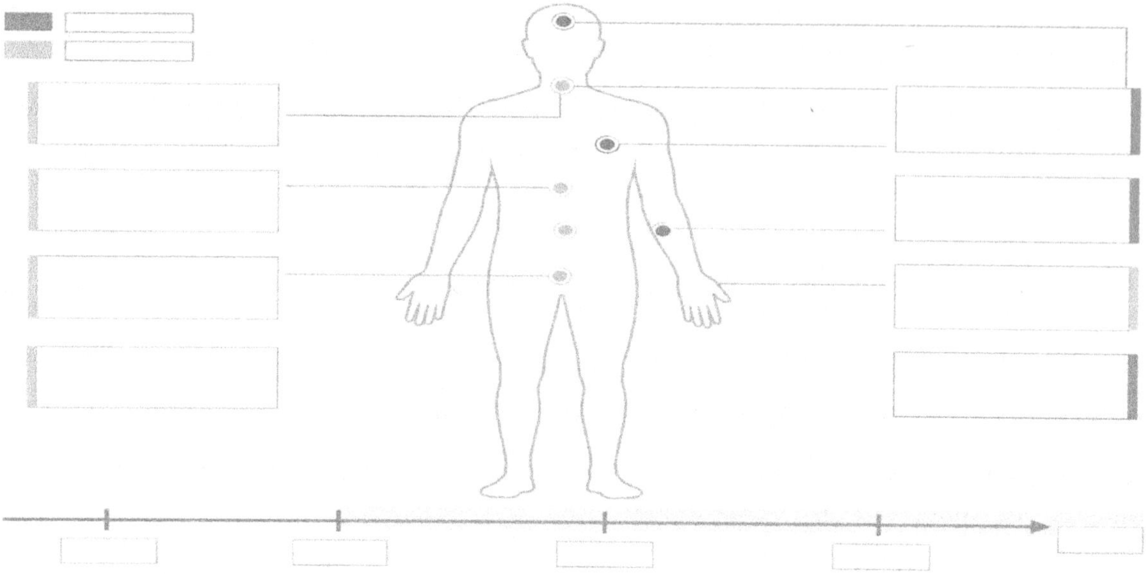

17.8.4 Management principles

Grade the severity using the standard toxicity criteria, since management is grade-dependent.

Mild events may be managed symptomatically with continued therapy under oncological supervision.

Moderate to severe events generally require withholding the checkpoint inhibitor and starting systemic corticosteroids at a dose proportionate to the grade, followed by a **slow taper over at least four to six weeks**, since rapid tapering causes relapse.

Escalate if there is no response within a defined short interval, conventionally two to three days, to a second-line immunosuppressive agent chosen according to the organ involved. Agent choice matters: the agent used for colitis is contraindicated in hepatitis, for example, and these decisions belong with oncology and the relevant organ specialist.

Endocrine events are the exception to the corticosteroid rule. Thyroid and adrenal events are managed with hormone replacement rather than immunosuppression, and checkpoint inhibitor therapy can frequently continue.

Contact the treating oncology team urgently in every case. They hold the treatment history, the tumour response status, and the decision about whether therapy can be resumed.

Consider prophylaxis against opportunistic infection in patients receiving prolonged high-dose corticosteroids, as Chapter 11, section 11.3.5, described.

Chapter Summary

- **Sequence matters.** Iodine after the thionamide in thyroid storm, hydrocortisone before thyroid hormone in myxoedema coma, and fluid before insulin in hyperosmolar states.
- **Check ketones in any unwell diabetic patient regardless of glucose**, because euglycaemic ketoacidosis occurs with sodium-glucose cotransporter-2 inhibitors and in

other settings. **Hypokalaemia during treatment is a leading cause of death**, and insulin should not be started below a threshold potassium.

- **The hyperosmolar state is treated with fluid first and corrected slowly**, because the adapted brain tolerates rapid osmolar change poorly.
- **Basal-bolus beats correction-scale-only prescribing**, never omit basal insulin in type 1 diabetes, and after every hypoglycaemic episode change something rather than simply treating it.
- **Thyroid storm is a clinical diagnosis** and hormone concentrations do not distinguish it. Iodine load from contrast is an under-recognised precipitant, and aspirin should be avoided.
- **Treat adrenal crisis on suspicion.** Hypotension refractory to fluids and vasopressors with hyponatraemia should prompt hydrocortisone before any test result.
- **Examine the blood film in every thrombocytopenia.** In heparin-induced thrombocytopenia, stopping heparin is insufficient, an alternative anticoagulant is required, platelets are contraindicated, and a vitamin K antagonist alone causes limb gangrene. In thrombotic thrombocytopenic purpura, the classical pentad is usually incomplete and waiting for it guarantees delay.
- **Prothrombin complex concentrate is preferred to plasma** for vitamin K antagonist reversal. **Platelet transfusion for antiplatelet-associated intracerebral haemorrhage worsens outcomes.** In massive haemorrhage, give tranexamic acid early, replace fibrinogen, and **give calcium**, which is the element most often forgotten.
- **In spinal cord compression, outcome depends on neurological status when treatment starts**, which makes back pain in a patient with malignancy the finding that matters. In superior vena cava obstruction, obtain tissue diagnosis first unless there is airway or cerebral compromise, because steroids can render lymphoma undiagnosable.
- **In tumour lysis, do not give calcium for asymptomatic hypocalcaemia and do not alkalinise the urine.**
- **Any new symptom in a patient who has received a checkpoint inhibitor is an immune-related adverse event until proven otherwise**, exclude infection concurrently, taper steroids slowly, and manage endocrine events with replacement rather than immunosuppression.

Review Questions

1. A patient on a sodium-glucose cotransporter-2 inhibitor is admitted with vomiting, tachypnoea, and a glucose of 9.8 millimoles per litre. The admitting team have excluded ketoacidosis on the basis of the glucose. State why this is wrong, what you would measure, and your management.
2. A patient with thyrotoxicosis develops fever, atrial fibrillation, and agitation two days after a contrast-enhanced computed tomography study. Set out your treatment in the correct order and explain why the order matters.
3. A patient on prophylactic low molecular weight heparin since admission has a platelet count that has fallen from 240 to 78 over eight days, with a new deep vein thrombosis. State your diagnosis, the four management rules, and the specific harm of two interventions you would avoid.

4. A patient with known metastatic prostate cancer reports two weeks of worsening mid-thoracic back pain, worse at night, with no weakness. State your assessment, the imaging you would request, and why the timing matters.
5. A patient who completed pembrolizumab four months ago presents with breathlessness, a mild troponin rise, and normal coronary anatomy on angiography. State the diagnosis you must consider, why it matters, and your immediate actions.

CHAPTER 18: Infection, Sepsis, and Antimicrobial Stewardship

Learning Objectives

After studying this chapter, the reader should be able to:

1. Apply current sepsis definitions and screening tools, and articulate the substantive criticisms of time-mandated care bundles.
2. Construct empiric antimicrobial therapy from an explicit assessment of source, host, acquisition setting, and local resistance.
3. Manage community-acquired, hospital-acquired, and aspiration pneumonia, including the role of corticosteroids and the evidence on duration.
4. Distinguish cellulitis from its mimics, and recognise necrotising infection and diabetic foot infection.
5. Distinguish urinary tract infection from asymptomatic bacteriuria and avoid the diagnostic anchoring that a positive urine culture produces.
6. Manage bacteraemia and endocarditis, including the specific obligations that accompany *Staphylococcus aureus* bacteraemia and the decision to remove a vascular catheter.
7. Recognise and manage bone, joint, and prosthetic joint infection.
8. Apply de-escalation, intravenous to oral switch, and evidence-based treatment durations.

Chapter Overview

Infection is the commonest reason for acute medical admission and antimicrobial prescribing is the commonest therapeutic act in hospitals. Chapter 11, section 11.7, argued that antibiotics are neither a diagnostic test nor a benign intervention. This chapter supplies the clinical content that makes that argument operational.

Four themes run through it.

Diagnosis before spectrum. The most consequential decision is not which antibiotic but whether the patient has a bacterial infection and where it is. A broad-spectrum agent prescribed for an uncertain diagnosis is a substitute for thinking, and it is a poor one.

Source control beats antimicrobial choice. An undrained abscess, an obstructed urinary tract, an infected prosthesis, and a colonised catheter will not resolve on antibiotics however carefully selected. Sections 18.4, 18.6, and 18.7 all turn on this.

Duration evidence has moved consistently in one direction. Across a wide range of infections, shorter courses have proved non-inferior to longer ones. The conventional durations were arbitrary, and the burden of justification now falls on the longer course. Section 18.8 assembles this.

Mandated protocols and clinical judgement are in genuine tension. Section 18.1 treats this honestly rather than pretending the question is settled, because hospitalists work within these mandates and should understand both what they achieve and what they cost.

18.1 Sepsis Definitions, Screening Tools, and the Hour-1 Bundle Critique

18.1.1 The current definitions

Sepsis is life-threatening organ dysfunction caused by a dysregulated host response to infection. The definition is deliberately physiological rather than microbiological, and it locates the danger in the host response rather than in the pathogen.

Organ dysfunction is operationalised in the consensus definition as an acute increase of two or more points in a validated organ failure score, which in practice means that a patient with infection and any new organ dysfunction has sepsis.

Septic shock is a subset with circulatory and cellular metabolic abnormality sufficient to increase mortality substantially, identified clinically by a requirement for vasopressors to maintain an adequate mean arterial pressure together with an elevated lactate despite adequate fluid resuscitation.

What changed and why it matters. The previous framework defined sepsis as infection plus a systemic inflammatory response, using criteria that were highly sensitive and poorly specific. Almost every patient with an infection, and a great many without, met them. Redefining sepsis around organ dysfunction was intended to identify the population at genuine risk of dying, and it succeeded at the cost of reduced sensitivity for early illness.

Severe sepsis was abandoned as a category, since under the new definition sepsis is by definition severe.

18.1.2 Screening tools and their performance

A screening tool and a definition are different instruments with different requirements, and conflating them has caused confusion.

A short bedside score combining respiratory rate, systolic pressure, and altered mentation was published alongside the definitions as a prompt for further assessment outside intensive care. Subsequent evaluation found its **sensitivity to be poor**, missing a substantial proportion of patients who went on to deteriorate, and current international guidance recommends **against** using it as a single screening tool.

Aggregate early warning scores, of the kind described in Chapter 4, section 4.5.3, generally outperform it for screening, as does the older inflammatory response criteria set, precisely because a screening tool should favour sensitivity.

The practical position for a hospitalist is that no score identifies sepsis reliably, that a patient with infection and any abnormal physiology deserves assessment rather than a score, and that the most sensitive instrument available remains a clinician or a nurse who thinks the patient looks unwell.

18.1.3 The bundle and its critics

Time-mandated care bundles for sepsis have been widely adopted and, in some jurisdictions, made mandatory by regulation. The best-known version specifies actions to be completed within one hour of recognition: measuring lactate, obtaining blood cultures before antimicrobials, administering broad-spectrum antimicrobials, beginning a weight-based crystalloid bolus for hypotension or elevated lactate, and starting vasopressors for hypotension not responding to fluid.

The case for the bundle is substantial. Observational data from large regulatory datasets have shown associations between more rapid completion of the antimicrobial element and lower mortality, with the association strongest in patients with septic shock. Delay in a patient with shock is unarguably harmful.

The case against mandating it in this form has been made by several professional bodies, some of which declined to endorse the one-hour version, and the criticisms deserve to be understood rather than dismissed.

The evidence is strongest for shock and weakest for undifferentiated possible sepsis. In the observational data, the mortality association with time to antimicrobial therapy was concentrated in patients with shock, and completion of the fluid bolus did not show the same association.

A one-hour mandate for antimicrobials creates pressure to treat before the diagnosis is established. A patient with fever and tachycardia who might have sepsis and might have pulmonary embolism, drug fever, or a flare of inflammatory disease receives broad-spectrum antimicrobials because the clock is running. The system-level consequence is substantial overtreatment, with all the harms catalogued in Chapter 11, section 11.7.1, and with the additional harm that the correct diagnosis is obscured.

A fixed weight-based fluid volume is inappropriate for some patients. A patient with heart failure, end-stage kidney disease, or established fluid overload may be harmed by a mandated bolus, and the prescription of a fixed volume irrespective of the individual contradicts the fluid stewardship principles of Chapter 12, section 12.2.5.

The current international guidance has moved toward this position, distinguishing patients with shock or a high probability of sepsis, for whom immediate antimicrobial therapy is recommended, from patients with possible sepsis without shock, for whom a period of rapid assessment and investigation before committing to antimicrobials is permitted.

The defensible practice is therefore: in a patient with septic shock or a convincing infective diagnosis with organ dysfunction, treat immediately and do not delay for anything except drawing cultures, which takes minutes. In a patient who is stable and in whom infection is one of several possibilities, use the available window to establish the diagnosis, and document the reasoning. Chapter 2's discipline applies here as everywhere.

18.1.4 Resuscitation

Fluid. Initial resuscitation with balanced crystalloid is standard. The conventional weight-based initial volume is a starting point derived from trial protocols rather than a physiological requirement, and current guidance grades it as a conditional recommendation on low-quality evidence. Subsequent fluid should be guided by dynamic assessment as in Chapter 12, section 12.1.3, rather than by protocol.

Restrictive and liberal strategies have been compared in randomised trials in septic shock without demonstrating a difference in mortality, which supports individualisation rather than either extreme.

Vasopressors should be started early rather than after exhaustive fluid loading, with noradrenaline as the first-line agent as described in Chapter 13, section 13.6.5, and with peripheral administration acceptable in the short term rather than delaying support to obtain central access.

Lactate is a marker of illness severity rather than a target in itself, and its clearance over hours carries more information than the initial value. Chapter 12, section 12.6.2, addressed the non-hypoperfusion causes.

Corticosteroids are recommended in patients with septic shock requiring ongoing vasopressor support.

Source control is the intervention that most often determines outcome and should be achieved as early as feasible. A patient with an undrained collection, an obstructed viscus, or an infected device will not improve on antimicrobial therapy alone.

18.1.5 What else looks like sepsis

A patient with fever, tachycardia, hypotension, and a raised inflammatory response does not necessarily have infection, and the conditions that mimic sepsis are treatable and are missed when the diagnosis is assumed.

Chapter 11, section 11.5.4, catalogued the non-infectious causes of fever, and several deserve restatement here because they present with the full physiological picture of sepsis: **pulmonary embolism**, which produces tachycardia, hypoxia, fever, and hypotension; **adrenal crisis**, whose hypotension is characteristically refractory to fluid and vasopressor and which is addressed in Chapter 17, section 17.4.1; **thyroid storm**; **acute pancreatitis**, which generates an intense systemic inflammatory response without infection in its early phase; **haemophagocytic lymphohistiocytosis**, which presents as a septic patient not responding to antimicrobial therapy with a strikingly high ferritin; **acute severe inflammatory disease**, including vasculitis and adult-onset Still disease; **toxicological syndromes** including serotonin syndrome and neuroleptic malignant syndrome; **transfusion reactions**; **mesenteric or other tissue infarction**; and **major haemorrhage**, which produces tachycardia and hypotension with a rising lactate and no infection at all.

The practical rule is that a patient not responding to appropriate antimicrobial therapy and source control within a reasonable interval has either an inadequately treated infection, an uncontrolled source, or a different diagnosis, and the third possibility must be actively considered rather than reached by exhaustion.

18.2 Empiric Therapy: The Source-and-Host Matrix

18.2.1 The questions that determine the prescription

Empiric prescribing done well is a structured judgement rather than a reflex, and seven questions determine the answer.

Where is the infection? The likely site determines the likely organisms and the required tissue penetration. If the site cannot be identified, that is itself important information, and broad empiric therapy in an unidentified source should be accompanied by an active search rather than substituting for one.

Who is the host? Neutropenia, transplantation, asplenia, corticosteroid and biologic therapy, cirrhosis, and advanced age all change the organism spectrum and the presentation. Chapter 11, section 11.3.5, developed this.

Where was it acquired? Community, healthcare-associated, or hospital-acquired, with the last two carrying substantially higher probability of resistant organisms.

What are the local resistance patterns? The institutional antibiogram, not a textbook, should determine empiric spectrum, and this varies markedly between institutions and between units within an institution.

What has this patient grown before? Prior cultures and known colonisation with resistant organisms are among the strongest predictors of the current organism and are frequently available in the record and not consulted.

Is there prosthetic material or a device? Biofilm-associated infection has different organisms, different antimicrobial requirements, and frequently requires removal.

How severe is the illness? Severity justifies broader initial cover, on the reasoning that the cost of an initially inadequate regimen is higher in a patient with shock than in a stable patient in whom the regimen can be adjusted tomorrow.

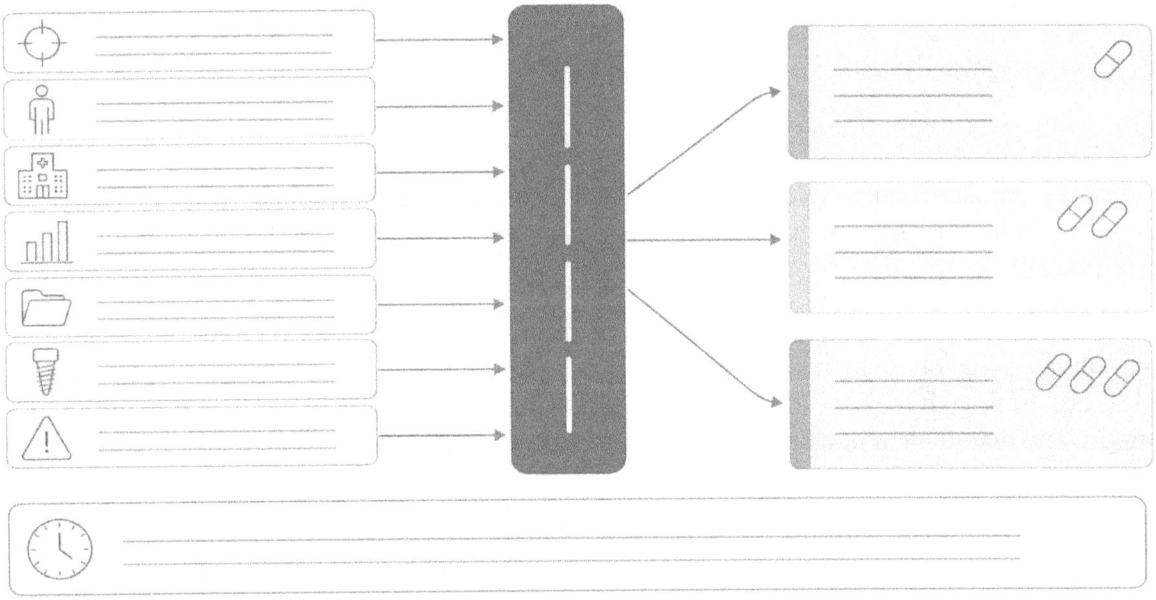

18.2.2 Choosing well within the spectrum

Take cultures before antimicrobials wherever this does not delay treatment, since a single dose substantially reduces yield, and the yield determines whether de-escalation will be possible. In septic shock this takes two minutes and should not be omitted.

Tissue penetration matters and is frequently ignored. Several sites are poorly penetrated by otherwise appropriate agents, including the central nervous system, bone, the prostate, the vitreous, and the interior of an abscess or a biofilm. An agent with excellent activity against the organism in vitro is useless if it does not reach it.

Pharmacokinetic and pharmacodynamic principles determine dosing strategy. Beta-lactam efficacy depends on the time that concentrations exceed the inhibitory concentration, which is the rationale for extended or continuous infusion in severe infection. Aminoglycoside efficacy depends on peak concentration, which is the rationale for once-daily dosing. Glycopeptide and fluoroquinolone efficacy depends on the ratio of total exposure to the inhibitory concentration.

Dosing in critical illness is frequently inadequate. Increased volume of distribution from fluid resuscitation and capillary leak lowers concentrations, and augmented renal clearance in younger patients with sepsis raises elimination. **Underdosing an antimicrobial in a septic patient because the creatinine is elevated is a specific and serious error**, as Chapter 16, section 16.4.4, argued.

Assess the allergy history properly. A large majority of patients labelled penicillin allergic are not, and the label leads to inferior alternative agents and worse outcomes. Chapter 11, section 11.7.3, addressed delabelling.

Combination therapy is justified for broadening spectrum in severe infection with uncertain organism, and is not justified as routine synergy for most infections. It should be de-escalated once the organism is known.

18.3 Pneumonia: Community-Acquired, Hospital-Acquired, and Aspiration

18.3.1 Community-acquired pneumonia

Diagnosis requires compatible symptoms and signs with radiographic infiltrate. The clinical diagnosis without imaging is unreliable, and radiographic changes may lag in dehydration and in early illness.

Severity assessment determines the site of care and the extent of investigation. Validated scores combining confusion, urea, respiratory rate, blood pressure, and age, or the more detailed severity index, are used, with the essential caveat that these predict mortality rather than the need for organ support, and that clinical judgement must override a reassuring score in a patient who looks unwell or has poor social support.

Microbiological investigation should be proportionate. In patients with mild disease managed as outpatients, routine investigation is not required. In severe disease, blood cultures, sputum culture, urinary antigen testing for pneumococcus and legionella, and respiratory viral testing are appropriate, and molecular respiratory panels are increasingly used.

Empiric therapy follows local guidance, generally a beta-lactam with or without a macrolide, or a respiratory fluoroquinolone, with the choice influenced by severity, comorbidity, recent antimicrobial exposure, and local resistance.

Corticosteroids in severe community-acquired pneumonia are a genuine change in practice. A randomised trial of hydrocortisone in patients with severe community-acquired pneumonia demonstrated a mortality reduction, and current guidance recommends their use in severe disease. Earlier trials were less clear, and the benefit appears concentrated in more severe illness. They should not be used routinely in non-severe pneumonia, and caution applies in influenza and in undiagnosed fungal infection.

Duration. Five days is adequate for most patients who have achieved clinical stability, and this is supported by strong randomised evidence. Longer courses do not improve outcomes.

Non-resolving pneumonia requires reconsideration rather than escalation. Ask whether the diagnosis is wrong, considering pulmonary embolism, heart failure, malignancy with obstruction, organising pneumonia, and vasculitis; whether there is a complication, principally empyema or abscess; whether the organism is resistant or unusual, including tuberculosis and fungal infection; and whether there is a host factor not previously recognised. Chapter 2, section 2.4.4, identified failure to improve as the most underused diagnostic signal.

Empyema requires drainage and is the commonest reason for failure to respond in a patient with a parapneumonic effusion. Sampling the fluid, rather than observing it, is the action that identifies it.

Follow-up imaging should be arranged in patients at risk of underlying malignancy, since a proportion of pneumonias are the presenting feature of lung cancer, and this is a common failure of the discharge process described in Chapter 3.

18.3.2 Hospital-acquired and ventilator-associated pneumonia

Definition rests on onset after a defined interval following admission, conventionally 48 hours, distinguishing it from community-acquired disease incubating on arrival.

Organisms are more likely to include Gram-negative bacilli including *Pseudomonas*, and resistant Gram-positive organisms, though the local antibiogram should determine empiric cover rather than a generic assumption.

Diagnosis is difficult and overdiagnosed. New infiltrates in a ventilated or hospitalised patient have many causes including atelectasis, pulmonary oedema, aspiration pneumonitis, and acute respiratory distress syndrome, and tracheal aspirate cultures grow colonising organisms routinely. Chapter 11, section 11.7.2, warned against treating the culture rather than the patient.

Duration. Seven days is adequate for most patients including those with ventilator-associated pneumonia, and this is supported by randomised evidence.

De-escalate as soon as culture results permit, which is the subject of section 18.8.

18.3.3 Aspiration

The essential distinction is between pneumonitis and pneumonia.

Aspiration pneumonitis is chemical injury from gastric contents, occurring within hours, producing fever, hypoxia, and infiltrates, and frequently resolving without antimicrobial therapy. Observation for the first day or so in a stable patient is a defensible approach, with antimicrobials started if the clinical picture does not improve or if features of infection develop.

Aspiration pneumonia is infection following aspiration of oropharyngeal contents, developing over days.

Anaerobic coverage is no longer routinely required for most aspiration pneumonia. The organisms are predominantly the same as in community-acquired pneumonia together with oral flora, and current guidance has moved away from mandatory anaerobic cover, which is reserved for lung abscess, necrotising pneumonia, and empyema.

The important intervention is preventive. Identify dysphagia with formal swallow assessment; attend to oral hygiene, which reduces pneumonia in several studies; position the patient upright; review sedating and anticholinergic medication; and recognise that gastrostomy feeding does not prevent aspiration pneumonia, since the aspirated material is frequently oropharyngeal secretions rather than food. Chapter 12, section 12.7.4, addressed the tube feeding decision in advanced dementia.

18.3.4 Viral respiratory infection

Viral pathogens account for a substantial proportion of lower respiratory tract infection in adults, and the practical questions for a hospitalist are whether a specific antiviral is indicated, whether antibacterial therapy can be withheld or stopped, and what infection control is required.

Test where the result would change management, which includes influenza during seasonal circulation, where antiviral therapy is indicated and is most effective when started early, and other pathogens where isolation, cohorting, or specific therapy would follow. Multiplex molecular panels return quickly and can support antibacterial de-escalation.

Bacterial coinfection at presentation is less common than antibacterial prescribing implies, and secondary bacterial infection characteristically develops later in the course after initial improvement. A patient with a positive viral test, a compatible clinical picture, and an unremarkable inflammatory response is a candidate for stopping antibacterials, which is a specific and underused application of section 18.8.2.

Do not withhold antibacterial therapy in a severely ill patient on the basis of a positive viral test, since coinfection occurs and the consequences of missing it are serious. The judgement rests on severity and on the overall picture rather than on the test alone.

Infection control requires prompt isolation according to the pathogen and local policy, which is a clinical action rather than an administrative one, since delayed isolation produces ward outbreaks that consume far more resource than the original case.

18.4 Skin, Soft Tissue, and Necrotising Infections

18.4.1 Cellulitis is overdiagnosed

A substantial proportion of patients admitted with a diagnosis of lower limb cellulitis do not have it, and the consequences are unnecessary antimicrobial exposure, missed alternative diagnoses, and prolonged admission.

The mimics, collectively termed pseudocellulitis:

Venous stasis dermatitis, which is the commonest. It is typically bilateral, chronic with acute exacerbations, associated with venous insufficiency and haemosiderin staining, itchy rather than painful, and afebrile.

Lipodermatosclerosis, producing induration and an inverted champagne bottle appearance.

Deep vein thrombosis, which produces unilateral swelling, warmth, and tenderness.

Acute gout and other crystal arthropathy, with periarticular erythema.

Contact dermatitis, in the distribution of the applied substance.

Lymphoedema with acute inflammation.

The single most useful discriminator is bilaterality. Bilateral lower limb cellulitis is very rare, and a patient with symmetrical bilateral erythema almost certainly has something else. Systematic assessment tools combining asymmetry, leucocytosis, tachycardia, and age have been developed to support this judgement.

Other features favouring true cellulitis: unilateral distribution, an identifiable portal of entry such as interdigital tinea, a wound, or an ulcer, an advancing margin, systemic features, and a raised inflammatory response.

18.4.2 Managing cellulitis

Classify by the presence of purulence. Non-purulent cellulitis is predominantly streptococcal and treated accordingly. Purulent infection, meaning abscess or infection with drainable pus, requires **incision and drainage as the primary treatment**, with antimicrobial therapy covering staphylococci including resistant strains where locally prevalent.

Practical measures that improve outcomes and are frequently omitted: elevate the affected limb; mark the margin of erythema with a pen and date it, which converts a subjective impression of progression into an observation; treat the portal of entry, particularly interdigital fungal infection, which prevents recurrence; and manage oedema, which is the principal risk factor for recurrence.

Anticipate initial worsening. Erythema frequently extends during the first day of effective treatment because of inflammatory response to bacterial killing, and this should not prompt escalation in a patient who is otherwise improving.

Duration is short, with five to six days adequate for uncomplicated infection.

18.4.3 Necrotising soft tissue infection

Chapter 8, section 8.2.4, addressed this in the postoperative context and the features are restated because the diagnosis is time-critical wherever it occurs.

Features prompting immediate surgical involvement: pain disproportionate to the visible findings, which is the earliest and most important; rapid progression over hours; systemic toxicity out of proportion to the local appearance; skin changes including bullae, dusky discolouration, and anaesthesia over the affected area; crepitus; and thin, watery, malodorous discharge rather than frank pus.

Scoring systems have inadequate sensitivity to exclude the diagnosis and should not be used to reassure. **Imaging should not delay surgical exploration** where suspicion is high; the diagnosis is made in theatre.

Management is emergency surgical debridement, which is the definitive treatment and must be repeated as required; broad-spectrum antimicrobial therapy with an agent that suppresses toxin production added for suspected streptococcal or clostridial infection; and aggressive resuscitation. Immunoglobulin is used in some centres for severe streptococcal disease.

18.4.4 Diabetic foot infection

Assess three things separately: the infection, the vascular supply, and the presence of bone involvement.

Grade the infection using a structured system, since the grade determines whether outpatient oral therapy or admission with parenteral therapy is appropriate.

Assess perfusion, since an ischaemic foot will not heal regardless of antimicrobial therapy and requires vascular assessment.

Assess for osteomyelitis, which changes the duration and frequently the management. A probe reaching bone through an ulcer substantially raises the probability, and magnetic resonance imaging is the imaging modality of choice. Bone biopsy provides the microbiological diagnosis where feasible.

Manage with a multidisciplinary team including diabetology, vascular surgery, podiatry, orthopaedics, and microbiology, since outcomes are demonstrably better with this model.

Offloading is as important as antimicrobial therapy and is frequently neglected in inpatients.

18.4.5 Two further soft tissue problems on the ward

Infected pressure injury. All pressure ulcers are colonised, and swab culture from the surface reflects colonisation rather than infection, which is why the practice of swabbing and treating produces repeated courses without benefit, as Chapter 11, section 11.7.2, described. **Infection is a clinical diagnosis**, indicated by advancing erythema, increasing pain, purulence, systemic features, or failure to heal despite adequate pressure relief and wound care. Where infection is present, deep tissue or bone sampling rather than surface swabbing provides the microbiology, and osteomyelitis should be considered in deep sacral and heel ulcers. Chapter 4, section 4.4.2, addressed prevention, which remains the main intervention.

Bite wounds, both human and animal, carry a distinctive polymicrobial flora including organisms not covered by many standard regimens, and require irrigation, consideration of primary closure, assessment of tendon and joint involvement particularly in hand injuries which have a high complication rate, and consideration of tetanus and rabies prophylaxis according to the exposure and local epidemiology.

18.5 Urinary Tract Infection Against Asymptomatic Bacteriuria

18.5.1 The distinction

Asymptomatic bacteriuria is the presence of bacteria in the urine without attributable urinary symptoms. It is common, increasing with age, near-universal in patients with long-term catheters, and, in almost all populations, it should be neither screened for nor treated.

The exceptions in which treatment is indicated are pregnancy and before urological procedures involving mucosal trauma. That is the complete list for practical purposes.

Treating asymptomatic bacteriuria does not prevent symptomatic infection and does cause harm: adverse drug effects, *Clostridioides difficile*, resistance, and, importantly, diagnostic anchoring that prevents the actual problem from being found.

18.5.2 The delirium trap

This deserves its own treatment because it is the commonest specific manifestation of the above and one of the commonest diagnostic errors in hospital medicine.

An older patient presents with confusion. A urine sample is sent, grows an organism, and the confusion is attributed to a urinary tract infection. Antimicrobials are started, and the search for the actual cause stops.

The reasoning is faulty because bacteriuria is highly prevalent in this population, so its presence carries almost no diagnostic information in a patient without urinary symptoms. Chapter 2, section 2.3.6, described base rate neglect; this is its most common clinical instance.

The correct approach is the systematic delirium assessment of Chapter 10, section 10.1.4, in which urinary infection is one possibility among many and is diagnosed only when urinary symptoms or signs are present, or when no other cause is found and the patient has systemic features of infection with no alternative source.

In a patient who cannot report symptoms, the diagnosis is genuinely difficult, and the correct response is to look harder for alternatives rather than to default to the urine. Fever with no other source, suprapubic or flank tenderness, and haemodynamic disturbance without another explanation are the features that support the diagnosis.

Pyuria does not establish infection. It is present in most catheterised patients and in many older patients with bacteriuria, and its absence is more useful than its presence, since a genuinely negative urinalysis makes urinary infection unlikely.

18.5.3 Diagnosing and treating urinary tract infection

Diagnosis requires symptoms: dysuria, frequency, urgency, suprapubic pain, new or worsening incontinence, flank pain or costovertebral angle tenderness, or fever without an alternative source.

Send urine culture in complicated infection, in men, in pyelonephritis, in healthcare-associated infection, and in treatment failure. Routine culture in uncomplicated cystitis in a young woman is not required.

Uncomplicated cystitis is treated with a short course of a narrow-spectrum agent selected by local resistance, with three to five days sufficient depending on the agent.

Pyelonephritis requires a longer course, with duration depending on the agent and the response, and requires imaging if the patient has not improved within a couple of days, to identify obstruction, abscess, or emphysematous change.

Obstruction with infection is a urological emergency requiring drainage, and antimicrobial therapy alone will not resolve it. This is the source control principle again.

Infection in men generally involves the prostate and requires an agent with prostatic penetration and a longer course.

Catheter-associated infection requires symptoms, not simply a positive culture. Where the catheter has been in place for a prolonged period and infection is diagnosed, replacing it improves outcomes. And the most effective intervention remains removing the catheter, as Chapter 4, section 4.4.4, argued.

Candiduria almost always represents colonisation and rarely requires treatment; removing or changing the catheter frequently resolves it.

18.5.4 Sepsis of urinary origin

Urinary tract infection is among the commonest sources of sepsis in hospitalised patients, and two features distinguish its management.

Obstruction converts a treatable infection into a surgical emergency. A patient with pyelonephritis and an obstructed system will not respond to antimicrobial therapy, deteriorates rapidly, and requires urgent decompression by ureteric stent or percutaneous nephrostomy. **Any patient with urinary sepsis who is not improving, or who is severely unwell at presentation, requires urgent imaging to exclude obstruction**, and urology should be involved at the point the possibility arises rather than after failure.

Emphysematous pyelonephritis, characterised by gas within the renal parenchyma, occurs predominantly in patients with diabetes, carries high mortality, and is diagnosed on cross-sectional imaging. Management combines antimicrobial therapy, drainage, and, in some cases, nephrectomy.

Renal and perinephric abscess should be considered in a patient with persistent fever despite appropriate therapy, and requires drainage.

A practical note on organism prediction. In a patient with recurrent urinary infection, prior instrumentation, or long-term catheterisation, the organism is frequently predictable from previous cultures, and reviewing those results before prescribing empirically is among the highest-yield actions available, as section 18.2.1 argued.

18.6 Endocarditis, Bacteraemia, and the Catheter Question

18.6.1 Interpreting a positive blood culture

Distinguish contamination from true bacteraemia using the organism identity, the number of culture sets positive, the time to positivity, and the clinical context. A common skin organism in one of several sets, in a patient without prosthetic material or a vascular device and without clinical sepsis, is usually contamination. The same organism in multiple sets, or in a patient with a device or prosthesis, is not.

Certain organisms are never dismissed as contaminants, notably *Staphylococcus aureus*, *Streptococcus* species associated with endocarditis, enterococci in the appropriate context, and *Candida*.

18.6.2 *Staphylococcus aureus* bacteraemia

This deserves separate treatment because it is common, carries substantial mortality, and has a defined set of management obligations that are frequently incompletely delivered.

Every episode requires:

Repeat blood cultures to document clearance, typically at 48 to 96 hours, since persistent bacteraemia defines complicated infection and changes duration and management.

Echocardiography, with transoesophageal imaging preferred in most patients because transthoracic imaging has inadequate sensitivity for endocarditis, particularly with prosthetic material.

Identification and removal of the source, including removal of infected vascular catheters and drainage of collections.

A search for metastatic foci, since seeding to bone, joints, the spine, the epidural space, and elsewhere is common and frequently silent.

Infectious diseases consultation, which has been repeatedly associated with improved adherence to these standards and with reduced mortality, and which should be routine rather than reserved for difficult cases.

Appropriate duration, with a minimum period of parenteral therapy for uncomplicated infection and a substantially longer course for complicated infection, defined by persistent bacteraemia, endocarditis, metastatic focus, prosthetic material, or delayed clinical response.

18.6.3 Infective endocarditis

Diagnosis uses established criteria combining microbiological, imaging, and clinical elements, recently updated to incorporate newer imaging modalities including cardiac computed tomography and nuclear imaging, particularly valuable in prosthetic valve infection.

Blood cultures should be taken as multiple sets from separate sites before antimicrobial therapy, since the diagnosis depends on them and a single dose of antimicrobial can render them negative for days.

Imaging begins with transthoracic echocardiography and proceeds to transoesophageal imaging, which has substantially better sensitivity for vegetations, abscess, and prosthetic involvement. A negative transthoracic study does not exclude the diagnosis.

Indications for surgery, which should be assessed early and by a multidisciplinary endocarditis team rather than after failure of medical therapy: heart failure from valvular dysfunction, which is the commonest indication; uncontrolled infection including abscess, fistula, and persistent bacteraemia despite appropriate therapy; and prevention of embolism in patients with large vegetations, particularly after an embolic event.

Partial oral therapy after an initial period of parenteral treatment has been shown to be non-inferior in stabilised left-sided endocarditis in randomised evaluation, which has changed practice in selected patients managed by specialist teams.

18.6.4 The catheter question

When must a vascular catheter be removed? This is among the most frequent practical questions in inpatient infection management.

Remove without attempting salvage in: infection with *Staphylococcus aureus*, *Candida*, *Pseudomonas*, or mycobacteria; tunnel infection or port pocket infection; septic thrombophlebitis; endocarditis; persistent bacteraemia despite appropriate therapy; and haemodynamic instability attributable to the line infection.

Salvage may be attempted in selected patients with limited access options and infection with less virulent organisms such as coagulase-negative staphylococci, using systemic therapy with antimicrobial lock therapy, and with a defined plan for removal if the patient does not respond.

Differential time to positivity, comparing cultures drawn simultaneously from the catheter and peripherally, supports a catheter source when the catheter culture turns positive substantially earlier.

A short-term peripheral or central catheter in a patient with unexplained bacteraemia should generally be removed rather than investigated, since it is easily replaced.

18.6.5 Two other bloodstream infections worth specific attention

Candidaemia carries high mortality and has a defined management set that parallels that of *Staphylococcus aureus* bacteraemia. It requires prompt initiation of appropriate antifungal therapy, **removal of vascular catheters** wherever feasible, repeat cultures to document clearance, **dilated ophthalmological examination** to identify endophthalmitis which is frequently asymptomatic and changes therapy, echocardiography where endocarditis is plausible, and infectious diseases involvement. Duration is counted from the first negative culture rather than from the start of therapy.

Enterococcal bacteraemia requires identification to species level and susceptibility testing, since management differs substantially, and warrants consideration of endocarditis, particularly with *Enterococcus faecalis*, community acquisition, and no identified alternative source.

In both, and in *Staphylococcus aureus* bacteraemia, the common error is treating the blood culture rather than the patient: giving a course of therapy without identifying the source, without documenting clearance, and without excluding endovascular or metastatic involvement.

18.7 Bone, Joint, and Prosthetic Infections

18.7.1 Vertebral osteomyelitis and discitis

Presentation is back pain, frequently without fever, with a raised inflammatory response, and with a subacute course over weeks. It is missed because back pain is common and the systemic features are muted.

Suspect it in a patient with new focal spinal pain and a raised inflammatory response, particularly with a history of bacteraemia, injecting drug use, a vascular catheter, recent spinal instrumentation, or immunosuppression. Chapter 16, section 16.6.3, noted the elevated risk in dialysis patients.

Investigate with magnetic resonance imaging of the whole spine, which is the imaging modality of choice, and with blood cultures, which are positive in a substantial proportion and may obviate biopsy.

Obtain a microbiological diagnosis before starting antimicrobials wherever the patient is stable, by blood culture or by image-guided biopsy, because treating empirically without an organism commits the patient to a prolonged broad course and to repeated uncertainty.

Epidural abscess is the complication that must not be missed. New neurological deficit, radicular symptoms, or bladder dysfunction in a patient with spinal infection requires urgent imaging and neurosurgical involvement, and the outcome depends on the deficit at the time of decompression, exactly as in the cord compression discussed in Chapter 17.

Duration is prolonged, conventionally around six weeks, and randomised evidence has shown that **oral therapy is non-inferior to intravenous therapy** for bone and joint infection in appropriately selected patients, which has substantially changed practice and reduced line-associated harm.

18.7.2 Septic arthritis

Aspirate the joint before giving antimicrobials. This is the single most important rule, because the diagnosis depends on synovial fluid analysis and culture and because a dose of antimicrobial substantially reduces yield.

Synovial fluid is sent for cell count and differential, Gram stain, culture, and crystal examination. A high leucocyte count with neutrophil predominance supports infection, and thresholds are guides rather than absolutes.

Crystals and infection coexist, and the presence of crystals does not exclude septic arthritis. Chapter 11, section 11.5.4, made this point from the fever perspective, and it bears repeating because it causes real harm in both directions.

Management is drainage, which may be by repeated aspiration, arthroscopic washout, or open procedure, together with antimicrobial therapy. Orthopaedic involvement should be immediate.

Gonococcal arthritis presents differently, with migratory polyarthralgia, tenosynovitis, and skin lesions, and requires specific testing.

18.7.3 Prosthetic joint infection

Classification by time from implantation informs the likely organism and the management strategy: early infection presenting within the first weeks, typically with virulent organisms; delayed infection over months, typically with low-virulence organisms such as coagulase-negative staphylococci and *Cutibacterium*; and late infection, usually haematogenous.

Diagnosis rests on clinical features, inflammatory markers, joint aspiration with cell count and culture, and, at revision, multiple periprosthetic tissue samples. **Do not aspirate through cellulitic skin**, and send multiple samples rather than a swab, which is inadequate.

Management strategies, decided by a specialist multidisciplinary team: debridement with implant retention and exchange of modular components, which is appropriate in early infection with a stable prosthesis and a susceptible organism; single-stage revision; and two-stage revision, which has the highest success rate in difficult cases.

Rifampicin has particular activity against staphylococcal biofilm and is used in combination, never as monotherapy because of rapid resistance, in patients with retained implants.

Suppressive therapy is used where surgery is not feasible.

A hospitalist encountering a patient with a prosthetic joint and bacteraemia should recognise the risk of seeding and involve orthopaedics, since haematogenous prosthetic infection is a recognised complication of any bacteraemia and particularly of *Staphylococcus aureus*.

18.8 Antimicrobial Resistance, De-escalation, and Duration Evidence

18.8.1 The stewardship framework

Chapter 11, section 11.7, made the case for restraint. This section addresses the operational elements.

Institutional interventions with evidence include prospective audit with feedback, in which prescriptions are reviewed and recommendations made to the prescriber; formulary restriction with preauthorisation for defined agents; institution-specific guidelines embedded in order sets, which work through defaults as Chapter 4, section 4.7.3, described; rapid diagnostic testing linked to stewardship intervention; and allergy delabelling programmes.

The measurement conventionally uses days of therapy per patient-days as the denominator-adjusted metric, alongside resistance rates and *Clostridioides difficile* incidence as balancing measures, in the sense of Chapter 4, section 4.2.1.

18.8.2 De-escalation

The antimicrobial timeout at approximately 48 to 72 hours is the single most valuable individual practice, as Chapter 11, section 11.7.3, described. Four questions: is there still evidence of infection, can the spectrum be narrowed, can the route be changed to oral, and when will treatment stop.

Narrowing is safe. Observational evidence does not support the concern that de-escalation worsens outcomes, and continuing broad-spectrum therapy once susceptibilities are known has no justification.

Stopping is also an option. Where the cultures are negative, the clinical course does not support bacterial infection, and an alternative diagnosis has emerged, stopping antimicrobials entirely is the correct action and requires the same deliberate decision as continuing.

Procalcitonin has been used to guide discontinuation, with evidence that protocols incorporating it can safely shorten duration in respiratory infection and sepsis. It should not be used to withhold initial therapy in a severely ill patient, and its value lies in supporting cessation rather than in diagnosis.

18.8.3 Intravenous to oral switch

Many agents have excellent oral bioavailability, and switching in a patient who is clinically improving, haemodynamically stable, and absorbing enterally removes catheter-associated risk, reduces cost, and frequently permits earlier discharge.

Criteria typically include clinical improvement, resolving fever, falling inflammatory markers, a functioning gastrointestinal tract, and an infection without a deep-seated focus requiring high tissue concentrations.

The exceptions where prolonged parenteral therapy remains standard are narrowing, and section 18.7.1 described the evidence that oral therapy is non-inferior even in bone and joint infection.

Outpatient parenteral antimicrobial therapy is appropriate where parenteral therapy is genuinely required and the patient is otherwise fit for discharge, and requires a defined service with monitoring arrangements.

18.8.4 Duration: the consistent direction of the evidence

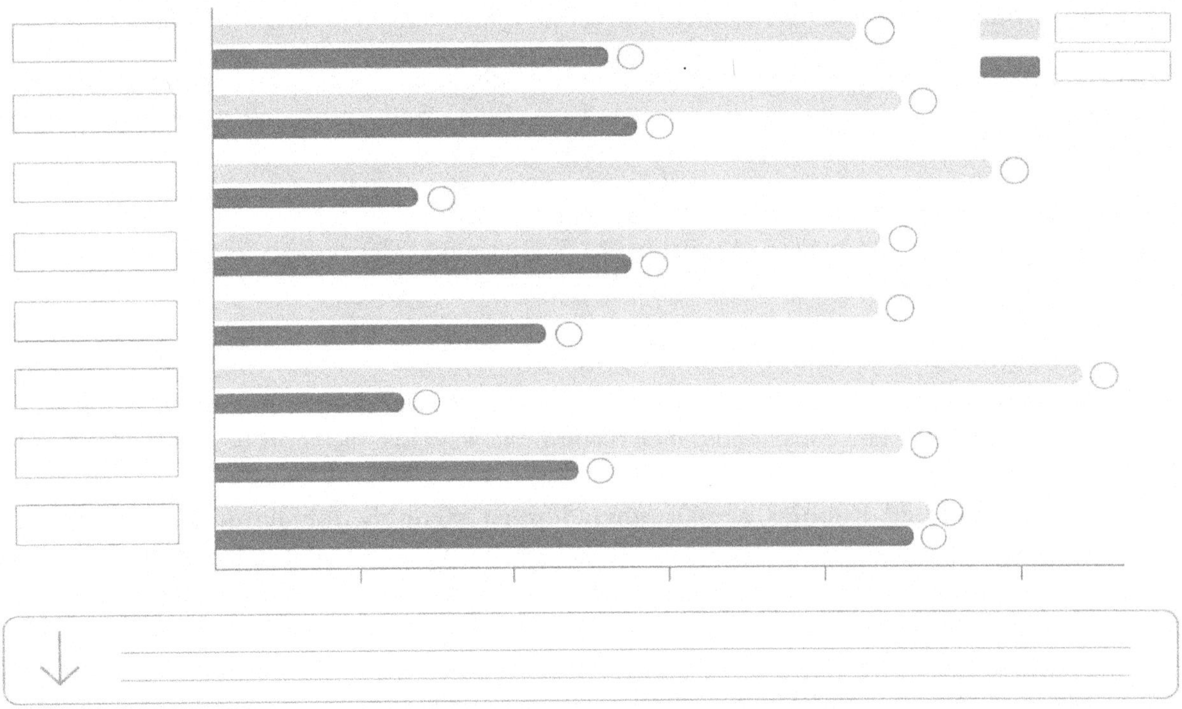

The trials of the past two decades have addressed duration systematically, and the direction has been consistent. Shorter courses have proved non-inferior in community-acquired pneumonia, hospital-acquired and ventilator-associated pneumonia, uncomplicated Gram-negative bacteraemia, pyelonephritis, intra-abdominal infection after adequate source control, cellulitis, and uncomplicated cystitis.

The general principle is that duration should be counted from the point of adequate source control rather than from the first dose, that clinical response should inform the decision, and that a course extended because the patient still has a catheter, or still has an abnormal chest radiograph, or because the prescriber is uneasy, is not justified.

Genuine exceptions requiring prolonged therapy include endovascular infection including endocarditis, bone and joint infection, prosthetic material infection, undrained collections, central nervous system infection, and infection in profoundly immunosuppressed hosts.

Specific durations should be taken from current guidance rather than from memory or from this book, since they continue to be revised.

18.8.5 Resistant organisms

Know the organisms that matter locally, which will include some combination of methicillin-resistant *Staphylococcus aureus*, vancomycin-resistant enterococci, extended-spectrum beta-lactamase and AmpC-producing Enterobacterales, carbapenemase producers, multidrug-resistant *Pseudomonas* and *Acinetobacter*, and increasingly *Candida auris*.

Screening and isolation policies are institution-specific and should be followed, recognising that contact precautions have costs including reduced clinical contact and adverse effects on patient experience, which is a balancing consideration rather than a reason to abandon them.

Where a resistant organism is identified, involve infectious diseases and microbiology early, since newer agents have specific indications and the choice frequently requires expertise beyond general prescribing.

The individual contribution to resistance is real but diffuse, which is precisely why it fails to influence prescribing, as Chapter 11, section 11.7.1, argued. The remedy is systems that make restraint the default rather than an act of individual virtue.

Chapter Summary

- **Sepsis is organ dysfunction from a dysregulated response to infection.** No screening score is reliable, and current guidance recommends against the short bedside score as a sole screening tool.
- **Time-mandated bundles are supported most strongly for septic shock and most weakly for undifferentiated possible sepsis.** In shock, treat immediately. In a stable patient with several possibilities, use the available window to establish the diagnosis and document the reasoning.
- **Empiric therapy follows from source, host, acquisition setting, local resistance, prior cultures, devices, and severity.** Take cultures first where this does not delay treatment, and **do not underdose an antimicrobial in a septic patient because the creatinine is elevated**.
- **Corticosteroids reduce mortality in severe community-acquired pneumonia.** Five days is adequate for most pneumonia, and failure to resolve requires reconsideration of the diagnosis rather than escalation of the antibiotic.
- **Aspiration pneumonitis is not pneumonia**, and routine anaerobic cover is no longer required for most aspiration pneumonia.
- **Bilateral lower limb cellulitis is very rare.** Mark the margin, elevate the limb, treat the portal of entry, and expect initial extension.

- **Do not treat asymptomatic bacteriuria**, and do not attribute delirium to a positive urine culture in a patient without urinary symptoms. Pyuria does not establish infection.
- ***Staphylococcus aureus* bacteraemia carries a defined set of obligations**: repeat cultures, echocardiography, source removal, a search for metastatic foci, infectious diseases consultation, and appropriate duration.
- **Aspirate a joint before giving antimicrobials**, obtain a microbiological diagnosis in vertebral osteomyelitis before treating, and remember that crystals and infection coexist.
- **Oral therapy is non-inferior to intravenous therapy in bone and joint infection**, and partial oral therapy is non-inferior in stabilised left-sided endocarditis.
- **The duration evidence points consistently toward shorter courses**, and the burden of justification now falls on the longer one.

Review Questions

1. A patient has a temperature of 38.6 degrees Celsius, a heart rate of 112, a normal blood pressure, and no identified source. The sepsis pathway requires antimicrobials within one hour. State your approach, the evidence you would cite, and what you would document.
2. A 79-year-old is admitted with confusion. A urine culture grows *Escherichia coli*. She has no urinary symptoms and no fever. Explain the reasoning error being made if this is treated as the diagnosis, and set out what you would do instead.
3. A blood culture from a patient with a peripherally inserted central catheter grows *Staphylococcus aureus*. List the six actions this obliges, and state which single one is most often omitted.
4. A patient with cellulitis of both lower legs, no fever, normal inflammatory markers, and chronic skin changes has been started on intravenous antibiotics. State your assessment, your differential, and your plan.
5. A patient with community-acquired pneumonia has completed five days of therapy, feels well, is afebrile, but has a persistent radiographic infiltrate. The team proposes a further week of antibiotics. State your position and your reasoning.

CHAPTER 19: Special Populations in the Hospital

Learning Objectives

After studying this chapter, the reader should be able to:

1. Apply a structured framework to the care of the older inpatient, including frailty assessment, deprescribing, and the prevention of hospital-associated disability.
2. Manage a pregnant patient on a medical service, accounting for altered physiology, shifted reference ranges, and the risks of both treatment and undertreatment.
3. Treat withdrawal states adequately, initiate medication for opioid use disorder in hospital, and apply harm reduction.
4. Care for patients with psychiatric comorbidity, manage agitation without restraint where possible, and respond appropriately to suicidal ideation in an inpatient.
5. Adapt clinical care to the patient with obesity, including drug dosing, equipment, and the specific needs of the post-bariatric patient.
6. Identify how structural factors shape inpatient outcomes, and adapt care for patients experiencing homelessness.
7. Use professional interpretation correctly and recognise language access as a patient safety issue.

Chapter Overview

Part V turns from organ systems to people. The populations in this chapter are not rare; between them they account for the majority of medical inpatients. What they share is that **standard care, delivered competently, produces worse outcomes for them than for other patients**, and the reasons are identifiable and largely correctable.

Four mechanisms recur throughout the chapter.

Physiological difference is not accounted for. Reference ranges, drug doses, and equipment calibrated to a notional average patient are wrong for the pregnant patient, the frail older patient, and the patient with obesity, and the errors are systematic rather than random.

Presentation is atypical and is read as absence of disease. The older adult without fever, the patient with serious mental illness whose physical symptom is attributed to their psychiatric diagnosis, and the patient who cannot describe their symptoms in the clinician's language are all at risk of the same failure.

Assumptions embedded in the plan do not hold. Chapter 3, section 3.7.1, established this for discharge, and it applies more broadly: a plan requiring refrigeration, literacy, transport, a stable address, or an intact cognitive apparatus fails when those are absent, and the failure is attributed to the patient.

Stigma changes clinical decisions measurably. This is not a matter of attitude but of documented differences in analgesia, in diagnostic effort, and in escalation. Chapter 1, section 1.7.2, described the evidence on documentation language, and it recurs in sections 19.3, 19.5, and 19.6.

19.1 The Older Adult: Frailty, Polypharmacy, Deprescribing, and the 4Ms Framework

19.1.1 What changes with age

The clinically relevant change is **reduced homeostatic reserve**: the capacity to respond to a stressor and return to baseline. Organ function at rest may be adequate while the capacity to increase it is not, which is why an older person may be entirely well until an apparently minor insult produces disproportionate decompensation.

Pharmacological changes are substantial and are the source of much preventable harm. Renal clearance falls, frequently without a rise in creatinine because muscle mass has fallen in parallel, as Chapter 16, section 16.1.2, described. Body composition shifts toward fat and away from water, which increases the volume of distribution of lipophilic drugs and prolongs their effect while reducing it for hydrophilic ones. Hepatic first-pass metabolism declines. And central nervous system sensitivity increases, so that a dose of a sedative or an anticholinergic that would be unremarkable in a younger patient produces delirium.

Presentation is altered. Fever is blunted, as Chapter 11, section 11.1.3, described. Pain may be less severe or absent in myocardial infarction and in abdominal catastrophe, as Chapter 9, section 9.3.1, described. And the presenting complaint is frequently a **geriatric syndrome** rather than an organ-specific symptom: falls, confusion, immobility, incontinence, or simply not coping.

The critical inference is that these syndromes are presentations of acute illness and require the same diagnostic effort as chest pain. Chapter 9, section 9.6.2, developed this for generalised weakness.

19.1.2 Frailty rather than age

Chronological age is a poor guide to physiological reserve and a poor basis for clinical decisions, and using it as one is both inaccurate and a form of discrimination.

Frailty is the appropriate measure, and Chapter 5, section 5.3.4, described the principal instruments. A brief judgement-based ordinal scale is practical for acute care, requires no equipment, and predicts mortality, length of stay, functional decline, institutionalisation, and delirium.

Assess and record frailty in every older inpatient, because it changes almost every subsequent decision: the risk of intervention, the likely benefit of preventive therapy, the appropriate intensity of investigation, the discharge destination, and the framing of goals-of-care conversations.

Comprehensive geriatric assessment, meaning a multidimensional multidisciplinary assessment of medical, functional, cognitive, psychological, and social domains with a coordinated plan, is the intervention with the best evidence in this population. Systematic review has found that older inpatients receiving it are more likely to be alive and living at home subsequently. Where a geriatric service exists, involve it; where it does not, the domains can still be assessed.

19.1.3 The 4Ms framework

A practical structure for the daily care of an older inpatient organises attention around four domains, which have the advantage of being memorable and of covering most of what matters.

What Matters. The patient's own goals, preferences, and priorities, including what outcomes they would accept and what they would not. This is placed first deliberately, because it determines whether the other three are being pursued in the right direction. Chapter 20 develops the conversation.

Medication. Whether each drug is necessary, whether the dose is appropriate for renal function and body composition, whether any drug is causing the presenting problem, and whether high-risk agents can be stopped. Section 19.1.4 develops this.

Mentation. Delirium prevention and detection, as in Chapter 10, section 10.1.5, together with assessment for underlying cognitive impairment and for depression, which is common and under-recognised.

Mobility. Maintaining and restoring the ability to move, addressed in section 19.1.5.

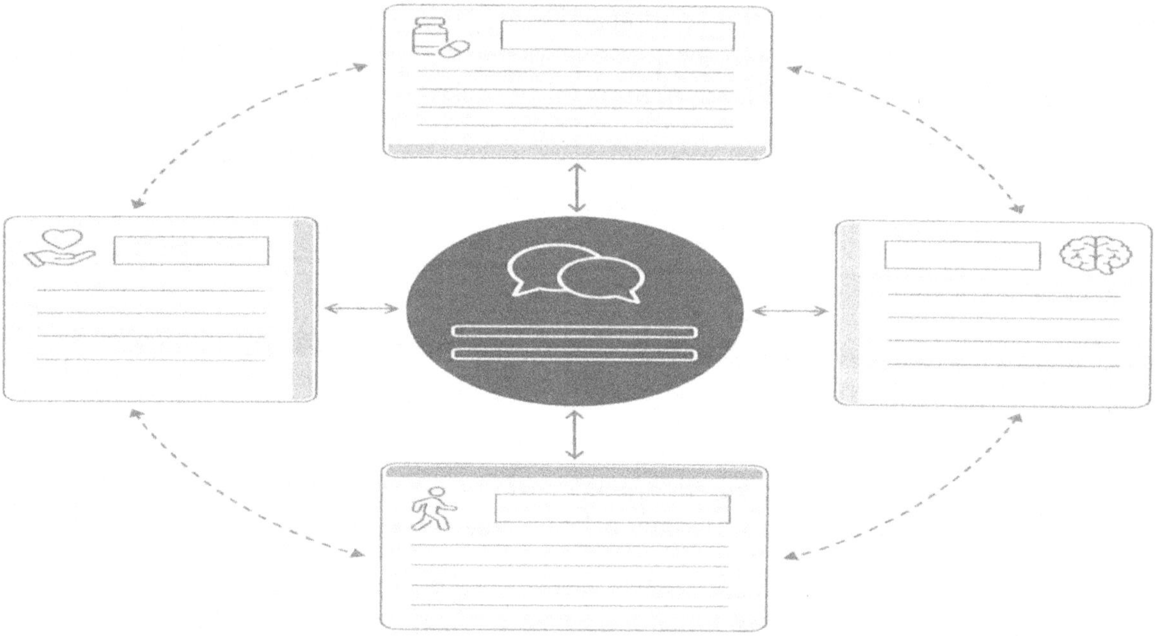

19.1.4 Polypharmacy and deprescribing

Polypharmacy is a risk factor in its own right, associated with adverse drug events, falls, delirium, hospitalisation, and mortality, partly through the individual drugs and partly through interactions and the burden of administration.

Explicit criteria identifying potentially inappropriate medications in older adults exist in several published forms and are useful as prompts rather than as prohibitions. The recurring high-risk categories are: benzodiazepines and other sedative-hypnotics; anticholinergics, whose cumulative burden across several apparently innocuous drugs is a major and under-recognised contributor to delirium and falls; antipsychotics; nonsteroidal anti-inflammatory drugs; some antihypertensives in the context of falls and orthostasis; sulfonylureas; and long-term proton pump inhibitors without indication.

The prescribing cascade deserves specific naming: a drug produces a side effect, the side effect is treated as a new condition with a second drug, which produces its own effect, and so on. Common examples are an antihypertensive causing ankle oedema treated with a diuretic, and an anticholinergic causing constipation treated with a laxative. Asking whether a new symptom might be caused by an existing drug is the interruption.

A structured deprescribing approach:

Compile the complete list, using the sources in Chapter 3, section 3.2.2, including preparations the patient does not consider medications.

Identify the indication for each drug, and flag those with none, those whose indication has lapsed, and those whose benefit horizon exceeds the patient's likely remaining life expectancy. This last consideration applies particularly to preventive therapies and requires the honest prognostic thinking of Chapter 20.

Prioritise by potential for harm rather than attempting to stop everything at once.

Taper where required, since abrupt withdrawal of benzodiazepines, opioids, beta-blockers, antidepressants, corticosteroids, and several other classes causes harm.

Monitor and document, and, critically, **communicate the change and the reasoning at discharge**, because a deprescribing decision made in hospital and not explained is routinely reversed by the next prescriber.

Hospitalisation is an opportunity for deprescribing because the whole regimen is visible to one clinician and the patient is observed. It is also a hazardous time to do it, since acute illness alters everything, so the judgement is to stop what is clearly harmful now and to propose the rest for outpatient review rather than attempting a complete rationalisation in a sick patient.

19.1.5 Hospital-associated disability

A substantial proportion of older patients lose the ability to perform at least one activity of daily living during a hospital admission, and a proportion never regain it. This loss is frequently unrelated to the illness that brought them in and is a consequence of the admission itself.

The mechanisms are immobility, which produces rapid loss of muscle mass and strength in older adults; tethering by catheters, drips, and monitoring; sedating medication; sleep deprivation; reduced nutritional intake; delirium; and a ward culture that treats bed rest as the default and mobilisation as an intervention requiring justification.

The interventions are unglamorous and effective: get the patient out of bed and walking daily, and record it; dress them in their own clothes; remove tethers; protect sleep; attend to nutrition, including ensuring that meals are within reach and that assistance is available; ensure glasses, hearing aids, and dentures are present and used; and involve therapy early rather than as a discharge formality.

Continence deserves specific attention. Urinary catheters are frequently placed for convenience and produce infection, immobility, delirium, and loss of continence that persists after removal. Toileting assistance is the alternative and requires staffing rather than equipment.

Bone health should be considered in any older patient admitted with a fall or a fracture, since a fragility fracture is a sentinel event predicting further fractures and is a treatable condition that is systematically under-addressed. Chapter 9, section 9.6.3, framed the fall as an event with a cause and a prediction.

19.1.6 Two further considerations in the older inpatient

Sensory impairment is prevalent, under-recognised, and trivially remediable. A patient without their glasses or hearing aids is functionally cognitively impaired: they cannot participate in a conversation about their care, cannot follow instructions, and are at markedly increased risk of delirium. **Establishing on admission whether the patient uses glasses, hearing aids, or dentures, and ensuring they are present and functioning, is a clinical action rather than a nursing courtesy**, and its omission is among the commonest contributors to a poor hospital course in this population.

Ageism in clinical decision making is documented and takes two opposite forms, both harmful. **Undertreatment** occurs when a beneficial intervention is withheld on the basis of chronological age rather than of physiological reserve and the patient's own goals, and a fit eighty-five-year-old may derive more benefit than a frail seventy-year-old. **Overtreatment** occurs when interventions are pursued without regard to the patient's frailty, prognosis, or stated priorities, frequently because no one has asked. The corrective for both is the same: assess frailty formally, establish what matters to the patient, and make the decision on those grounds explicitly rather than on an unexamined assumption about age. Chapter 20 develops the conversation.

19.2 The Pregnant Patient on a Medical Service

19.2.1 The governing principle

Pregnant patients admitted under medical services receive worse care than their non-pregnant counterparts for a reason that is well documented and should be stated plainly: **clinicians systematically undertreat, underinvestigate, and delay, out of concern for the fetus, and this harms both the patient and the fetus.**

Maternal death reviews in several countries have repeatedly identified failure to investigate, failure to treat, and failure to escalate as contributory, with the underlying pattern being an assumption that a symptom is a normal feature of pregnancy.

The correct framing is that the best treatment for the fetus is a well mother, and that a necessary investigation or treatment should be given, with the risk minimised where possible, rather than withheld.

Involve obstetrics early in any pregnant patient admitted for a medical reason, and involve them in the plan rather than notifying them of it.

19.2.2 Physiological changes and shifted reference ranges

Applying non-pregnant reference ranges is a systematic source of error. The principal changes:

System	Change in pregnancy	Practical consequence
Cardiovascular	Plasma volume and cardiac output rise; systemic resistance and blood pressure fall, with a mid-pregnancy nadir; heart rate rises	A blood pressure that appears normal may be elevated for pregnancy; tachycardia is common but should not be dismissed
Haematological	Plasma volume rises more than red cell mass, producing dilutional anaemia; a prothrombotic state develops	Haemoglobin thresholds differ; thromboembolic risk is markedly elevated
Renal	Glomerular filtration rate rises substantially	A creatinine in the normal non-pregnant range may represent significant impairment
Respiratory	Progesterone-driven hyperventilation produces a compensated respiratory alkalosis; functional residual capacity falls	Carbon dioxide and bicarbonate ranges are lower; oxygen desaturation occurs faster
Gastrointestinal	Gastric emptying is delayed and sphincter tone reduced	Aspiration risk is increased
Positional	The gravid uterus compresses the inferior vena cava when supine beyond the middle of pregnancy	Left lateral tilt is required for examination, imaging, and resuscitation

The most consequential of these in practice are the renal and respiratory changes, because a creatinine and a bicarbonate that look normal may both be markedly abnormal for pregnancy.

19.2.3 Investigation

Do not withhold necessary diagnostic imaging. The radiation dose from almost all diagnostic studies, including computed tomography of the chest and abdomen, falls well below the threshold associated with fetal harm, and the risk of a missed diagnosis substantially exceeds it. Where a choice exists, prefer the modality with less ionising radiation, shield where practical, and discuss with radiology, but **do not omit the study**.

Iodinated contrast may be used where necessary. **Gadolinium** is generally avoided in pregnancy.

Diagnosing pulmonary embolism requires a modified approach, since standard clinical decision rules and D-dimer thresholds perform differently. Pregnancy-adapted algorithms exist and should be used, and where imaging is required, both computed tomographic pulmonary angiography and ventilation-perfusion imaging are acceptable with different dose profiles to breast and fetus.

19.2.4 Treatment

Prescribing should use a current teratogenicity reference rather than memory, since the field changes and the information is specific.

Agents generally avoided include angiotensin converting enzyme inhibitors and receptor blockers, warfarin, most direct oral anticoagulants, valproate, methotrexate, tetracyclines, and retinoids.

Anticoagulation in pregnancy uses low molecular weight heparin, which does not cross the placenta.

Many chronic conditions require continued treatment, and stopping antiepileptic, antipsychotic, antiretroviral, or immunosuppressive therapy because a patient is pregnant frequently causes more harm than the drug. These decisions require specialist input rather than unilateral cessation.

19.2.5 Conditions to recognise

Venous thromboembolism is a leading cause of maternal death, and the threshold for investigation should be low.

Sepsis progresses rapidly in pregnancy and the physiological reserve masks it early. Maternal sepsis, including from genital tract sources, should be considered in any unwell pregnant or recently pregnant patient.

Pre-eclampsia and its variants present with hypertension, proteinuria, and organ dysfunction including hepatic, renal, haematological, and neurological involvement. **It can present or worsen postpartum**, up to several weeks after delivery, and a recently delivered woman presenting with headache, visual disturbance, epigastric pain, or hypertension must be assessed for it. Magnesium sulphate is used for seizure prophylaxis and treatment, and definitive treatment is delivery.

Peripartum cardiomyopathy presents with heart failure in late pregnancy or the months after delivery, and is frequently attributed to normal postpartum breathlessness.

Ask about recent pregnancy in any woman of reproductive age, since the postpartum period carries specific risks that will not be considered if the pregnancy is not known about.

19.2.6 Resuscitation modifications

Cardiac arrest in pregnancy beyond the middle of gestation requires **manual left uterine displacement or left lateral tilt** to relieve aortocaval compression, since chest compressions are ineffective without it, and **resuscitative hysterotomy should be initiated early** if there is no return of circulation, since it benefits both the mother, by relieving compression, and the fetus. This requires the obstetric and neonatal teams to be summoned at the moment the arrest is called rather than after.

19.3 Substance Use Disorder: Withdrawal, Medication Initiation, and Harm Reduction

19.3.1 The framing that determines the outcome

Patients with substance use disorder have high rates of premature discharge, readmission, and post-discharge mortality, and the largest single modifiable contributor is **inadequate treatment of withdrawal and pain**, which makes leaving a rational decision from the patient's perspective.

Substance use disorder is a medical condition, and the hospital admission is frequently the only sustained contact the patient has with the health system, which makes it an opportunity rather than an inconvenience. Chapter 1, section 1.7.2, described the evidence that stigmatising documentation alters subsequent analgesic prescribing, and this population is where that effect is most consequential.

19.3.2 Alcohol withdrawal

The timeline is predictable and should be anticipated rather than discovered: autonomic features including tremor, anxiety, sweating, and tachycardia begin within the first hours; perceptual disturbance and alcoholic hallucinosis, characteristically with preserved orientation, follow; withdrawal seizures occur in a window during the first day or two; and delirium tremens, with global confusion, marked autonomic instability, and hallucinations, develops later, typically after the second day, and carries significant mortality when untreated.

Predict severity. A history of prior withdrawal seizures or delirium tremens is the strongest predictor, together with the quantity and duration of use, the time since the last drink, prior detoxification episodes, and concurrent illness. Validated prediction instruments exist and should be used on admission so that prophylaxis and monitoring are matched to risk.

Benzodiazepines are the treatment, and this is the one situation in which the general caution about benzodiazepines in Chapter 10, section 10.1.6, does not apply. **Symptom-triggered dosing guided by a validated withdrawal scale is superior to fixed-schedule dosing**, producing less total drug and shorter treatment.

An important limitation of symptom-triggered protocols is that they depend on the patient being able to report symptoms. In a patient with delirium, intubation, communication difficulty, or another cause of confusion, a subjective scale is invalid and may either over-treat or under-treat dangerously. In these patients, an objective assessment scale or a structured protocol with specialist input should be used instead, and this is a common and important error.

Refractory withdrawal, requiring escalating benzodiazepine doses without control, warrants phenobarbital or another agent with critical care involvement.

Thiamine must be given parenterally and in adequate dose, before any glucose-containing fluid, for the reasons in Chapter 10, section 10.6.3.

Attend to the associated problems: hypoglycaemia, electrolyte disturbance particularly magnesium, phosphate, and potassium, alcoholic ketoacidosis, liver disease, malnutrition, and the risk of refeeding syndrome described in Chapter 12, section 12.7.

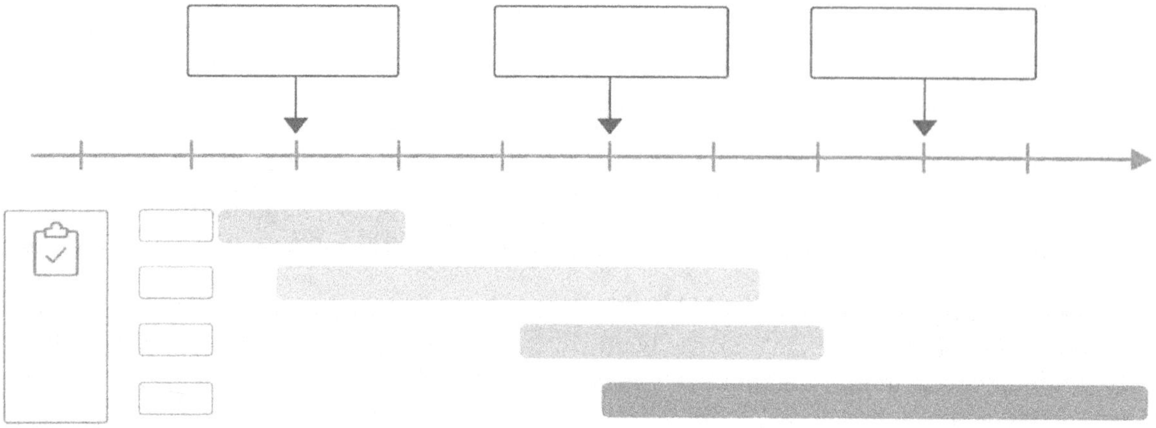

19.3.3 Opioid use disorder

Withdrawal is not usually life-threatening and is the reason patients leave. Treating it adequately is therefore both humane and the intervention that keeps the patient in hospital long enough to treat the condition that brought them in.

Medication for opioid use disorder should be initiated in hospital rather than referred for after discharge. Randomised evidence has shown that in-hospital initiation with linkage to outpatient care improves engagement in treatment compared with referral alone.

Buprenorphine is a partial agonist with a ceiling effect on respiratory depression. Traditional induction requires the patient to be in moderate withdrawal before the first dose, assessed with a validated scale, to avoid precipitated withdrawal. **Low-dose initiation protocols**, in which small doses are overlapped with continued full agonist use, have been developed and are increasingly used, particularly in the context of high-potency synthetic opioids where traditional induction is more difficult. Local protocols and addiction specialist input should guide the approach.

Methadone is a full agonist requiring linkage to a licensed programme for continuation, with provisions in most jurisdictions permitting its use for withdrawal management during an admission. Confirm the dose with the dispensing programme rather than relying on the patient's report, and be aware of QT prolongation and interactions.

Continue existing medication for opioid use disorder during admission and perioperatively, as Chapter 8, section 8.7.4, described, and do not attempt tapering during an acute admission.

Treat pain adequately. Patients on maintenance therapy have a baseline requirement that treats their disorder and provides no analgesia for new injury, and acute pain must be treated in addition to it, frequently at higher doses than in opioid-naive patients. Use multimodal and regional approaches preferentially.

19.3.4 Harm reduction

Harm reduction accepts that a patient may continue using and seeks to reduce the associated harm, which is both effective and, for many patients, the only realistic goal in the short term.

Naloxone at discharge, with training for the patient and a household member, is the highest-priority intervention. **The period immediately after discharge carries markedly elevated overdose risk**, because tolerance falls during a period of reduced or absent use in hospital while the patient's usual dose does not change.

Testing for human immunodeficiency virus, hepatitis B and C, and, where indicated, tuberculosis, with linkage to treatment. Hepatitis C is curable and the admission is an opportunity to begin the pathway.

Vaccination, wound care, and safer injecting supplies or referral to services providing them, according to local availability and law.

Recognise the complications of injecting, including skin and soft tissue infection, endocarditis, epidural abscess, and septic emboli, as Chapter 18 described, and maintain a low threshold for investigating them.

Plan for discharge against medical advice rather than treating it as a rupture. Provide prescriptions, a return threshold, harm reduction supplies, and an explicit statement that the patient may return without judgement, as Chapter 3, section 3.7.3, argued.

19.3.5 Other substances

Benzodiazepine and sedative withdrawal can be life-threatening and requires a taper rather than abrupt cessation, with a longer-acting agent substituted where appropriate.

Stimulants have no established pharmacotherapy for the disorder. Acute management addresses agitation, hyperthermia, and cardiovascular and cerebrovascular complications, as Chapter 17 and Chapter 10, section 10.6.4, described.

Nicotine withdrawal is common, under-treated, and contributes to agitation and to discharge against advice. Offer replacement therapy routinely.

Gabapentinoids and other agents are increasingly used and their withdrawal is under-recognised.

19.4 Psychiatric Comorbidity, Agitation, and the Suicidal Inpatient

19.4.1 Physical health in serious mental illness

People with serious mental illness die substantially earlier than the general population, and the excess mortality is driven predominantly by physical disease that is under-detected and under-treated rather than by suicide, important though that is.

Diagnostic overshadowing is the mechanism: a physical symptom in a patient with a psychiatric diagnosis is attributed to that diagnosis. Chapter 2, section 2.4.4, listed it among the structural risk factors for diagnostic error, and this population is where it operates most strongly.

The corrective is to apply the same diagnostic standard as to any other patient, and to be explicitly suspicious of the reflex that a symptom is psychosomatic or attention-seeking. A patient with schizophrenia who reports abdominal pain requires the assessment of Chapter 9, section 9.3, not reassurance.

The concept of medical clearance is unhelpful when it means a cursory examination to permit psychiatric admission. What is required is a proper assessment for medical causes of the psychiatric presentation, which is a diagnostic task rather than an administrative one. Chapter 10 covers the differential.

19.4.2 Psychotropic medications and their complications

Several agents produce complications that hospitalists must recognise.

Antipsychotics cause QT prolongation with arrhythmia risk, extrapyramidal effects, metabolic effects, and neuroleptic malignant syndrome as described in Chapter 10, section 10.6.4. In older adults with dementia they are associated with increased mortality.

Lithium has a narrow therapeutic index. Toxicity is precipitated by dehydration, acute kidney injury, and interacting drugs including nonsteroidal anti-inflammatory agents, diuretics, and angiotensin system inhibitors. **Any patient on lithium who becomes acutely unwell requires a level and consideration of holding the drug**, and lithium is dialysable.

Clozapine requires particular vigilance. Agranulocytosis mandates monitoring; myocarditis occurs early in treatment; and **severe constipation with ileus is a recognised cause of death** and requires active prevention and treatment, connecting to Chapter 15, section 15.8. Critically, **if doses are missed for more than a short interval, the drug must be retitrated from a low dose** rather than resumed at the previous dose, and an admission with vomiting or nil by mouth status is a common cause of unplanned interruption.

Serotonergic agents, addressed in Chapter 10, section 10.6.4.

Catatonia is under-recognised in general hospitals, presents with immobility, mutism, negativism, posturing, and refusal of food and fluids, may complicate psychiatric and medical illness, responds to benzodiazepine challenge, and can progress to a malignant form with autonomic instability. It is frequently mistaken for depression, delirium, or non-cooperation.

19.4.3 Agitation

Prevention comes first. Most agitation in general hospitals is a consequence of delirium, pain, withdrawal, fear, unmet need, sensory impairment, or the environment, and addressing these prevents more agitation than any drug.

Verbal de-escalation is the first-line intervention and is a learnable technique: approach calmly with adequate personal space, one person speaking, simple short statements, acknowledgement of the person's concern, offering choices where possible, and identifying the unmet need. It is effective in a substantial proportion of episodes and should be attempted before pharmacological or physical measures.

Pharmacological management, where necessary, should use the oral route where the patient will accept it, a single agent at the lowest effective dose, with the choice determined by the likely cause: benzodiazepines for withdrawal states, antipsychotics for psychosis, and caution in delirium where Chapter 10, section 10.1.6, applies. **Monitoring after administration is mandatory**, since over-sedation, respiratory depression, aspiration, falls, and cardiac effects all occur.

Physical restraint causes harm, including injury, delirium, deconditioning, and death, and should be a last resort with a documented rationale, the shortest possible duration, continuous monitoring, and frequent review. Its use should be reported and reviewed institutionally.

After the episode, review what precipitated it and what would prevent recurrence, and, where appropriate, discuss it with the patient afterwards, since patients frequently find these episodes distressing and remember them.

19.4.4 The suicidal inpatient

Suicidal ideation may be the reason for admission, may emerge during an admission, or may be disclosed incidentally, and a hospitalist will encounter all three.

Ask directly. Asking about suicidal thoughts does not increase risk, and it is the only way to identify it. The question should be asked plainly and without euphemism in any patient with depression, with a recent significant loss or diagnosis, with substance use disorder, or where staff or family have expressed concern.

Risk stratification instruments should not determine management. Structured tools have poor predictive value for individual patients, classifying large numbers of low-risk patients who go on to harm themselves and large numbers of high-risk patients who do not. They may support a structured assessment; they must not be used to justify a lower level of observation in a patient the clinician is concerned about, and this misuse is documented and harmful.

What should be done instead is a clinical assessment and formulation covering the nature of the thoughts, whether there is intent and planning, the presence of protective factors, previous attempts which are the strongest single historical predictor, current mental state, substance use, and the acute stressors, combined with collateral information.

Immediate management:

Ensure the patient's immediate safety according to institutional policy, which will specify levels of observation and the circumstances requiring continuous supervision. The level should be determined by clinical assessment rather than by a score.

Arrange environmental risk assessment by staff trained to perform it, following the institution's protocol.

Obtain urgent psychiatric assessment, and treat any underlying medical or psychiatric condition, including delirium, which is a common and reversible contributor.

Involve family or supporters with the patient's consent where possible, both for collateral information and because their involvement is protective.

Undertake safety planning with the patient before discharge, which is a structured, collaborative process with evidence of benefit, and which includes discussion of restricting access to means, conducted with the patient and where appropriate the family.

Recognise that the period after discharge carries markedly elevated risk, and ensure that follow-up is arranged within days rather than weeks, that it is communicated, and that the patient knows how to seek help urgently.

Document the assessment, the reasoning, and the plan, rather than only the conclusion, as Chapter 10, section 10.7.3, required for capacity.

Attend to the staff. Caring for a patient who has attempted or completed suicide is distressing, and the second victim considerations of Chapter 4, section 4.6.2, apply directly.

Legal frameworks governing detention and treatment without consent are jurisdiction-specific and must be known locally. Capacity assessment, as in Chapter 10, section 10.7, is frequently relevant and is distinct from the question of whether detention criteria are met.

19.5 The Patient with Obesity and Metabolic Disease

19.5.1 Physiological considerations

Respiratory. Functional residual capacity and expiratory reserve volume are reduced, particularly when supine, which produces the atelectasis physiology described in Chapter 6, section 6.6.3, and shortens the safe apnoea time during intubation. Obstructive sleep apnoea and obesity hypoventilation syndrome are common and frequently undiagnosed, and Chapter 6, section 6.6.5, addressed their perioperative implications. Obesity hypoventilation specifically produces chronic hypercapnia and requires the controlled oxygen approach of Chapter 14, section 14.2.2.

Cardiovascular. Increased blood volume and cardiac output, a higher prevalence of hypertension, heart failure with preserved ejection fraction, and atrial fibrillation. **Blood pressure measured with a cuff that is too small reads falsely high**, which is a common and consequential measurement error, and an appropriately sized cuff must be used.

Thromboembolic risk is elevated, and prophylaxis dosing may require adjustment.

Examination is limited, with reduced reliability of abdominal, cardiac, and respiratory examination, which raises the threshold for imaging and lowers the threshold for point-of-care ultrasound, itself technically more difficult.

19.5.2 Practical care

Drug dosing requires attention to whether the agent is hydrophilic or lipophilic and to which weight descriptor the dosing recommendation uses. Total body weight, ideal body weight, and adjusted body weight give substantially different doses, and using the wrong one produces systematic under or overdosing. **Involve pharmacy**, particularly for antimicrobials, anticoagulants, and chemotherapy.

Equipment and environment must be arranged in advance rather than discovered at the point of need: appropriately rated beds, chairs, hoists, and commodes; appropriately sized cuffs and gowns;

and awareness of weight and bore limits for imaging modalities, which should be checked before a study is requested rather than after the patient has been moved.

Vascular access is frequently difficult and ultrasound guidance should be used early rather than after repeated failed attempts.

Pressure injury risk is elevated, including in skin folds, and Chapter 4, section 4.4.2, applies.

Mobility and rehabilitation require early therapy involvement and adequate staffing for safe handling, and delays here produce the hospital-associated disability described in section 19.1.5.

19.5.3 Stigma and its measurable effects

Weight stigma in healthcare is well documented and has measurable consequences: symptoms attributed to weight without investigation, delayed diagnosis, reduced examination, and avoidance of healthcare by patients who anticipate poor treatment.

The clinical corrective is to apply the same diagnostic process as to any other patient, to avoid attributing a new symptom to weight without excluding other causes, and to attend to language in speech and documentation, per Chapter 1, section 1.7.2.

19.5.4 The post-bariatric patient

Patients who have undergone bariatric surgery present specific problems that are frequently unfamiliar to general physicians.

Know the procedure, since the anatomy and its consequences differ substantially between operations, and obtain the operative details.

Micronutrient deficiencies are common and require monitoring and supplementation, including thiamine, vitamin B12, iron, folate, vitamin D and calcium, and, in some procedures, fat-soluble vitamins and copper. **Thiamine deficiency after bariatric surgery, particularly with vomiting, causes Wernicke encephalopathy** and should be treated on suspicion as in Chapter 10, section 10.6.3.

Internal hernia is a surgical emergency presenting with intermittent or severe abdominal pain, and **computed tomography may be normal or only subtly abnormal**, so a patient with a history of bypass surgery and significant abdominal pain requires urgent bariatric surgical assessment rather than reassurance from a normal scan.

Avoid nonsteroidal anti-inflammatory drugs, which carry a high risk of marginal ulceration.

Medication absorption may be altered, and extended-release preparations may be inappropriate.

Post-bariatric hypoglycaemia occurs, typically postprandially and some time after surgery, and is distinct from dumping syndrome.

19.5.5 Related metabolic conditions

Metabolic dysfunction-associated steatotic liver disease, the current terminology for what was previously described as non-alcoholic fatty liver disease, is highly prevalent and progresses to cirrhosis in a proportion. It should be recognised as a cause of abnormal liver enzymes and of cirrhosis in patients without alcohol use, and Chapter 15 applies once decompensation occurs.

Glucagon-like peptide-1 receptor agonists are now widely prescribed for both diabetes and weight management, and hospitalists will encounter them frequently. Relevant effects include gastrointestinal symptoms, delayed gastric emptying with the perioperative implications described in Chapter 7, section 7.1.3, pancreatitis, and gallbladder disease.

19.6 Structural Determinants, Disparities, and the Unhoused Patient

19.6.1 What determines outcomes

A substantial proportion of variation in health outcomes is attributable to factors outside the clinical encounter: housing, income, education, food security, transport, employment, immigration status, and the structural conditions that distribute these unevenly.

For a hospitalist, the practical relevance is not sociological but operational. These factors determine whether a discharge plan will work, whether a medication will be taken, whether follow-up will be attended, and whether the patient will return. Chapter 3, section 3.5.1, noted that social factors predict readmission more powerfully than most measures of inpatient care quality.

19.6.2 Disparities within the hospital

Documented differences in inpatient care by race, ethnicity, language, and socioeconomic status include differences in analgesia provision, in time to treatment, in diagnostic effort, and in the language used in documentation. Chapter 1, section 1.7.2, described evidence that negative descriptors appear disproportionately in the records of some patient groups and that such language alters subsequent clinicians' decisions.

One example deserves specific attention because it is a direct measurement problem. Pulse oximetry has been shown to overestimate arterial oxygen saturation more frequently in patients with darker skin pigmentation, producing occult hypoxaemia in which a reassuring reading conceals genuine desaturation. The clinical implications are immediate: a saturation reading in a patient with darker skin carries a greater probability of overestimating the true value, the threshold for arterial or venous blood gas measurement should be correspondingly lower, and trends and clinical assessment should be weighted more heavily than a single reading. This is a technical limitation of the device rather than a matter of clinician attitude, and it affects the acute decisions in Chapter 14 directly.

Race-based clinical algorithms have been reconsidered across several specialties. The removal of the race coefficient from kidney function estimating equations, noted in Chapter 16, section 16.1.3, is the most prominent example, and others remain under review. The general principle is that race is a social rather than a biological category and its use as a proxy in clinical calculation requires specific justification.

19.6.3 The patient experiencing homelessness

Mortality is markedly elevated and life expectancy substantially reduced, with a pattern of premature ageing such that a patient in their fifties may have the comorbidity profile of a much older person. Frailty assessment as in section 19.1.2 is appropriate at younger ages in this population.

Tri-morbidity, meaning the coexistence of physical illness, mental illness, and substance use disorder, is common and means that addressing one problem without the others frequently fails.

Prior negative experience of healthcare is common, and patients may present late, may be wary, and may leave early. The clinical response is to establish trust deliberately, to address pain and withdrawal promptly as section 19.3 argued, and to avoid the language and behaviour that confirms the expectation.

Practical management, developed in Chapter 3, section 3.7.2, and summarised: ask about housing routinely rather than assuming; simplify the medication regimen to once-daily dosing without refrigeration where possible; provide medications in hand rather than a prescription; arrange medical respite care where it exists and document its absence as an unmet need where it does not; use the admission for vaccination, screening, dental and foot care, and wound care; involve social work early rather than on the day of discharge; and avoid discharge to the street at night or in extreme weather without exhausting alternatives.

Specific clinical problems to consider: foot pathology, which is common and frequently severe; hypothermia and cold injury; skin infestation; tuberculosis and other communicable disease with public health implications; the sequelae of violence and of traumatic brain injury; and the consequences of prolonged untreated chronic disease.

19.6.4 Screening for social needs

Screen only if you can act. Identifying food insecurity, transport difficulty, or housing instability and then doing nothing about it is worse than not asking, because it signals that the disclosure was pointless. Where screening is undertaken, it must be linked to a pathway with social work, community services, and, where they exist, community health worker or navigator programmes.

Immigration status and fear of consequences affect presentation and disclosure in some populations, and clinicians should be aware of local law regarding information sharing and should be able to state clearly what will and will not be shared.

19.7 Language, Culture, and Interpretation as Clinical Safety Issues

19.7.1 Language access is a safety issue, not a courtesy

Patients with limited proficiency in the language of care experience longer stays, more adverse events, poorer comprehension of their diagnosis and treatment, lower satisfaction, and worse outcomes. The mechanism is straightforward: the history is the principal diagnostic instrument, consent depends on understanding, and the discharge plan depends on communication.

Professional interpretation improves outcomes, including comprehension, adherence, and satisfaction, and reduces adverse events.

Ad hoc interpreters produce more errors of clinical consequence. Studies comparing professional with ad hoc interpretation, including by family members and by bilingual staff without interpreter training, have found substantially higher rates of errors with potential clinical consequence in the latter. **Children should never be used as interpreters**, for reasons of accuracy, confidentiality, and the burden placed on the child.

Family members may still have a role in supporting the patient and providing collateral history, and this is different from using them as the channel for clinical information.

19.7.2 Using an interpreter well

The technique is learnable and improves the encounter substantially.

Brief the interpreter before the encounter about its purpose, particularly for difficult conversations.

Address the patient directly, in the second person, maintaining eye contact with the patient rather than with the interpreter.

Speak in short segments and pause for interpretation, rather than delivering a long passage.

Use plain language and avoid idiom, metaphor, and humour, which interpret poorly and generate confusion.

Allow more time, approximately double, and schedule accordingly rather than compressing the encounter.

Check understanding with teach-back, as in Chapter 3, section 3.4.4, which is more important rather than less when interpretation is involved.

Use interpretation for the encounters that matter most: the initial history, consent for procedures, the communication of a serious diagnosis, goals-of-care discussions, and discharge instructions. These are precisely the encounters where the temptation to proceed without interpretation is greatest because of time pressure.

Provide written material in the patient's language where available, and document that an interpreter was used and by what mode.

Patients who are deaf or hard of hearing require sign language interpretation where that is their language, and written notes and lip reading are not adequate substitutes for important conversations.

19.7.3 Culture and the individual

Cultural humility is a more useful stance than cultural competence. The latter implies a body of knowledge about groups, which invites stereotyping; the former implies an ongoing willingness to ask, to acknowledge one's own limits, and to treat the individual as the authority on their own beliefs and preferences.

Ask rather than assume. Variation within any group exceeds variation between groups, and a patient's individual practice may differ substantially from what is described in a reference text about their community.

Areas where practical accommodation is frequently required: dietary restrictions and their interaction with hospital catering; religious observance including prayer times, fasting and its interaction with medication and diabetes management, and religious days; modesty requirements and preferences regarding the gender of the examining clinician, which can usually be accommodated with notice; and expectations about family involvement in decision making, which may differ from an individual-autonomy model and which should be negotiated with the patient rather than assumed in either direction.

Practices around serious illness, death, and the body vary considerably and matter enormously to families. Asking early, before the situation is urgent, permits accommodation, and Chapter 20 addresses this directly.

Where a cultural expectation conflicts with clinical safety or with the patient's own expressed wishes, the conflict should be addressed openly with the patient, and the patient's own decision, where they have capacity, governs.

Chapter Summary

- **Standard care produces worse outcomes for these populations for identifiable and correctable reasons**: unaccounted physiological difference, atypical presentation read as absence of disease, plans that assume capacities the patient lacks, and stigma that measurably changes clinical decisions.
- **Use frailty rather than age.** Assess and record it, apply a four-domain framework centred on what matters to the patient, and recognise geriatric syndromes as presentations of acute illness requiring full diagnostic effort.
- **Hospital-associated disability is caused by the admission**, principally through immobility, tethering, sedation, and sleep deprivation, and is prevented by unglamorous daily actions.
- **In pregnancy, undertreatment harms both patient and fetus.** Do not withhold necessary imaging. Non-pregnant reference ranges are misleading, particularly for creatinine and bicarbonate. Consider pre-eclampsia in a recently delivered woman.
- **Inadequately treated withdrawal and pain are the main modifiable drivers of premature discharge** in substance use disorder. Symptom-triggered benzodiazepine protocols require a patient who can report symptoms and are invalid in delirium. **Initiate medication for opioid use disorder in hospital**, and provide naloxone at discharge, since post-discharge overdose risk is elevated by reduced tolerance.
- **Diagnostic overshadowing drives the excess physical mortality in serious mental illness.** Know the specific hazards of lithium and clozapine, recognise catatonia, and prevent agitation rather than treating it.
- **Suicide risk stratification instruments must not determine level of observation.** Ask directly, formulate clinically, ensure safety per institutional protocol, undertake safety planning, and arrange follow-up within days, since the post-discharge period carries elevated risk.
- **In obesity, an undersized cuff reads falsely high**, drug dosing depends on which weight descriptor the recommendation uses, and a normal computed tomogram does not exclude internal hernia after bypass surgery.
- **Pulse oximetry overestimates saturation more often in patients with darker skin pigmentation**, which is a device limitation requiring a lower threshold for blood gas measurement.

- **Professional interpretation is a safety intervention.** Ad hoc interpreters produce more clinically significant errors, children should never interpret, and the encounters most often conducted without an interpreter are the ones where it matters most.

Review Questions

1. An 86-year-old woman is admitted with a urinary tract infection and by day four is unable to transfer independently, having walked into the hospital. Explain what has happened, name the mechanisms, and state what should have been done differently from day one.
2. A woman at 26 weeks of gestation presents with pleuritic chest pain and breathlessness. The team is reluctant to obtain imaging. State your position, the evidence, and how you would proceed.
3. A patient with alcohol dependence is admitted with pneumonia and is confused on day two. He is on a symptom-triggered benzodiazepine protocol. Explain why this protocol may now be unsafe and what you would do instead.
4. A patient discloses suicidal ideation to a nurse. A risk assessment tool scores them low risk, and the team proposes routine observation. State your position and set out your management.
5. A patient who speaks little English requires consent for a procedure. A bilingual healthcare assistant is available and the ward is busy. State what you would do and why.

CHAPTER 20: Palliative Care, Ethics, and the Dying Patient

Learning Objectives

After studying this chapter, the reader should be able to:

1. Deliver the primary palliative care skills expected of every hospitalist, and identify when specialist involvement is needed.
2. Prognosticate using functional status and illness trajectory, and communicate prognosis honestly under uncertainty.
3. Conduct a goals-of-care conversation using a structured framework, and avoid the errors that most often derail one.
4. Manage the principal symptoms at the end of life, including pain, breathlessness, nausea, delirium, and secretions.
5. Apply advance directives correctly, support surrogate decision makers, and act for the incapacitated patient without one.
6. Withdraw life-sustaining therapy safely, respectfully, and with adequate symptom control.
7. Use ethics consultation appropriately, respond to disputes about non-beneficial treatment, and recognise moral distress.
8. Recognise dying, care for the patient in the final hours, and support the family before and after death.

Chapter Overview

This is the last chapter of the book, and it addresses the part of hospital medicine that most determines how patients and families remember the whole of it.

A substantial proportion of deaths occur in hospital, and hospitalists are therefore among the clinicians most frequently present at the end of life. Yet the skills involved are the least systematically taught of any in this book, and the consequence is a recognisable pattern of poor deaths: prognosis never discussed, dying recognised only in the final hours, symptoms undertreated because of unfounded fears about opioids, families asked to make decisions they were never prepared for, and interventions continued because no one held the conversation that would have stopped them.

Four principles run through the chapter.

Palliative care is not the same as end-of-life care. It is the management of symptoms and the alignment of treatment with the patient's goals, and it is appropriate concurrently with disease-directed treatment from the point of serious diagnosis. Trial evidence in advanced cancer has shown that early palliative care improves quality of life and mood, and in one landmark trial was associated with longer survival despite less aggressive treatment.

Recognising dying is a diagnosis, with signs, with consequences for management, and with the same obligation to communicate as any other diagnosis. Failure to make it is the single largest cause of poor death in hospital, because everything else follows from it.

These conversations are procedures. They have indications, preparation, a technique that can be taught and improved, complications when done badly, and a defined product. Treating them as a matter of innate personality or of finding the right words in the moment is the reason they go badly.

Uncertainty is not a reason for silence. Clinicians avoid discussing prognosis because they cannot be precise. Patients and families consistently report wanting honest information including its uncertainty, and the alternative to an uncertain conversation is not a certain one but an absent one.

20.1 Primary Palliative Care Skills for Every Hospitalist

20.1.1 Primary and specialist palliative care

Primary palliative care comprises the skills every clinician caring for seriously ill patients should possess: basic symptom management, communication about prognosis and goals, identification of psychosocial and spiritual distress, and recognition of dying.

Specialist palliative care addresses complexity beyond that: refractory symptoms, complex psychological or existential distress, difficult family conflict, and complicated decision-making.

The distinction matters practically because specialist services are finite, and a model in which every serious illness conversation is referred both overwhelms them and deskills the clinicians who see the patient daily. The hospitalist who knows the patient and the family is frequently better placed to hold the conversation than a consultant meeting them for the first time.

Triggers for specialist referral include symptoms not responding to first-line management; requests for hastened death; complex existential or spiritual distress; significant family conflict or an impasse in decision-making; complex prognostic uncertainty affecting a major decision; and the need for specialised interventions.

20.1.2 The domains of assessment

Serious illness produces distress across four domains, and assessing only the first produces incomplete care.

Physical. Systematic symptom assessment rather than waiting for symptoms to be reported. Patients under-report, particularly symptoms they believe are inevitable or that they fear will lead to reduced treatment. A structured enquiry covering pain, breathlessness, nausea, appetite, bowels, sleep, and fatigue takes two minutes and finds a great deal.

Psychological. Depression and anxiety are common, are distinguishable from appropriate sadness, and are treatable. Depression in serious illness is under-diagnosed because low mood is assumed to be understandable, and the discriminating features are anhedonia, hopelessness, worthlessness, and guilt rather than sadness alone.

Social. Who is at home, who provides care, what the financial consequences are, and what the caregiver's own state is. **Caregiver strain is a clinical problem** with consequences for the patient's outcome and for the caregiver's own health, and asking about it is part of the assessment.

Spiritual and existential. This is the domain most often omitted and is frequently the source of the greatest distress. It is not confined to religious belief, and the useful questions concern what gives the person's life meaning, what they are most worried about, what they hope for, and whether there is anything left unresolved. Brief structured approaches to this enquiry exist and are learnable. Chaplaincy is a clinical service, not a religious one, and referral does not require the patient to hold a faith.

20.1.3 The skills themselves

The remaining sections of this chapter address these individually: prognostication in section 20.2, communication in section 20.3, symptom management in section 20.4, decision-making in sections 20.5 and 20.6, and recognition of dying in section 20.8.

One further skill deserves naming here: the ability to sit with distress without fixing it. Much of what patients and families express in serious illness is not a question requiring an answer but an emotion requiring acknowledgement. The reflex to respond to distress with information is the commonest single error in these conversations, and section 20.3.4 addresses it directly.

20.2 Prognostication: Tools, Accuracy, and Honest Uncertainty

20.2.1 How clinicians perform

Two findings from the prognostication literature should shape practice.

Clinicians are systematically over-optimistic. Studies of physician prediction of survival in terminally ill patients have found substantial overestimation, in one influential study by a factor of several times, with error in the optimistic direction predominating.

The error increases with the closeness of the relationship. Physicians who have known the patient longer are less accurate and more optimistic, which is counterintuitive and important: the clinician who feels best placed to prognosticate may be least reliable.

Clinicians also avoid communicating prognosis even when they have formed one, and when they do communicate it they tend to give a more optimistic figure than they privately believe.

The practical implications are to anchor estimates to objective markers rather than to impression, to be aware of the optimistic bias and correct for it, and to recognise that reluctance to communicate is a separate problem from inaccuracy and requires a separate remedy.

20.2.2 Functional status is the strongest general predictor

Across most serious illnesses, **the trajectory of functional decline predicts survival better than any laboratory measure or disease-specific variable.**

Structured performance status scales, whether the simple ordinal scales used in oncology or the more detailed palliative performance measures, capture this and should be recorded. The specific observations that carry most information are: how much of the day the patient spends in bed or a chair, and how that has changed over recent weeks; whether they can perform self-care; oral intake and its change; and level of consciousness.

A patient whose functional decline is measured in months has a prognosis of months. A patient declining week by week has a prognosis of weeks. A patient declining day by day has a prognosis of days. This heuristic is imprecise and is more useful than most formal tools for framing a conversation.

Disease-specific prognostic models exist for heart failure, chronic obstructive pulmonary disease, liver disease, dementia, and several malignancies. They are useful for populations and imprecise for individuals, with the limitations described in Chapter 5, section 5.3.1, applying fully.

The surprise question, asking oneself whether one would be surprised if this patient died within the next year, has modest predictive accuracy. Its value is as a **trigger for further thought and for advance care planning** rather than as a prediction, and used that way it is a useful screening instrument.

20.2.3 Illness trajectories

Four characteristic trajectories describe the great majority of deaths, and recognising which applies to a patient explains both the prognostic difficulty and the appropriate planning.

Sudden death from an unexpected event, with high function until the moment of death. Planning here is necessarily general and takes the form of advance care planning while well.

Progressive illness with a short terminal decline, characteristic of many cancers. Function is relatively preserved until a period of weeks to a few months before death, when it declines steeply. This trajectory is the most predictable and is the one around which hospice services were originally designed.

Organ failure with intermittent exacerbations, characteristic of heart failure, chronic obstructive pulmonary disease, and end-stage liver and kidney disease. Function declines gradually with acute deteriorations from which the patient partially recovers, and **death may occur during any exacerbation**, including one that appears no worse than several the patient has survived. This is the hardest trajectory to prognosticate and the one where conversations are most often deferred, because there is always a plausible reason to wait until the patient is out of the current crisis.

Prolonged dwindling, characteristic of frailty and dementia, with slow decline over years from an already low baseline, and death frequently precipitated by a minor event such as an infection or a fall.

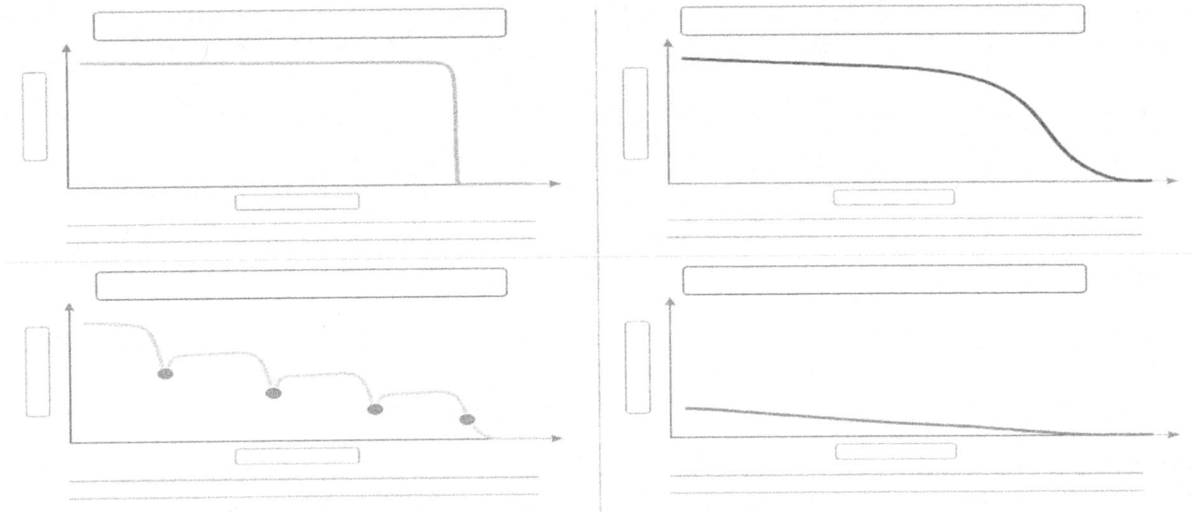

20.2.4 Communicating prognosis

Ask permission before giving prognostic information, and establish what the patient already understands and what they want to know. Preferences vary substantially, and some patients wish detailed information while others prefer that it be given to a family member. Asking directly resolves this.

Use ranges rather than numbers. Hours to days, days to weeks, weeks to months, months to a year or two. These convey the magnitude accurately without a false precision that will be either wrong or interpreted as a promise.

Acknowledge the uncertainty explicitly and state that the range is what is known rather than an evasion.

Pair the possibilities. Preparing for the worst while hoping for the best is a formulation that permits both to be held simultaneously, and it gives the patient permission to plan without abandoning hope.

Check what was understood, since prognostic information is frequently not retained after a first hearing, and expect to repeat the conversation.

Revisit it. Prognosis changes, and a conversation held at diagnosis does not serve for the whole illness.

20.3 Goals-of-Care Conversations: Frameworks and Common Errors

20.3.1 What the conversation is for

A goals-of-care conversation establishes what the patient values and what outcomes they would find acceptable, in order that treatment decisions can be aligned with those values.

It is not a code status discussion, and treating it as one is the most consequential structural error in this domain. Beginning with a question about cardiopulmonary resuscitation inverts the logic:

it asks the patient to choose an intervention before establishing what they are trying to achieve, and it presents an isolated technical decision without context.

The order is: understanding, then values, then recommendation, then specific decisions.

20.3.2 A structured framework

Several validated frameworks exist and share a common structure. The sequence below draws on them.

Prepare. Know the clinical facts including the prognosis, know who should be present, arrange an appropriate space and adequate time, and ensure interpretation is arranged where needed, as Chapter 19, section 19.7.2, required.

Establish understanding first. Ask what the patient and family understand about the situation. This takes a minute, identifies misunderstandings that would otherwise derail everything that follows, and frequently reveals that the patient understands more than the team assumed.

Ask permission and give the headline. Deliver the key information in a short, plain sentence and then stop. The instinct to continue talking is strong and should be resisted, since nothing said in the following thirty seconds will be heard.

Expect and respond to emotion. This is the pivot of the conversation and is addressed in section 20.3.4.

Map the values. Ask what matters most to the patient now, what they are hoping for, what worries them most, what abilities or experiences are essential to them, and what they would not want. These questions elicit the material on which the recommendation will be built.

Align and recommend. Reflect back what has been heard, and then **make a recommendation** based on it. This is discussed in section 20.3.3.

Plan. State specifically what will and will not be done, what will happen next, and when the conversation will be revisited. Document it in the patient's own words where possible.

20.3.3 Make a recommendation

Presenting a menu of options and asking the family to choose is a failure of the clinician's role. It transfers a burden the family is not equipped to carry, is associated with lasting psychological harm in surrogates, and produces decisions less aligned with the patient's values than a clinician recommendation informed by them.

The clinician's expertise is in what the interventions can and cannot achieve. The patient's and family's expertise is in what the patient values. **The recommendation is the product of combining the two**, and making it is the clinician's job.

The formulation is: "From what you have told me about what matters to your mother, I would recommend that we focus on keeping her comfortable and at home, and that we do not put her through another admission to intensive care. How does that sound to you?"

This does not remove choice. The family retains the ability to disagree, and the recommendation can be revised. It removes the burden of originating the decision.

Time-limited trials are a valuable middle option where the prognosis is genuinely uncertain: an agreement to provide a specified intensive treatment for a defined period with defined markers of improvement, and to reassess at the end. The value depends on the endpoint being specified in advance, since without it the trial has no end.

20.3.4 Responding to emotion

The commonest error in these conversations is responding to an emotional statement with medical information.

A family member says "I just can't believe this is happening." The clinician, meaning well, explains the pathophysiology again. The emotion is left unaddressed, the family concludes that the clinician has not understood, and the conversation stalls. This is described in the communication literature as a missed empathic opportunity and it is very common.

The alternative is a brief empathic response before any further information: naming the emotion, expressing understanding, showing respect for what the person is doing, offering support, or exploring further. These responses take seconds, and after them the conversation can proceed.

Clinicians talk too much in these encounters. Observational studies consistently find that clinicians occupy the majority of the speaking time, and that greater clinician talk time is associated with lower family satisfaction and poorer understanding. **Silence is an active technique.** After delivering serious information, waiting is more useful than filling thc space.

20.3.5 Other common errors

"Do you want us to do everything?" This question is unanswerable, since no family will say no to everything, and it frames the choice as one between care and abandonment.

"There is nothing more we can do." This is never true and is heard as abandonment. There is always something to be done, and stating what it is preserves the relationship.

Jargon, including terms that clinicians do not recognise as jargon such as comfort care, palliative, aggressive, and even terminal.

Asking the family what they want, rather than asking what the patient would have said, which is the correct question and is discussed in section 20.5.3.

Presenting artificial nutrition, hydration, and ventilation as neutral defaults rather than as treatments with indications, burdens, and outcomes.

Deferring the conversation until a crisis, at which point it is held at three in the morning with a covering clinician who has never met the family, under time pressure, with the patient unable to participate. This is the most common failure of all, and it is a systems failure as much as an individual one.

20.3.6 Discussing resuscitation specifically

When the conversation reaches specific interventions, several points improve it.

Discuss it in the context of the goals already established, not as an isolated question.

Give outcome information honestly. Survival to discharge after in-hospital cardiac arrest is far lower than public perception, which is shaped substantially by television portrayals, and it is lower still in patients with metastatic malignancy, multiple organ failure, or poor functional status. Patients and families frequently revise their preference when given accurate figures.

Frame it as a recommendation where the intervention would not achieve an outcome the patient values, rather than as a choice offered neutrally.

Distinguish resuscitation from other treatments explicitly. A decision not to attempt resuscitation says nothing about antibiotics, admission to hospital, or any other intervention, and families frequently assume it means the withdrawal of all treatment. State plainly what will continue.

Record the decision where it will be found, and ensure it travels with the patient, as section 20.5.2 discusses.

20.4 Symptom Management at the End of Life

20.4.1 Pain

Assess it properly, including the site, character, and pattern, and distinguish nociceptive from neuropathic components, since the latter responds poorly to opioids alone and requires adjuvant therapy.

Titrate opioids against the symptom. Use a regular baseline dose with a breakthrough dose available, conventionally a defined fraction of the total daily dose, and review the number of breakthrough doses used in order to adjust the baseline. There is no maximum dose when titrating to symptom; the correct dose is the one that relieves the pain without unacceptable adverse effects.

Route conversion and opioid rotation require accurate use of equianalgesic conversion, with the essential caveat that **incomplete cross-tolerance means the calculated equivalent dose of a new opioid should be reduced substantially**, conventionally by a quarter to a half, when switching agents. Errors here cause both under-treatment and serious over-sedation, and the conversion should be checked against a current reference and with pharmacy rather than from memory.

Renal impairment requires attention to the accumulation of active metabolites, and morphine and codeine are poor choices, as Chapter 16, section 16.4.4, noted.

Adjuvants matter: agents for neuropathic pain; corticosteroids for pain from oedema, capsular stretch, or nerve compression; bisphosphonates and radiotherapy for bone pain; and non-pharmacological approaches including positioning and heat.

Address the fear. Patients and families frequently resist adequate analgesia because of fears about addiction, tolerance, and hastening death. These should be raised proactively and answered: addiction is not a meaningful concern in this context, tolerance is managed by titration, and opioids titrated to symptom do not shorten life. This conversation prevents more suffering than any prescription.

20.4.2 Breathlessness

Low-dose opioids are the evidence-based pharmacological treatment for breathlessness in advanced illness and are effective at doses well below those required for analgesia. This is the single most useful and most under-used intervention in this section.

Benzodiazepines have a role where anxiety is a prominent component, as a second-line addition rather than as the primary treatment.

Oxygen benefits hypoxaemic patients and does not benefit non-hypoxaemic ones. Randomised evidence has found that in patients with refractory breathlessness who are not hypoxaemic, oxygen is no better than medical air, and a fan directing airflow across the face is as effective and considerably less encumbering. Prescribing oxygen reflexively to a breathless patient who is not hypoxaemic tethers them to a mask and a machine for no benefit.

Non-pharmacological measures: positioning upright, airflow from a fan or open window, reducing exertion, breathing techniques, and addressing the anxiety that both results from and worsens breathlessness.

Treat reversible contributors where the treatment is proportionate: effusion, anaemia, bronchospasm, infection, and heart failure.

20.4.3 Nausea and vomiting

Choose the antiemetic by mechanism, which is more effective than sequential empirical trials.

Consider: chemical and drug-related causes including opioids, hypercalcaemia, and uraemia, acting on the chemoreceptor trigger zone; gastric stasis and outlet obstruction; bowel obstruction; vestibular causes; raised intracranial pressure; and anxiety.

The corresponding agents differ in receptor profile and should be selected accordingly, with a prokinetic for gastric stasis, a dopamine antagonist for chemical causes, an antihistaminic and antimuscarinic agent for vestibular causes, corticosteroids for raised intracranial pressure and for bowel obstruction, and a somatostatin analogue for high-output obstruction. Combining agents with the same mechanism adds toxicity without benefit.

Malignant bowel obstruction can frequently be managed medically without a nasogastric tube, using a combination of antisecretory, antiemetic, and analgesic agents, and surgical or stenting options should be considered where appropriate.

20.4.4 Delirium and terminal restlessness

Delirium is common at the end of life and is distressing to families, who frequently interpret it as pain or as the patient's suffering.

Look for reversible contributors first, and the highest-yield are urinary retention, constipation, uncontrolled pain, opioid toxicity, and medications. Opioid-induced neurotoxicity presents with myoclonus, hyperalgesia, and delirium, and is treated by rotation and dose reduction rather than by escalation.

Non-pharmacological measures as in Chapter 10, section 10.1.5, with familiar presence, orientation, and a calm environment.

Where distress persists, an antipsychotic may be used for symptom control, recognising the limitations described in Chapter 10, section 10.1.6, that these agents treat agitation rather than delirium.

Explain it to the family, since without explanation they will interpret restlessness as pain and request escalating analgesia that will not help.

20.4.5 Respiratory secretions

Noisy breathing from upper airway secretions in the dying patient is common in the final hours.

The most important intervention is explanation. The evidence indicates that this does not cause distress to the patient, who is typically deeply unconscious, and the distress is the family's. Explaining what is happening, and that it does not mean the patient is drowning or choking, relieves most of the suffering it causes.

Practical measures are repositioning, stopping or reducing artificial hydration where it is contributing, and gentle mouth care. Suction is generally not helpful and can be distressing.

Antimuscarinic agents are widely used and their evidence of benefit is modest. They do not clear existing secretions and are more effective if given early, and they carry anticholinergic effects. They are reasonable but should not be presented as the main answer.

20.4.6 Other symptoms and anticipatory prescribing

Mouth care is among the most neglected and most valued interventions. A dry mouth causes real suffering, is easily relieved, and is a task families can perform, which gives them something meaningful to do.

Constipation requires anticipation with every opioid, as Chapter 15, section 15.8.3, argued.

Anorexia and reduced intake are expected. Explain to families that reduced eating is a consequence of dying rather than a cause of it, and that forced feeding does not help and may harm, connecting to Chapter 12, section 12.7.4.

Anticipatory prescribing is the practice of ensuring that medications for the common terminal symptoms are prescribed and available before they are needed, so that a symptom arising at night does not require locating a prescriber. A standard set covers pain, breathlessness, nausea, agitation, and secretions, with route and doses appropriate to the patient. **This is one of the highest-value actions a hospitalist can take for a dying patient**, and its omission is a frequent cause of an uncomfortable death.

20.5 Advance Directives, Surrogates, and the Incapacitated Patient

20.5.1 The instruments and what each does

Terminology and legal effect vary substantially between jurisdictions, and clinicians must know their local framework. The general categories:

An advance decision to refuse treatment, in some jurisdictions legally binding where it is valid and applicable to the situation that has arisen, in which a person with capacity records a refusal of specified treatment in specified circumstances.

An advance statement of preferences and values, which is not binding but which informs decisions made on the patient's behalf and is frequently more useful in practice, since it addresses values rather than attempting to anticipate specific scenarios.

An appointed proxy decision maker, variously called a healthcare proxy, an attorney for health and welfare, or a durable power of attorney, who is authorised to make decisions on the person's behalf when they lack capacity.

Portable medical orders, which differ importantly from advance directives in that they are clinician orders, actionable immediately, signed by a clinician after discussion with the patient, and designed to travel with the patient between settings. They exist under various names in different systems.

20.5.2 The limitations

Advance directives have not delivered what was hoped, and knowing why prevents over-reliance on them.

Completion rates are low, and among patients who have completed one, **the document is frequently unavailable at the moment it is needed**.

They may not anticipate the actual situation. A document specifying refusal of ventilation in the event of irreversible illness does not resolve the question of ventilation for a potentially reversible pneumonia.

Stated preferences change with circumstance and with experience of illness, and preferences expressed while well predict later preferences imperfectly.

The reframing that follows is that the value of advance care planning lies less in producing a document than in **preparing the patient and the surrogate for in-the-moment decision making**: identifying who will decide, ensuring that person understands the patient's values, and giving them permission to exercise judgement rather than to follow a script.

The practical corollary for a hospitalist is to establish who the surrogate is, to ask whether any documentation exists and to obtain it, and to have the values conversation rather than relying on a form.

20.5.3 Supporting surrogate decision makers

The standards of decision making, in the order in which they apply: the patient's own previously expressed wishes where these are known and applicable; substituted judgement, meaning what the patient would have decided, which requires the surrogate to set aside their own preference; and, where neither is available, the patient's best interests.

Surrogate decision making causes lasting psychological harm. Family members who make these decisions have high rates of anxiety, depression, and post-traumatic symptoms persisting for months. Reducing that burden is a clinical obligation, and three practices do so.

Frame the question correctly. Ask "what do you think your father would say if he were sitting here with us?" rather than "what do you want us to do?" This is not a semantic difference. The first asks the surrogate to report; the second asks them to choose, and it is the second that produces guilt.

Make a recommendation, as section 20.3.3 argued.

Share the responsibility explicitly. Say that this is a decision the team is making together with the family based on what the patient valued, and that the family is not deciding alone. Say, where it is true, that the illness is causing the death rather than the decision.

Where a surrogate insists on treatment inconsistent with the patient's known wishes, explore the reason rather than confronting it. The reason is usually guilt, a promise made, family conflict, mistrust, or an unrealistic expectation created by an earlier conversation, and each has a different response.

20.5.4 The patient without a surrogate

Patients who lack capacity and have no available surrogate present a recognised difficulty, and institutions should have a defined process.

Search properly first, since a friend, neighbour, or distant relative frequently exists and is not found because no one looked.

Follow the local framework, which may involve an independent advocate, a defined institutional committee, a second physician opinion, or a court process depending on the jurisdiction and the decision.

Document the search and the reasoning, and recognise that the standard applied is the patient's best interests informed by whatever is known of their values, including from prior records and from anyone who knew them.

20.6 Withdrawal of Life-Sustaining Therapy and the Terminal Wean

20.6.1 The ethical framework

Withholding and withdrawing a treatment are ethically equivalent. A treatment that would not be started need not be continued, and the widely held intuition that stopping is worse than not starting is psychologically real and ethically unfounded. Its practical importance is that clinicians who accept it become reluctant to start treatments that might later need stopping, which harms patients by making time-limited trials less available.

There is no obligation to provide a treatment that cannot achieve its intended goal, and section 20.7 addresses disputes about this.

Withdrawal of life-sustaining treatment is distinct from euthanasia. The intention is to cease an intervention that is no longer serving the patient's goals, and the cause of death is the underlying disease. Where jurisdictions permit assisted dying, that is a separate matter governed by its own legal framework, and clinicians should know their local law.

20.6.2 Preparing

Ensure the decision is settled and shared among the team and the family before proceeding, and that the reasoning is documented.

Prepare the family for what will happen. Describe the expected sequence, the possible sounds and appearance, and the uncertainty about timing, which may be minutes or considerably longer. Families who are unprepared interpret normal events as suffering.

Time it to permit those who wish to be present to arrive, within reason, and ask who should be there.

Address the environment: privacy, space for family to sit, and removal of unnecessary equipment.

Discontinue what is no longer serving comfort: monitoring and alarms, which distract the family from the patient and provide no information that will change anything; blood tests; observations; and non-comfort medications and infusions, including vasopressors, antibiotics, and nutrition, with each addressed explicitly rather than left running.

Prescribe symptom medications in advance and have them at the bedside, so that they can be given immediately rather than sought after distress appears.

Remove restraints and, where present, arrange **deactivation of an implantable defibrillator**, as Chapter 13, section 13.4.5, noted, since shocks during dying are distressing and avoidable.

20.6.3 The terminal wean and extubation

Both terminal extubation, in which the tube is removed, and terminal weaning, in which support is reduced progressively, are acceptable practices, and the evidence does not establish the superiority of either. Extubation permits the family to see the patient's face and permits the patient to speak if able, which many families value; weaning may allow more gradual titration of symptom control.

Give symptom medication before, not after, reducing support. Anticipating distress is the standard, and waiting to see whether the patient becomes distressed before treating is not.

Titrate sedation and analgesia to comfort, with no fixed maximum when titrating to symptom, and document the intent, which is relief of distress.

Neuromuscular blocking agents must not be used, and where one has been given it must have worn off or been reversed before support is withdrawn. A paralysed patient cannot display distress, which makes symptom assessment impossible and is ethically impermissible.

Manage the airway problems that arise: secretions as in section 20.4.5, and stridor, for which corticosteroids and adrenaline nebulisation may be considered in advance if it is anticipated.

Stay. The clinician's presence at the moment of withdrawal, and shortly afterwards, matters greatly to families and is frequently omitted because it is uncomfortable.

20.6.4 Withdrawal of other therapies

Dialysis withdrawal is a common and appropriate decision in patients for whom it no longer serves their goals, as Chapter 16, section 16.5.6, discussed. Death typically follows over a period of days to a week or two, permitting time for family to gather and for hospice arrangements, and symptoms are generally manageable.

Artificial nutrition and hydration are medical treatments subject to the same considerations, as Chapter 12, section 12.7.4, established.

Mechanical circulatory support raises specific and complex issues requiring specialist involvement.

Organ donation should be considered where applicable, with the approach made by trained donation specialists and, importantly, **only after the decision to withdraw has been made and communicated**, so that the two conversations are not conflated.

20.7 Ethics Consultation, Futility Disputes, and Moral Distress

20.7.1 When to seek ethics consultation

Common indications include disagreement between the team and the family or between team members about goals; uncertainty about capacity or about the authority of a surrogate; requests for treatment the team considers non-beneficial; questions about the interpretation of an advance directive; and situations where the clinically indicated course conflicts with a legal or institutional constraint.

A practical structure for analysing such a case, widely used and easily remembered, considers four domains: the medical indications, meaning what the treatment can achieve; the patient's preferences, actual or substituted; quality of life as the patient would assess it; and contextual features including family, resources, law, and institutional factors. Working through these systematically frequently resolves the case without formal consultation.

Ethics consultation should be available to anyone, including nursing staff and families, and not gated by the attending physician, since the situations most needing it are frequently those in which the attending is a party to the disagreement.

20.7.2 Disputes about non-beneficial treatment

The term futility should generally be avoided, because it conflates two different claims. **Physiological futility**, meaning that an intervention cannot achieve its physiological effect, is rare and uncontroversial. What is usually meant is that the achievable outcome is not worth the burden, which is a **value judgement**, and one on which the clinician's view has no special authority.

Professional consensus has moved toward the term **potentially inappropriate treatment**, and toward a **process-based approach to resolution** rather than unilateral refusal.

The process, in sequence: intensive communication to understand the family's reasoning; a second medical opinion; ethics consultation; an offer to transfer care to another clinician or institution willing to provide the treatment; institutional review; and, only after these are exhausted and in accordance with local law and policy, a decision to decline the treatment.

Most disputes resolve with communication, and the underlying causes are identifiable: **mistrust**, which in patients from communities with a documented history of poor treatment by medical institutions is a rational response rather than an obstacle, and which requires acknowledgement rather than argument; **unrealistic expectations** created by earlier optimistic communication from clinicians; **religious belief**, including hope for a miracle, which is best explored with chaplaincy involvement and which frequently coexists with a willingness to accept limits; **family conflict and guilt**, in which the demand for treatment is about the family's relationships rather than the patient; and **grief and denial**, which take time.

The response to all of these is exploration rather than argument. Asking what the family is hoping for, what they are worried about, and what they understand, will do more than restating the prognosis.

20.7.3 Moral distress

Moral distress is the experience of knowing the right course of action while being constrained from taking it. Chapter 1, section 1.6.2, distinguished it from burnout and made the point that treating it as a resilience deficit both fails and insults.

In end-of-life care it is common, arising from providing treatment believed to be causing suffering without benefit, from being unable to relieve suffering, from participating in decisions one disagrees with, and from repeatedly witnessing poor deaths that better systems would have prevented.

Its effects accumulate. Repeated episodes produce a residue that lowers the threshold for the next, and moral distress is associated with burnout, with attrition, and with disengagement from precisely the patients who need most.

What helps: structured debriefing after difficult deaths; forums in which the distress can be named without it being treated as a performance problem; ethics education and availability; genuine mechanisms for staff to raise concerns and see them acted upon; and, most importantly, **addressing the structural causes**, since the distress is usually a correct perception of a real problem rather than a failure of coping.

Nursing staff experience it at higher rates than physicians, in part because they are present continuously and have less decision-making authority, and their perspective is frequently the earliest indicator that something in the plan is wrong.

20.8 Care of the Dying Patient and Their Family in the Final Hours

20.8.1 Recognising dying

This is a diagnosis and should be made explicitly. The failure to make it is the largest single cause of a poor death in hospital, because every subsequent action depends on it: symptom management, cessation of futile interventions, communication with the family, and the opportunity for people to say what they need to say.

The signs, which develop over days and then hours: profound weakness and becoming bed-bound; reduced or absent oral intake; difficulty swallowing, including of medication; increasing sleep and reduced consciousness; disorientation and reduced attention; mottling of the skin, particularly the knees and feet; cool peripheries; reduced urine output; changes in breathing pattern including periodic breathing and long pauses; and upper airway secretions.

Diagnostic uncertainty is common and is not a reason to defer the conversation. It is entirely possible to say that the patient appears to be dying, that this may be wrong, and that the plan will be reviewed, while beginning comfort-focused care.

Communicate it plainly. "I think he is dying" is the sentence, and it should be said rather than implied. Families frequently report afterwards that no one told them, when in fact several clinicians used indirect language that was not understood.

20.8.2 What changes

Stop what is not contributing to comfort: observations, blood tests, monitoring, blood glucose testing, most medications, intravenous fluids where they are not helping, and antibiotics where they are not.

Review every medication and stop those not serving comfort, converting essential symptom medications to a route the patient can receive, which is usually subcutaneous.

Ensure anticipatory medications are prescribed and present, as section 20.4.6 required.

Decide about hydration individually. Neither routine administration nor routine withdrawal is correct. Artificial hydration may relieve thirst in some patients and may worsen secretions and oedema in others, and the decision should be explained to the family whichever way it goes, since withdrawal is frequently interpreted as abandonment.

Attend to mouth care, pressure areas, positioning, and continence, which are the interventions that now matter.

Arrange privacy and space, and relax visiting restrictions.

Ask about spiritual, religious, and cultural needs, and about specific practices around dying and the body, which vary considerably and are far easier to accommodate if asked about in advance. Chapter 19, section 19.7.3, addressed this.

20.8.3 Supporting the family

Explain what they will see and hear, including the breathing changes and the secretions, and that these do not indicate suffering.

Explain that reduced intake is expected and is a part of dying rather than a cause of it.

Tell them that hearing may persist, and give them explicit permission to talk to the patient, to touch them, and to say what they want to say.

Give them something to do. Mouth care, moistening the lips, and simply being present are meaningful, and families who feel useless afterwards report it as a source of lasting distress.

Address the question of presence at the moment of death. Many families feel they must not leave. Tell them that it is not possible to predict the moment, that many people die when their family has briefly stepped out, and that this is common and does not represent a failure. This single reassurance prevents a great deal of subsequent guilt.

Consider children, who are frequently excluded and who generally do better when prepared and included in an age-appropriate way, with support.

Ask whether they want anyone contacted, including a religious representative.

20.8.4 After death

Verify and certify according to local requirements, and identify whether the death requires referral to a coroner, medical examiner, or equivalent, which varies by jurisdiction and circumstance.

Care for the body respectfully and in accordance with the family's cultural and religious practices, which should have been established beforehand, and which may include requirements about who may touch the body, positioning, timing, and washing.

Offer the family time with the person without being hurried, and be clear that they may return.

Handle belongings with care, which sounds minor and is remembered.

Provide bereavement information and a named contact, and where the institution offers a bereavement follow-up call or meeting, arrange it. Families frequently have questions that emerge only after some weeks.

Offer a condolence, in whatever form is appropriate. A letter or a call from the clinician who cared for the patient is remembered by families for years and takes ten minutes.

Complete the documentation and the communications, including informing the primary care clinician promptly, which is frequently delayed and which results in avoidable distress when a letter or appointment arrives for a person who has died.

20.8.5 Caring for the team

Debrief, particularly after difficult or unexpected deaths, and particularly for junior staff and for nursing staff who provided the direct care.

Acknowledge the death within the team. A ward on which deaths pass without acknowledgement teaches its staff that this is ordinary, which is the beginning of the depersonalisation described in Chapter 1, section 1.6.

Recognise your own response. Clinicians who care for dying patients regularly accumulate grief that is rarely given anywhere to go, and Chapter 4, section 4.6.2, and Chapter 1, section 1.6, both apply.

Chapter Summary

- **Palliative care is not end-of-life care.** It is concurrent with disease-directed treatment, and early involvement in advanced illness improves quality of life and mood.
- **Clinicians are systematically over-optimistic about prognosis**, more so the better they know the patient. **Functional trajectory is the strongest general predictor**, and the four illness trajectories explain why organ failure is the hardest to prognosticate and the one in which conversations are most often deferred.
- **Communicate prognosis in ranges, acknowledge uncertainty explicitly, and revisit it.** Uncertainty is a reason to be honest, not a reason to be silent.
- **A goals-of-care conversation is not a code status discussion.** Establish understanding, give the headline and stop, answer emotion with empathy rather than information, map values, and then **make a recommendation**. Asking a family to choose from a menu transfers a burden that causes lasting harm.
- **Low-dose opioids treat breathlessness**, and oxygen does not help the non-hypoxaemic patient. **Anticipatory prescribing** is among the highest-value actions for a dying patient. Explanation is the principal treatment for terminal secretions.
- **Advance directives underperform**, and the value of advance care planning lies in preparing the surrogate rather than in producing a document. Ask what the patient would say, not what the family wants.
- **Withholding and withdrawing are ethically equivalent.** Give symptom medication before reducing support, never use neuromuscular blockade, and stay.
- **Avoid the word futility.** Most disputes about non-beneficial treatment resolve through exploration of the underlying cause, which is usually mistrust, unrealistic expectation, religious belief, guilt, or grief, and each requires a different response.
- **Moral distress is a correct perception of a real problem**, not a failure of coping, and it accumulates.
- **Recognising dying is a diagnosis**, and saying it plainly is the action on which everything else depends.

Review Questions

1. A patient with advanced heart failure has had four admissions in six months, each time recovering to a lower baseline. The team plans to discharge him without discussing prognosis, reasoning that he improved again. State what trajectory this represents, why the conversation is being deferred, and what you would do.
2. A daughter says "I just can't believe this is happening" when told her mother is dying. Give two responses, one that would be a missed empathic opportunity and one that would not, and explain the difference.

3. A family asks you to "do everything" for a patient with metastatic malignancy, multiorgan failure, and a poor functional baseline. Set out your approach, including what you would explore before responding, and what you would eventually recommend and how.
4. A patient is to be extubated with a comfort-focused plan. List the actions you would take before the tube is removed, and state the one agent that must not be present.
5. A patient dies overnight on your ward. List what you would do in the following twenty-four hours for the family, for the record, and for the team.